PARENTS' AND TEACHERS' GUIDES: 22

Maintaining Three Languages

The Teenage Years

Xiao-lei Wang

MULTILINGUAL MATTERS
Bristol • Buffalo • Toronto

Library of Congress Cataloging in Publication Data
A catalog record for this book is available from the Library of Congress.
Wang, Xiao-Lei - author.
Maintaining Three Languages: The Teenage Years/Xiao-lei Wang.
Parents' and Teachers' Guides: 22
Includes bibliographical references and index.
1. Teenagers–Language. 2. Multilingualism. 3. Language acquisition–Parent participation.
4. Sociolinguistics. I. Title.
P120.Y68W36 2015
404'.20835–dc23 2015023399

British Library Cataloguing in Publication Data
A catalogue entry for this book is available from the British Library.

ISBN-13: 978-1-78309-448-6 (hbk)
ISBN-13: 978-1-78309-447-9 (pbk)

Multilingual Matters
UK: St Nicholas House, 31-34 High Street, Bristol BS1 2AW, UK.
USA: UTP, 2250 Military Road, Tonawanda, NY 14150, USA.
Canada: UTP, 5201 Dufferin Street, North York, Ontario M3H 5T8, Canada.

Website: www.multilingual-matters.com
Twitter: Multi_Ling_Mat
Facebook: https://www.facebook.com/multilingualmatters
Blog: www.channelviewpublications.wordpress.com

Copyright © 2016 Xiao-lei Wang.

All rights reserved. No part of this work may be reproduced in any form or by any means without permission in writing from the publisher.

The policy of Multilingual Matters/Channel View Publications is to use papers that are natural, renewable and recyclable products, made from wood grown in sustainable forests. In the manufacturing process of our books, and to further support our policy, preference is given to printers that have FSC and PEFC Chain of Custody certification. The FSC and/or PEFC logos will appear on those books where full certification has been granted to the printer concerned.

Typeset by Deanta Global Publishing Services Limited.
Printed and bound in Great Britain by the CPI Books Group.

Maintaining Three Languages

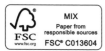

PARENTS' AND TEACHERS' GUIDES

Series Editor: Colin Baker, *Bangor University, UK*

This series provides immediate advice and practical help on topics where parents and teachers frequently seek answers. Each book is written by one or more experts in a style that is highly readable, non-technical and comprehensive. No prior knowledge is assumed: a thorough understanding of a topic is promised after reading the appropriate book.

Full details of all the books in this series and of all our other publications can be found on http://www.multilingual-matters.com, or by writing to Multilingual Matters, St Nicholas House, 31-34 High Street, Bristol BS1 2AW, UK.

Contents

	Acknowledgements	vii
1	Introduction	1
2	Heritage-Language Maintenance and Multilingual Development in the Teenage Years	25
3	Multilingual Sound System Development During Adolescence	55
4	Multilingual Word and Meaning Development During Adolescence	74
5	Multilingual Word- and Sentence-Structure Development During Adolescence	106
6	The Development of Multilingual Knowledge and Usage During Adolescence	133
7	Multilingual Literacies Development During Adolescence	168
8	Developing Multiple Identities During Adolescence	214
9	Multilingual Childrearing and Family Welfare	241
10	Pulling It Together: Concluding Thoughts	264
	Appendix: Examples of Standardised Language Assessments	291
	Glossary	293
	Author Index	305
	Subject Index	313

Acknowledgements

First and foremost, I want to thank my two sons Léandre and Dominique for giving me the possibility of producing this and other books. You have inspired me to write about multilingual development. Although your father and I initiated your multilingual journey in the very beginning of your lives, you have been enthusiastic travellers the whole way. It is truly a joy listening to you speaking in different languages. You have not only taught me what it means to be multilingual, but have also made me marvel at a human being's fascinating linguistic capability.

All of Léandre and Dominique's multilingual achievements and other accomplishments would not have been possible without my husband Philippe's collaboration and efforts. I was lucky to meet you in the communal kitchen on the campus of the University of Chicago 26 years ago. Together, we have raised two intelligent, kind, eloquent, humorous and wonderful children.

I also appreciate Multilingual Matters for providing me, for the third time, with a great platform to promote multilingualism in the home context. In addition, all the staff I have worked with at Multilingual Matters are indeed first-class professionals.

I am genuinely in debt to you, Professor Colin Baker for your thoughtful and encouraging comments on three of my books with Multilingual Matters. In fact, it was through you that I learnt how to write for parents. It was also through you that I learnt the art of making constructive comments.

I am thankful to the many parents who sent me appreciative and encouraging emails about my previous books and generously shared with me their own multilingual childrearing experiences.

Finally, I am forever grateful to my graduate research assistants: Anna Michelle Grimaldi, Amanda Albano, Brigita Dedivanaj-Shkreli and Courtney Klein for your help at different stages of the book and for being there with me throughout the process of writing the book.

Xiao-lei Wang
Basel, Switzerland, July 2015

1 Introduction

On a frigid winter night a few years ago, our family was chatting while dipping bread into a fondue *caquelon* (pot). I complained, in English, to my husband Philippe about an unpleasant meeting I had attended that afternoon. Philippe, in French, told a joke he just read in *Le Chat*[1] (The Cat) to our two sons, Léandre and Dominique. The two boys nattered about their schoolmates, in French, and poked fun at each other, in Spanish, while I, in Chinese, asked the boys about their day in school. Our family was carrying on our usual dinner-table conversation.

As we were enjoying the last bit of *la religieuse* (the cheese crust on the bottom of the fondue pot), our older son Léandre, who was 15 years old at the time (15; 7; 24),[2] told me, in Chinese, about a physical fight between him and a classmate in the school library that day. While Léandre was sensationally recounting the event, I noticed that he had a slight bruise on his neck. I became worried and pressed him for more details. Sensing something serious in our conversation from my anxious tone of voice and facial expressions, Philippe interrupted our conversation and eagerly asked Léandre in French what had happened before Léandre had time to finish telling me his story in Chinese. Léandre grimaced from annoyance, complaining loudly, in Chinese first and then in French, that he was fed up with having to always repeat the same story twice and having to always decide to whom to respond first. In this case, both his father and mother wanted to know the story at the same time and he had to decide whom to address first and in what language. He went on carping about his father not learning enough Chinese to understand our conversation. Truth be told, if we had an English-speaking guest at our dinner table that night, he would have to repeat the same story three times, and if his former babysitter Carmen was around, he might have to tell it a fourth time in Spanish.

This was the first time I heard this resentment from Léandre. Although I was somewhat taken back by his strong reaction to the way our family had always communicated, I knew deep down that his frustration and defiance was understandable. After all, Léandre was a teenager! In the midst of questioning everything else in his life, it was reasonable for him to also question his family's communication routine that he had taken for granted before.

Need for A Book About Adolescent Heritage-Language Maintenance and Multilingual Development

The vignette you just read about Léandre's grouse epitomises adolescence, commonly referred to as the teenager years. Up until that night, he seemed to be quite content with our family communication routine; that is, negotiating more than one language on a daily basis was normal for him. However, the moment finally came for him to openly challenge 'his way of life'. Léandre's reaction was not his alone. In fact, I have heard many similar stories from parents who expressed their disbelief when they first heard their teens' disgruntlements about speaking their heritage language(s). For example, Marija, mother of 14-year-old Nikola, who was brought up speaking Croatian, Polish, and French in Belgium, wrote:

> He told us to our face one day that he would stop talking to me in Croatian and to his father in Polish. He said that he always hated talking about the same thing twice…He said that he felt embarrassed to speak Croatian and Polish when his friends were around…His friends told him that he sounded strange when he spoke to us…He was going to only speak French from now on…We were speechless to hear his comments…But, what can we do? We don't know how to make him speak our languages and it has to be his choice…[3]

Similarly, Lijin, whose family lives in the United States, felt frustrated with his helplessness in motivating his daughter to maintain her heritage language, Chinese. He wrote:

> My daughter spoke Chinese to my wife and me when she was a child. She was quite happy with that. But, when she was about twelve, she began to speak English to us. When we spoke Chinese to her, she kept answering in English. We tried and tried, but she still refused to speak Chinese with us. Eventually, we got tired of this daily struggle and we just stopped trying…I cannot win the battle anyway. I wish I could find support somewhere to help my daughter keep up with her Chinese. It is really a pity that kids like my daughter lose their ancestral language…they will regret when they grow up.[4]

Likewise, when I was invited by *L'association des familles franco-chinoises de Pékin* (the French-Chinese Parent Association in Beijing) to give a talk on multilingual parenting in 2012, a mother, who travelled all the way from Tianjin to the French Embassy in Beijing when she read the announcement about my talk in *Aujourd'hui la Chine* (China Today), asked me one pressing question: what should she do to help her daughter keep up with her French in China before she lost it?

Obviously, these anecdotes indicate that when children turn into teenagers, parents are faced with the enormous challenge of continuing to help their children maintain their heritage language(s), and these parents desperately need support.

In recent years, there have been a burgeoning number of parenting books and articles about how to raise multilingual[5] young children; however, few books or resources are available for parents of multilingual adolescents.[6] In particular, there are few books that have offered parents of teenagers detailed accounts of the challenges which they might face in everyday heritage-language maintenance, as well as useful strategies that are grounded in research and parental self-reflection.

The teenage years are a unique and fascinating period in human life and this is also a period of exploration and rebellion. How to motivate teens to maintain their heritage language(s) in the home environment is a concern for many parents. Thus, I feel compelled to write a book about multilingual adolescent parenting, sharing successful stories as well as challenges. My overarching goal in writing this book is to help parents provide their teens with an optimal learning environment that is conducive to heritage-language development.

Multilingual Necessity and Advantages in the 21st Century

In our increasingly globalised world, knowing more than one language is a necessity and an asset. The Universal Declaration issued by the United Nations Educational, Scientific, and Cultural Organization (UNESCO) urges us whenever possible to foster 'the learning of several languages from the earliest age...' Similarly, the European Union (EU) also encourages linguistic diversity and has created an official position to promote multilingualism (i.e. the European Commissioner for Multilingualism).

There are many advantages associated with being multilingual. Below are a few examples.

Cognitive advantages

Although multilinguals share universal learning characteristics with their monolingual counterparts, they may diverge from monolinguals in their cognitive (intellectual) abilities as a result of being exposed to more than one linguistic system. Knowing more than one language involves much more than simply knowing more than one way of speaking. Ellen Bialystok, a well-known psychologist, has explained that because the mind of a multilingual speaker is exposed to more than one set of linguistic details and conceptual representations, a multilingual speaker is able to entertain possibilities that a monolingual speaker has no need to consider.[7] Moreover, brain research shows that multilinguals have greater tissue density in the areas of the brain related to language, memory and attention, and that those people who were exposed to an additional language prior to age five have the highest levels of brain tissue density.[8] As such, multilinguals may possess several cognitive advantages.

Selective attention

One of the multilingual cognitive advantages is selective attention. **Selective attention**, also called attention control, means that when more than one language coexists, one of the languages must be constantly inhibited to prevent ongoing intrusion.[9] This may explain why people who speak more than one language are better at problem solving, because tackling a problem successfully requires focusing on some aspects of the information and ignoring the others. For example, when monolingual and bilingual young adults were asked to perform a visual search task by determining whether a target shape was present amid distractor shapes, bilinguals were significantly faster than monolinguals in identifying the target in the more difficult conjunction search, thus demonstrating better control of visual attention.[10]

Mental flexibility and creativity

Another multilingual cognitive advantage is elastic thinking. Because multilinguals regularly switch between different languages, they may possess an added mental flexibility and creativity,[11] notwithstanding counterevidence with adults.[12] Colin Baker, an expert in multilingualism, used the following example to illustrate how the knowledge of two words – one in English and one in Welsh – for a single idea (a school) could enhance one's concept of *school*. In Welsh, the word *ysgol* not only means *school* but also *ladder*. Thus, a Welsh-English bilingual has an added dimension of the word *school*; that is, school is a place to learn, and it functions as a ladder for one's knowledge. Such cognitive flexibility can be manifested, for example, in multilingual children's superior storytelling skills, because they are less bound by words and are more elastic in their thinking as a result of knowing more than one language.[13]

I can cite many instances where my own children Léandre and Dominique demonstrated exceptional mental flexibility and creativity in problem solving, both in their schoolwork and in their daily lives. For example, once I asked Philippe to carve a dead tree trunk in the woods into a big container for planting lettuce. The problem, however, was that the trunk was heavy to move from the woods to our terrace, and there was no access in the woods for a vehicle to move the trunk mechanically. While we were scratching our heads for a solution to the problem, Léandre came to our aid by proposing that we put the tree trunk in the lake and drag it along the shore. It was an instant success! While I cannot be absolutely sure that this anecdote has anything to do with Léandre being multilingual, what I can say for certain is that using multiple languages on a daily basis does help Léandre and Dominique see more than one way of doing things (see Box. 1.1 for more examples of flexibility).

Novel conceptual combination

Individuals who are exposed to more than one language and culture tend to have more than one set of cultural tools with which to interpret the world. These tools can foster competent behaviours in multiple cultures. For instance, an individual who has extensive knowledge and experiences in cultures A and B may be able to retrieve ideas from cultures A and B spontaneously, place them in juxtaposition, and integrate the two into a novel idea through creative insight. This process is referred to as **novel conceptual combination**, which has been shown to have beneficial effects on creative conceptual expansion.[14] I have witnessed many examples where Léandre and Dominique demonstrated this novel conceptual combination in their daily problem solving, in their music composition, in their writing, and in their academic work in school. You will read some of them later in the book.

Box 1.1 Examples of Flexibility

Example 1:

When I asked Léandre (14; 7; 0) to proofread one of my manuscripts, he was flexible enough to accept the spelling of foreign names such as *Mrs. Andersson*. He kept these foreign names as they were, with a clear understanding that names could be spelt differently in different languages. However, one of my monolingual English-speaking graduate assistants changed all the foreign names to English spellings, such as changing *Mrs. Andersson* to *Mrs. Anderson*.

Similarly, once I wrote a paper for a UK publisher using the UK spelling and punctuation convention. When Léandre (14; 7; 3) proofread my manuscript, he got the idea of UK spelling and punctuation spelling quickly and adapted to the UK spelling and punctuation convention in his proofs.

Example 2:

In St. Ambrogio's Basilica, Milan (Italy), a French-speaking woman spoke French to the doorkeeper and told him that she did not have change for the tickets, despite the fact that the doorkeeper did not understand French. The doorkeeper ignored her. We did not have change for the tickets either. However, Léandre and Dominique greeted the doorkeeper in Italian and made an effort to use the Italian words they knew (they even made up a few Italian words using their knowledge of Spanish and French). The doorkeeper not only let us in, he also stood up and showed us where to look to find St. Ambrogio's pictures and he also showed us where we could see the treasures. The doorkeeper's reaction to Léandre and Dominique was a direct consequence of their flexibility of adaptation to a new linguistic environment and to the person with whom they were communicating.

Knowledge transfer

It is now generally recognised that multilinguals have an advantage in knowledge transfer from their heritage language to the mainstream language and vice versa. Compared with monolinguals, multilinguals can benefit greatly from knowledge acquired in their multiple languages to enrich their learning and understanding. For instance, Dominique accumulated knowledge about the Qin (秦) Dynasty (221–206 BC) in Chinese history (through the stories I read to him as well as a visit to Xi'an in China) and the West Roman Empire (27 BC–476 AD) (through the stories read to him by his father as well as visits to various Roman relics in Europe). By the time he studied world history in high school, his understanding of the two historical periods was more in-depth compared to most of his peers as a result of his knowledge transfer from his heritage-language resources.

However, a caveat must be mentioned about these multilingual cognitive advantages; that is, the aforementioned multilingual advantages are not automatically or equally associated with multilingualism, and it is likely that more proficient multilinguals are able to show these characteristics more readily than less proficient multilinguals.

Linguistic advantages

Aside from the cognitive benefits, multilinguals also have advantages in terms of their linguistic abilities.

Metalinguistic skills

Being multilingual helps an individual develop the ability to think and talk about one's language, which is called **metalinguistic ability**.[15] Individuals with more than one language generally tend to have a metalinguistic advantage when compared to their monolingual counterparts. For instance, Léandre commented that French homophones such as *Livre-lui une livre de livres* (deliver him a pond of books) is an interesting linguistic phenomenon. You will see many such metalinguistic examples from Léandre and Dominique later in Chapter 6.

Linguistic intuition

Multilinguals may have better intuitive inklings in their heritage language than non-heritage-language learners. Box 1.2 shows a good example. A friend of mine, who is a nonnative Chinese speaker, once tried to impress me by sending me a Chinese message using Google Translate.

This message is obviously not from someone who has native intuition about Chinese; the Google-translated Chinese you just read is quite amusing and does not make much sense. However, children who acquire Chinese early in life, such as Léandre and Dominique, tend to have a better sense of the language. Even though they sometimes may not know how to write it, they do have a better linguistic hunch to judge what sounds authentic and what does not. Over the years, Léandre has managed many times to send me Chinese messages by using Google Translate. In fact, it was Léandre who, as a young child at the time, first drew my attention to this website. He apparently used this site often when he wanted to impress me with literary Chinese. He usually wrote the messages in English first, then translated them into Chinese using Google Translate, revised the Google-translated messages, and made them read like authentic Chinese. For a while, I was led to believe that he knew how to write Chinese very well. Despite the apparent 'cheating', I do give Léandre credit for having the ability to make the botched Chinese in Google Translate read like authentic literary Chinese. This is the kind of linguistic knowledge that heritage-language-speaking children intuitively have that non-heritage-language learners such as my friend seem to lack.

Box 1.2 Writing Example of A Non-Heritage-Language Speaker

Original Message in Chinese (through Google Translate)

亲爱的小雷,
你好吗?我希望一切都受到惩罚,这是这么长时间我都没有听你的。我接受选举委员会的xxxx是不是从至少看到自己盎司每年剥离的唯一理由!看你来了,如果不及早比晚。
谢谢。

Literal Translation in English

Dear friend little thunder (This is the wrong word for my name. My name is 'early morning blossom' in Chinese.),

How are you? I hope all is punished, it is such a long time I have not hearing yours. I accept election to xxxx committee the only reason see myself every year be taken the right of! See you coming, if it not early than later. Thanks.

Intended Message

Dear Friend Xiao-lei,

How are you? I hope all is fine. I have not heard from you for a long time. The only reason I accepted the nomination for xxxx committee is that I don't want to miss the opportunity to see you at least once a year. Look forward to seeing you.

Thank you.

Linguistic breadth

Multilinguals also tend to have a linguistic breadth in their linguistic knowledge, and they can readily draw upon their linguistic resources. For example, when looking for a name for his band, Léandre (17; 11; 27) came up with many interesting words such as *alloys*. To me, his choice of the word *alloys* is especially intriguing. It embodies what his band was: a blend of its players in a racial sense (White, Black, Asian and racially mixed), a blend of instruments (e.g. guitar, base and drum), and a blend of different music genres (heavy metal, rock, and classic). Although the band did not use this particular name and used another name Léandre proposed, his monolingual bandmates did appreciate Léandre's breadth of word knowledge in coming up with a name for the band.

Linguistic resources

When Léandre (14; 7; 22) was a high-school freshman, he was able to proofread for me. He was far better at making comments and detecting errors than some of my graduate assistants because of his linguistic abilities in more than one language.

Also, in 9th grade, Dominique (14; 4; 12) used his linguistic and cultural resources to come up with an interesting comment for his English class. He commented on a quote in the Bible (Mark 1; 17), 'Follow me, and I will make you become fishers of men.' He observed that 'In French, the word for *fisherman* (*pêcheur*) is very similar to the word for *sinner* (*pécheur*), with only the accent difference on the *e*...'

Linguistic faculty

Exposing children to more than one language early in life facilitates new language learning. Researchers found that bilinguals learning a third language tend to outperform monolinguals learning a second language.[16] This is perhaps because bilinguals are more experienced language learners who have potentially developed more language learning strategies than monolinguals and have a larger linguistic and intercultural repertoire at their disposal.[17]

I can affirm the fact that knowing more than one language can facilitate additional language learning by using Léandre and Dominique as examples. If you had the pleasure of hearing Léandre speak Spanish (which he acquired in middle school and further developed in high school and college) and German (which he acquired in college), you would be impressed. In fact, when Léandre was in 10th grade (15; 2; 24), his Spanish teacher commented that his Spanish accent was like that of a native speaker. In eleventh grade, the Spanish teacher told Léandre that his Spanish was too good for him to stay in her class. Our neighbour and Léandre's former babysitter Carmen, who was from Ecuador, also commented that Léandre and Dominique speak very good Spanish. Similarly, you would be impressed by how quickly Dominique 'picked up' Spanish and imitated Arabic and Italian. As a result of growing up simultaneously with English, French, and Chinese, our two children have a language faculty that has certainly contributed to their ease in learning additional languages.

Also, Léandre and Dominique's speed in learning additional languages is astounding. I was so envious of how quickly Léandre beat me in learning German. When Léandre took a German course during his freshman year of college, I decided to learn German too. We started at the same time; however, I was still at the stage of *'Hallo, wie geht's?'* (Hello, how are you?), while Léandre had already advanced and was able to carry on a conversation in German. When Léandre came home for Thanksgiving (about two months into his German learning), he could easily converse with our German guest and received her compliments. Both Philippe and I were pleasantly surprised when Léandre (18; 8; 27) sent us his multimedia German class project, in which he commented on a painting about Egypt. In addition to his multimedia talent (the music and visual effect he created in the presentation), he sounded very much like a real German narrator. Indeed, one would have been impressed with this young man, who had only been studying German for five to six months at that point.

Other advantages

Besides the cognitive and linguistic advantages, being multilingual can also benefit an individual in many other aspects of his or her life.

Facilitation in academic success

Proficiency in more than one language has been shown to be associated with high academic achievement. Individuals who have the ability to switch between two or more languages also exhibit higher cognitive functioning than those who abandon one of their heritage languages.[18] Research shows that when children were encouraged to further develop their home language, the skills they built in that language helped their mainstream language literacy development. In fact, the longer children receive reinforcement in their home language, the better they learn their mainstream language. The most promising way to enable children's long-term academic success is to promote both home language and mainstream literacy development.[19]

Again, Léandre and Dominique's experiences can provide testimony for this. They both have done very well in their academic subject areas from kindergarten to college. Most importantly, Léandre and Dominique's home language attainment did not hinder the development of their mainstream language, English. Throughout their K-12[20] schooling, both Léandre and Dominique's English Language Arts standardised test scores, including on the SAT, are always between the 98th and 100th percentile, and they both received the highest English score (5, which means extremely well qualified to receive college credit) on their high school Advance Placement (AP) tests.[21] Dominique in particular is well-versed in English writing. His composition in junior high was used as a sample for other students (16; 9; 01). All things considered, I am confident that their multilingual upbringing did not hinder their academic success and mainstream language advancement.

Access to heritage family and culture

Research shows that children who speak their parents' heritage language(s) enjoy better relationships with their families[22] and are less likely to be alienated from their parents and relatives.[23] Having knowledge about their heritage language(s), children and adolescents have an advantage in accessing their heritage culture and communicating with their heritage family. I always feel very fortunate that Léandre and Dominique can communicate well with their Chinese monolingual grandparents. I cannot image how much cultural information Léandre and Dominique would have missed if they did not know Chinese. The Skype conversations and visits with their Chinese grandparents are a valuable heritage-cultural resource for Léandre and Dominique. I was so pleased to observe Léandre (17; 11; 8) carry out conversations in Chinese with his grandparents' friends in the community clubhouse in Shanghai, which was such a cultural education for Léandre.

In addition to having access to their heritage family and relatives, knowledge of heritage languages also helps children and adolescents access their heritage cultures. For instance, understanding French has helped Léandre and Dominique to benefit from many of the museums in Switzerland and has enhanced their cultural identification to their heritage country. Similarly, understanding Chinese has allowed both of them to deepen their knowledge of many of the historical events that their school world history class only covered superficially.

Benefits in life

Being multilingual also has lots of advantages in life, whether in terms of worldview, travel, career, personality adjustment or mental health.[24] Anyone who knows more than one language probably can corroborate this claim. The fact that multilinguals, such as Léandre and Dominique, can read books and newspapers, as well as watch news and films in several languages, makes them more versatile and helps them to approach things from multiple perspectives. Being multilingual, one certainly has the privilege of accessing different sources of information. Many times, I have observed how the same issue was reported differently on CNN (English), TV5 Monde (French), CCTV (The People's Republic of China), ETTV (Taiwanese 东森新闻) and Deutsch Weila (German). If one receives information from just one source, what diverse views one would miss. Being multilingual definitely helps a person take different perspectives on issues, see things from different angles, and think more critically.

Knowing more than one language is also convenient because it makes life easier. Elsewhere,[25] I told a story about a car trip to a conference in Utrecht (the Netherlands) from Neuchâtel (Switzerland). Our French rental car displayed a French message on the front screen that the suspension was broken and service was needed immediately. Pressed for time to reach Utrecht that same evening, Philippe and I were worried that we would not have time to have the car repaired before the conference. While driving, Philippe asked Dominique to read the French vehicle manual and figure out whether the message displayed on the front screen was indeed true. After studying the manual, Dominique concluded that if we restarted the car, the suspension would adjust itself. As a result, we were able to arrive at our Utrecht conference on time. Dominique's ability to read French was obviously handy. Similarly, when we travel in Europe, we always lease a new car from Peugeot in France because we can get discounts as university professors who live outside of Europe. Each year, we rent a newer car model. Léandre and Dominique are always in charge of reading the instruction manual and briefing Philippe on the new gadgets in the vehicle. This always helps Philippe to understand the new features of the car, such as speed limiters for avoiding exceeding the speed limit.

Likewise, being multilingual certainly helps widen one's range of information sources. For example, one summer I was very busy and did not have time to plan a family trip. I put Léandre (14; 11; 0) in charge of researching ferry and hotel prices for our trip to Ireland, Northern Ireland, and Scotland. He researched all kinds of multilingual websites. In the end, Léandre found us ferry prices (from Cherbourg, France to Rosslare, Ireland; and from Belfast, Northern Ireland, to Scotland) and hotel prices that were unbeatable. Thanks to his multilingual abilities, Léandre saved us quite a bit of money on that family trip.

Social acceptance

Moreover, multilingualism can increase a person's social circle to include friends from many parts of the world. When travelling to another country, being able to speak the language really helps bring people together and facilitates communication, exchange and socialisation. For instance, being able to speak other languages such as French, Chinese, Spanish and German has helped Léandre make friends with international students in college. Similarly, because he was able to speak French, Dominique was accepted immediately by the soccer players in a soccer club in the French-speaking part of Switzerland when he participated in their training one summer.

Career advantages

Being multilingual has career advantages as well. For example, Carlos, my acquaintance, who is trilingual in Spanish, Portuguese and English, had a competitive advantage when being interviewed for a bank job compared with other applicants because of his multilingual ability. The bank hired him over hundreds of other applicants because of his multilingual ability, as they needed someone who could work with an increasing Latino population in the area.[26] Nowadays, globally minded companies are looking for people who can speak more than one language. Personally, I know a family member who was paid substantially more than her monolingual coworkers because of her multilingual skills.

Identity and self-esteem

The process of acquiring a language entails more than developing knowledge and skills about a language for communication; it is a process of making that language part of oneself (one's identity). In fact, identity is constructed by and in a language.[27] Research has shown that people who are proficient in their heritage language tend to have higher self-esteem, are more confident in achieving goals, feel they have more control over their lives, and have more ambitious plans for the future.[28]

Given all the advantages mentioned above and many others that I have not mentioned, it is definitely worthwhile to raise multilingual children and adolescents. As Stephen Krashen, an expert in second-language learning, commented, 'Heritage language development appears to be an excellent investment. For a small effort… the payoffs are enormous.'[29] Another well-known multilingual expert, Colin Baker, also echoed that multilingualism has more advantages than drawbacks.[30] Having discussed the multilingual advantages, I would like to caution that multilingual advantages do not have a single effect, but rather may interact with other variables such as a person's **aptitude** (mental ability), motivation and attitudes.

About the Book

In my previous book *Growing up with Three Languages: Birth to Eleven*,[31] I documented the simultaneous trilingual development of my two sons, Léandre and Dominique. I shared with readers how my husband and I, who are from different cultural, linguistic, and ethnic-racial backgrounds, successfully raised two children with their heritage languages[32] outside our native countries. Using daily observations, I illustrated how the two boys each negotiated multiple cultures and languages and developed a multilingual identity. An encouraging message coming from that book is that it is possible to raise multilingual children when parents are the major source of the heritage-language input as long as parents provide unconditional support and use suitable strategies.

As a sequel to my earlier book, this book is about how Léandre and Dominique kept up with their three languages in the home context during adolescence (from ages 12 to 19). In reflecting on how our family travelled together over the difficult terrains of multilingual maintenance in the United States, this book shares the successful strategies my husband and I used to support our teens' multilingual development and the way in which they negotiated their multilingual lives and continued to develop more empowered multilingual identities.

My unique vantage

I believe that I have a unique vantage point in writing this book. First, as a mother who has experienced success raising multilingual children and adolescents, I am not just talking the talk of raising multilingual children and adolescents; I have actually walked the walk of rearing them. My daily interactions with my own multilingual children from their births until their adolescence has enabled me to understand and articulate more fully what it means for children to grow up simultaneously with multiple languages, as well as what it takes for parents to support them in their heritage-language development.

Second, as a parent in a family with mixed racial backgrounds and cultural heritages (my husband is White and from Switzerland; I am an Asian, born and raised in the People's Republic of China; and we live in the United States), I am concerned that in the multilingual parenting advice literature, families with vastly different linguistic and parental cultural values are rarely addressed. This type of family is on the rise due to globalisation; thus, it is important to discuss how parents with diverse backgrounds can negotiate their differences and overcome challenges while raising multilingual children.

Third, as a mother with a minority background who also raised her children with her minority heritage language (Chinese) in the United States, I can shed a different light on the complexity of raising children with a minority language that is sometimes devalued by the larger society. Additionally, I understand how this societal bias can influence the maintenance of the minority language and the development of multilingual identities.

Fourth, as a university professor and an interdisciplinary researcher, I have updated knowledge in the field of multilingual development. I have been teaching and conducting research in areas such as child and adolescent development, language and literacy development, multilingual development, and parent-child interactions. My interdisciplinary experiences have enriched my perspective on many aspects of multilingual development, including heritage-language development; that is, I regard multilingual development not just from the linguistic viewpoint but also from other angles.

Finally, as a multilingual advocate, I frequently work with parents of multilingual children and adolescents. Therefore, I can add an insightful spin to the discussion of multilingual childrearing by including these parents' voices.

Unique features of the book

Deviating from the approaches of the traditional parent advice book, this book will take a few unique stances.

Treating parents as active and intelligent readers

Unlike most parenting advice books, in which parents tend to be treated as passive readers and are rarely provided with access to original sources, this book takes a different approach by considering parents as active and intelligent readers. To this end, readers are provided with original research sources, such as references, and further readings are also suggested at the end of each chapter for those interested in pursuing the topics discussed. In the same vein, some jargon and technical terminologies regarding multilingualism are deliberately introduced to empower readers to access research literature directly if they wish to do so. When jargon and technical terms are introduced, they are bolded (as you have probably noticed) with an explanation either before or after the bolded terms or in the endnotes. You can also see the definitions of bolded terms in the glossary at the end of the book. Based on my interactions with parents, those who take the time to look for reading materials on multilingual childrearing topics are already motivated, and they want to have more information about certain topics. The e-mails I have received from parents suggest that some parents want to read the first-hand information about multilingual research instead of having it interpreted by parenting book authors.

Situating multilingual and heritage-language development in other developmental contexts

This book does not consider adolescents' multilingual development as an isolated linguistic phenomenon; rather, it addresses multilingual development concurrently with other aspects of adolescents' life such as biological, cognitive, and social development. Situating adolescent multilingual development in other contexts encourages parents to consider taking an approach that aims to cultivate a *whole* person rather than just a *multilingual* person.

Providing a general picture of adolescent language development

Before discussing the specific heritage-language development characteristics in Chapters 3, 4, 5, 6 and 7, I begin with a general overview of adolescent language development. The purpose of doing so is not to use monolingual adolescent language development as a yardstick to measure heritage-language development; instead, it provides a broader picture for you to see how certain language features are typically developed during adolescence. By knowing the general language development pattern, you can decide how to plan your strategies to support your children's heritage-language development. Even though your heritage-language-learning teens may not reach the same level as their native speaking peers who live in the native language speaking environment, it is always useful for you to understand the important areas on which you might focus your effort. For example, when I understood that Chinese-speaking adolescents who lived in a Chinese dominant environment usually mastered certain **measurement words** or **classifiers** (words used along with numerals to define the quantity of a given object such as one 篇 essay), I deliberately taught these Chinese measurement words in my daily interactions with my two children.

Considering heritage-language development in the *discourse* framework

Multilingual development is not just about developing multiple languages; it is also involves understanding how a language (discourse) is used in different cultures. The word *discourse* has been commonly referred to as language exchanges (e.g. conversations). Linguist Paul Gee considers this definition too narrow. He has proposed broadening the definition of *discourse* by capitalising the word *Discourse* and differentiating it from the common rendering of the word *discourse*.[33] The capitalised **Discourse or the big D** highlights different cultural, social and linguistic groups' practices in using language that is based on their beliefs and values.

In accordance with the Discourse framework (or the big D idea), this book emphasises that acquiring multiple languages does not just mean learning multiple grammatical rules; rather, it means that multilingual learners also learn how these languages are used to communicate different worldviews. Understanding heritage-language development from the big D perspective allows us to broaden the scope of multilingual development discussion to include topics beyond just linguist forms and functions.

Addressing heritage-language childrearing and its impact on multilingual family welfare

Multilingual and heritage-language childrearing is already a complex endeavour, and on top of that, parents from multilingual families often come from different cultural backgrounds. As a result, the multilingual childrearing process may affect the coherence and wellbeing of multilingual families.[34] Until recently,[35] this topic had been largely neglected in the published literature. This book takes this matter of multilingual family wellbeing seriously and devotes an entire chapter (Chapter 9) to addressing this topic in an effort to help parents avoid unwanted consequences.

Utilising interdisciplinary information

This book utilises information from multiple fields such as linguistics, literacy, psychology and education. Thus, the recommended strategies provide you with a comprehensive understanding of what multilingual childrearing, especially multilingual adolescent development, involves.

Providing useful language development measures

To help you view your adolescent's current heritage-language development in terms of words, grammar and language use, this book includes some practical and simple language and literacy measures that can be implemented when appropriate. By understanding your children's current heritage-language development levels, you can focus on those areas that need more support.

Reader-friendly writing style

After the publication of my book *Growing Up With Three Languages: Birth to Eleven*, many readers told me that they liked my personal narrative writing style. To keep the same style, I have tried my best to strike a balance between scholarly rigour and reader accessibility. To increase readers' enjoyment, I have included many interesting and meaningful personal anecdotes. I suppose that readers will probably enjoy a book with real-life anecdotes rather than a dry advice book that presents information out of context.

Data used in this book

Unlike the data sources used in my book *Growing Up With Three Languages: Birth to Eleven*, which were based mainly on a large corpus of video-recoded data, the data used in this book are based on several sources, including daily observational notes, regular video-recorded data and audio-recorded data. As young children, Léandre and Dominique were fine with me videotaping them in the daily context. In general, both children were quite comfortable with videotaping until the end of elementary school, when they were each about eleven. Staring from middle school, Dominique became more conscious of the videotaping. One time, when his friend came to have lunch with us, I set up my camera (as usual) to record their natural conversations. Dominique (12; 2; 4) told his friends 'Don't say anything. My mom is video-recording.' Léandre also occasionally protested that he did not feel comfortable being videotaped all the time. As a result of the children's increasing consciousness of being video-recorded, I negotiated with them that I would videotape them only on special occasions such as birthdays, holidays, vacations abroad and guest visits, and I would replace videotaping with on-the-spot note-taking at other times.

Some readers may question whether or not the teens behaved naturally when they were conscious of being videotaped. Based on my years of videotaping data collection experiences, it should not be a concern as long as the videotaped data are handled well. I usually ignored the first 10 minutes of data and used the data 10 minutes into the recording (in a two-hour recording), because I noticed how my children revealed their 'true colours' a few minutes after the camera started rolling. I have also found that I acted natural in these recording, even though I was supposed to be very conscious about my own taping. You would be shocked to hear what I revealed in those video recordings, saying and doing things that I would not do or say if I knew that others would hear.

This new way of documenting my sons' multilingual development turned out to be quite effective from the data collecting perspective. Because the contexts of the videos have been similar over the years (e.g. birthdays, holidays, vacations abroad, selected guest visits), I was better able to compare **lexicon** (words), **syntax** (sentences), and other areas of growth and change throughout the years. Moreover, by taking the on-the-spot notes, I could immediately reflect on (I call it coding) what had been said immediately and follow up, or clarify, with the children if necessary.

I want to note that even though Dominique and Léandre sometimes felt uncomfortable being treated as research subjects in their teen years, they have been, for the most part, willing participants in my research. For example, when Dominique (16; 6; 28) saw me leaving the dinner table and writing down something in my notebook, he asked what example I was writing down. I said it was not about him. He replied, 'Oh, what I said was not a good example?' Also, he (17; 0; 18) insisted that I should study why he mistook Léandre's pronouncing *er* (which sounds like Chinese *one* and *two*) when explaining the rules in German to Chinese 一 (one) and 二 (two).

Brief Update on the Two Main Characters Featured in the Book

Since the publication of the book *Growing Up With Three Languages: Birth to Eleven*, many readers have asked what happened to the trilingual development of our two children. In addition, some have asked for updates on what they have been doing since the book was published. Here is a brief update.

Léandre

Our older son Léandre is a happy-go-lucky young man. His zany humour is contagious. We call him Mr Bean[36] in the family. There is not one day that goes by that he doesn't tell jokes. When he (16; 2; 2) saw a few bikers passing by in our neighbourhood, he said to them, 'France is that way!' Also, when I reminded him in a text message that my birthday was the next day, saying, 'What's special about tomorrow?' He replied, 'It is Chairman Wang's birthday,' obviously referring to my background in communist China and replacing Chairman Mao with Chairman Wang.

Léandre reluctantly played bass in his school orchestra throughout elementary, middle school and high school and hated playing piano as a child; however, he is now an enthusiastic electronic and classic guitar player. He even has his own band and composes his own music. The band occasionally gives performances and produces CDs and other recordings. He is also very good at fundraising. In each fundraising event in which he has participated, he has always raised the most money by using some interesting strategies. We call him the 'Capitalist Benefiting Social Causes.'

Léandre is an intelligent young man. He consistently scored between the 98th and 100th percentile on all standardised tests, including the SAT, from kindergarten to 12th grade, which suggests that being multilingual is definitely not a drawback, if not advantageous. However, being a smart person, Léandre is also a procrastinator. He almost always does his work at the last minute. He even has a theory about it. He often reasoned with us that when he does his work first, it takes him two hours to do what he can do in 20 minutes. If he played first, that would leave him little time to do his work and would force him to do it completely focused, whereas if he started early he would idle and waste time and end up having no time to play at all. He calls himself an 'active' or 'reasoned' procrastinator. He believes and often tries to convince others that this type of procrastination is productive and healthy.

Léandre is now attending a university in the United States. He is triple majoring in economics, international studies, and German. He acquired three languages (English, French and Chinese) simultaneously from birth and learnt and mastered Spanish in middle and high school with additional input from his babysitter and Spanish-speaking friends. He acquired advanced German in college, in addition to having solid knowledge of Swiss-German dialect; and he has elementary knowledge of Portuguese. He has been teaching himself Russian sporadically and plans to formally study Russian. Léandre has a genuine interest in world languages and he is a keen observer of language differences (a real linguistic in the everyday context!).

Léandre gets along well with people, and he is happy wherever he goes. I remember that I was tearing up when I said good-bye to him when we dropped him off at his university for the first time, worrying how he would cope with the new college life because he had literally never been separated from us. He left us happily; two minutes later, I saw him walking with a group of new friends. I attribute his easy adjustment to a different environment to his security attachment, because we have spent time with him instilling our heritage languages, and he left us easily.

He has not finalised his future career plan yet, and I suspect it will take him a long time to decide what to do, as this seems to be his personality. However, the indication is that he might do something international and utilise his multilingual assets.

Dominique

Dominique is also doing exceptionally well in his academics, scoring between the 98th and 100th percentile on all his standardised tests and the SAT. For example, he had the highest grade in his 11th grade English Regent's Test, earning a score of 100%. As a young child, Dominique already exhibited exceptional creativity. Throughout adolescence, his creativity developed further in many areas. For instance, during his sophomore year in high school, Dominique (15; 3; 5) was running for sophomore class president. He made an advertisement by replacing the image of Washington on the one-dollar bill with his own photo. I suspect that his creative flier was partially responsible for winning him the seat.

Dominique is also attending a university in the United States. He continues to be an active and talented soccer (football) player. However, in the last couple of years, his passion for soccer has petered out a bit, and he is now very passionate about musical composition. His genre of music is somewhat avant-garde, but he is in the process of defining it. He claims that he will compose music that most people will enjoy. He also likes to rap. He is a fan of Snoop Dog, Mobb Deep, Dr Dre, Kanye West, Ice Cube, Mos Def, Tupac Shakur, the Notorious B.I.G, Dumbfoundead and Grand Corps Malade, to name just a few. Dominique's rap lyrics often demonstrate his linguistic talent in multilingual word playing.

Besides the three languages he grew up with (French, Chinese and English), Dominique is also fluent in Spanish, which he acquired in middle and high school and practised often with a friend's mother, who used to be his babysitter. He also has passing knowledge of Portuguese and Swiss German. He is interested in Arabic and plans to formally learn it soon. Dominique is a creative writer. He definitely has a talent for writing. He began to write screenplays in middle school as a hobby, and some of them are really fantastic. In high school, his composition was chosen by one of his AP English teachers as a model for his peers.

Dominique is also a caring and spiritual person, and he shows concern for global issues, such as the environment. For example, he picks up garbage on his way home. We call him 'the garbage man' in our community. He is also keen on social justice. After visiting the White House as a young child, he said, 'If I were president, I would give money to everyone.' When driving to France when he was a teenager (17; 0; 2), he imitated the accent of French president François Hollande, repeating the same idea. He was named the socialist in the family. Recently, he told me that he wanted to major in international studies, environmental studies and Portuguese so that he can pursue humanitarian work in Brazil. However, he does have a penchant for changing his mind frequently.

The following revelation on the definition of *universe* occurred one day during dinner and seems to personify Léandre and Dominique metaphorically:

Léandre (15; 3; 6): Universe is logic and possibility.
Dominique (13; 4; 10): Universe is a song.

Overview of the Book

This book contains 10 chapters.

In Chapter 1, the introduction chapter you just read, the pressing need for supporting adolescent multilingual development, especially heritage-language development, is briefly addressed. This chapter also showcases the advantages of multilingualism with various examples. My unique background as an author and the content of the book, as well as its unique features, are discussed. The chapter concludes with a description of how the data used in the book were collected, an update of the two main characters featured in the book, and an overview of the chapters.

Chapter 2 begins with a discussion of adolescent physical, cognitive, social and identity development characteristics. It then identifies the challenges of continuing multilingual development, especially heritage-language development, during life's most interesting period: adolescence. It concludes with useful strategies to help you maximise your chances of raising multilingual teens.

Chapter 3 focuses on heritage-language **phonological** (sound system) development during adolescence. It pinpoints the specific heritage-language phonological development characteristics as well as challenges and provides supporting strategies to help adolescents further develop their heritage-language phonological skills.

Chapter 4 discusses heritage-language **lexical-semantic** (words and meanings) development during adolescence. It focuses on the specific heritage-language lexical-semantic development features and provides supporting strategies to help adolescents further develop their heritage-language lexical-semantic skills.

Chapter 5 provides an overview of the general **morphological** (word structure) and **syntactic** (word order or sentence) developmental trend during adolescence. It focuses on the specific heritage-language morphosyntactic development features as well as challenges, and it provides supporting strategies to help adolescents further develop their heritage-language morphosyntactic skills. Please note that this chapter is more technical than other chapters. You can directly go to the section on strategies if you do not want to be bothered with the technical terms.

Chapter 6 provides an overview of the general characteristics of **pragmatic** (language use) and metalinguistic (the ability to think about language) achievements during adolescence. It presents the specific heritage-language pragmatic and metalinguistic development characteristics as well as challenges and provides supporting strategies to help adolescents further develop their heritage-language pragmatic and metalinguistic skills (e.g. awareness of the rules of the word structure).

Chapter 7 outlines the general literacy development characteristics during adolescence. It also identifies heritage-language literacy developmental uniqueness. It suggests how to motivate adolescents to continue with their heritage-language and literacy development when they are undergoing many changes in their lives. It also offers effective strategies that facilitate the development of self-motivated language and literacy learning behaviours. In addition, digital-mediated skills and critical literacy skills are identified as necessary multilingual literacy skills. Suggestions are made about how to choose stimulating language and literacy materials, carry out engaging family activities, and monitor adolescents' heritage-language literacy progress. It also recommends strategies that can foster adolescents' sustainable interest in furthering language and literacy development throughout their lives. Please note that this chapter is a lot longer than other chapters because literacy encapsulates all the areas in language development discussed in Chapters 3, 4, 5 and 6.

Chapter 8 examines how multilingual upbringing impacts multilingual adolescents' identity development. It demonstrates how multilingual adolescents navigate and negotiate their complex linguistic, cultural, and personal experiences. Suggestions are made about how to support multilingual adolescents' healthy identity development.

Chapter 9 underscores the importance of multilingual family welfare in the process of raising multilingual adolescents. It begins by examining the four indicators of multilingual family cohesion (parental congruence on childrearing, quality of family communication, time allocated for heritage-language learning and leisure and parental expectations of their offspring's heritage-language achievement). In this chapter, I share my own family anecdotes and discuss the issues that arise as a result of multilingual practices that may potentially threaten the welfare of the multilingual family. It concludes by providing practical strategies to help adolescents continue their multilingual development without sacrificing family wellbeing.

In Chapter 10, the main points conveyed throughout the book are recaptured with several important take-away messages. Readers are left with a positive message: Although it is challenging to raise multilingual adolescents (and multilingual children in general), it is possible as long as parents use adequate supporting strategies. Moreover, the book touches upon some complex issues regarding multilingual childrearing, such as how single parents and monolingual parents can promote multilingual development in adolescence and how parents can continue to support their children's heritage and multilingual development when they leave home for college or other independent living.

A Few Cautionary Comments

Before you read the rest of the book, I would like to make a few cautionary comments about the rearing of multilingual children and adolescents.

First, few studies to date have examined the specific phonological, lexical, semantic, syntactic and pragmatic features of heritage-language speaking adolescents, much less how these features interact in the heritage-language reading and writing process. Thus, when you consider the strategies I propose in the following chapters, you may want to cautiously test them in your own family.

Second, multilingual language development should not only include the so-called 'standard' languages but should also include dialects, creoles and manual languages, such as signed languages. Although this book is not able to cover all of these different types of communication forms due to space limits, the strategies that will be discussed may also be useful if your teens are learning dialects, **creoles**[37] or signed languages in addition to their mainstream language(s).

Third, because this book is about my own children, the accounts discussed certainly cannot do justice to the richness and diversity in multilingual families. However, this is not the point of the book. The point is to use my two children as a basis for addressing the issues and strategies involved in adolescent continued multilingual development. The purpose is not to describe what will happen to all multilingual adolescents, but to describe what could happen, given the use of some strategies. In other words, by sharing our successes, failures, frustrations and challenges in our childrearing process, you can compare them to your own experiences and find the best way to raise your children with more than one language. As Mitsuyo Sakamoto commented, 'Successful stories of raising children with heritage language(s) have to be told because they can support and validate what parents are doing now and demonstrate what can be done in the future.'[38]

Thus, this book is not meant to be a panacea for parenting multilingual adolescents, nor does it attempt to show all of the ways to raise multilingual adolescents. Rather, it intends to discuss the complex process of raising multilingual adolescents through personal experience and anecdotes. In such a way, the goal of this book is to inspire you and encourage you to reflect on your own multilingual adolescent–raising practices.

Fourth, many people tend to have a somewhat incomplete notion about the effects of multilingualism; they either idolise it or vilify it. I want to stress that multilingualism affects individuals differently. Some multilinguals may develop particularly strong intellectual and linguistic abilities as a byproduct of multiple language leaning and use.[39] Other multilinguals may have relatively weaker abilities in their respective languages, because input in or exposure to each language is not evenly distributed.[40] It is important to have a realistic view of multilingual effects and understand that there is no guarantee that being multilingual will result in benefits that are associated with multilingualism as described earlier in the chapter, nor does it suggest that multilingualism is the cause of all the problems. Thus, not all multilinguals will function superbly or equally well; rather, the multilingual effects on an individual depend on many complex factors, including the individual child or adolescent's sociolinguistic environments, parental support, aptitude, motivation and personality.

Finally, and most importantly, this book is definitely not about raising 'super' children. I have observed a recent frenzy over raising multilingual children and want to emphasise that it is not my intention to follow that trend. In essence, this book is my reflective account of my family's story of multilingual development and maintenance.

Recommended Readings

Bialystok, E., Craik, F.I.M. and Luk, G. (2012) Bilingualism: Consequences for mind and brain. *Trends in Cognitive Sciences* 16, 240–50.
Bialystok, E. and Hakuta, K. (1994) *In Other Words*. New York: Basic Books.
Cummins, J. (2000) *Language, Power and Pedagogy: Bilingual Children in the Crossfire*. Clevedon: Multilingual Matters.

Notes and References

1. *Le Chat* is a series of cartoons by the popular Belgium humourist, writer, illustrator, actor and comic Philippe Geluck.
2. In conventional language research literature, children's age is described as year; month; and day. So if a child is 15 years, 9 months, and 10 days old, their age is shown as (15; 9; 10). Going forward in the text, the ages of children will be described in this way.
3. E-mail communication on 28 May 2011. Pseudonyms were used for the teen at the request of his mother.
4. E-mail communication on 3 November 2013.
5. Traditionally, people who speak more than one language are labelled based on the number of languages they speak: bilingual (two languages), trilingual (three languages) or quadralingual (four languages). However, some researchers suggest that it may be more accurate to use the word *multilingual* to describe people who know more than one language. Charlotte Hoffmann suggested that the term *multilingual* is a more authentic term than *bilingual* or *trilingual* because it clearly distinguishes the macrolinguistic level (bilingual or trilingual) from the microlinguistic level (monolingual) [see Hoffmann, C. (2001). Toward the description of trilingual competence. *International Journal of Bilingualism*, 5(1), 1–17]. Moreover, Marilyn Martin-Jones and Kathryn Jones (2000) provided additional reasons why it may be more accurate to use the term *multilingual* than *bilingual*. First, many people have more than two spoken or written languages and language varieties within their communicative repertoire. These include the languages and literacies associated with their cultural inheritance, the regional variety of dialects spoken in their local neighbourhoods and some form of 'standard' language (such as 'standard' English). Second, the term *multilingual* signals the multiplicity and complexity of the communicative purposes that have come to be associated with different spoken and written languages within a group's repertoire. Third, the term *multilingual* takes into account the fact that in any linguistic minority household or local group (for example, among speakers of Welsh, Gujarati or Cantonese), there are multiple paths to the acquisition of the spoken and written languages within the group repertoire, and people have varying degrees of expertise in these languages and literacies. Finally, the term *multilingual* is more useful than the term *bilingual* because it focuses attention on the multiple ways in which people draw on and combine the codes in their communicative repertoire when they speak and write [see Martin-Jones, M. and Jones, K.E. (2000). Multilingual literacies. In M. Martin-Jones and K. Jones (eds) *Multilingual literacies: Reading and writing different worlds* (pp. 1–15). Amsterdam: John Benjamins]. In this book, unless the specific numbers of languages are actually referred to (*bilingual* or *trilingual*), the word *multilingual* is used as a generic term.
6. With the only exception of the book by Caldas, S.J. (2006) *Raising Bilingual-Biliterate Children in Monolingual Cultures*. Clevedon: Multilingual Matters Ltd.
7. Bialystok, E. and Hakuta, K. (1994) *In other words*. New York: Basic Books.
8. Mechelli, A., Crinion, J.T., Noppeney, U., O'Doherty, J., Ashburner, J., Frackowiak, R. and Price, C.J. (2004) Neurolinguistics: Structural plasticity in the bilingual brain. *Nature* 431, 757.
9. Bialystok, E. and Martin, M.M. (2004) Attention and inhibition in bilingual children: Evidence from the dimensional change card sort task. *Developmental Science* 7 (3), 325–39.
10. Friesen, D.C., Latman, V., Alejandra Calvo, A. and Bialystok, E. (2014) Attention during visual search: The benefit of bilingualism. *International Journal of Bilingualism*.

¹¹ Bialystok, E., Craik, F.I.M. and Luk, G. (2012) Bilingualism: Consequences for mind and brain. *Trends in Cognitive Sciences* 16, 240–50. Poulin-Dubois, D., Blaye, A., Coutya, J. and Bialystok, E. (2011) The effects of bilingualism on toddlers' executive functions. *Journal of Experimental Psychology*, 108, 567–79.

¹² Paap, K.R. and Greenberg, Z.I. (2013) There is no evidence for a bilingual advantage in executive processing. *Cognitive Psychology* 66, 232–58.

¹³ Baker, C. (2011) *Foundations of Bilingual Education and Bilingualism*. Bristol: Multilingual Matters.

¹⁴ Hong, Y.-Y., Wang, C., No, S. and Chiu, C.-Y. (2007) Multicultural identities. In S. Kitayama and D. Cohen (eds) *Handbook of Cultural Psychology* (pp. 323–45). New York: Guilford Press

¹⁵ Bialystok, E. (2007) Acquisition of literacy in multilingual children: A framework for research. *Language Learning* 57 (1), 45–77.

¹⁶ Dibaj, F. (2011). Vocabulary learning: A comparison of learners of English as a second and third Language. *Australian Review of Applied Linguistics* 34 (2), 19–215.

¹⁷ Cenoz, J. (2011) The influence of bilingualism on third language acquisition: Focus on multilingualism. *Language Teaching* 46 (1), 71–86.

¹⁸ García, E. (1983) *Early Child Bilingualism, With Special Reference to the Mexican-American Child*. Albuquerque: University of New Mexico Press.

¹⁹ Cohen, A.D. and Horowitz, R. (2002) What should teachers know about bilingual learners and the reading process. In J.H. Sullivan (ed) *Literacy and the Second Language Learner*, vol. 1. Greenwich, CT: Information Age.

²⁰ K-12 is the US school system, meaning kindergarten to 12th grade or the end of high school.

²¹ In US high schools, college-level courses are offered. After finishing the courses, students can take AP tests for college credit.

²² Oh, J.S. and Fuligni, A.J. (2010) The role of heritage language development in the ethnic identity and family relationships of adolescents from immigrant backgrounds. *Social Development* 19, 202–20.

²³ Tabors, P.O. (1997) *One Child, Two Languages: A Guide for Preschool Educators of Children Learning English as a Second Language*. Baltimore: Brookes.

²⁴ Portes, A. and Rumbaut, R.G. (2001) *Legacies: The Story of the Immigrant Second Generation*. Berkeley: University of California Press.
Rogler, L.H., Cortes, R.S. and Malgady, R.G. (1991) Acculturation, mental health status among Hispanics. *American Psychologist* 46, 585–97.

²⁵ Wang, X.-L. (2011) *Learning to Read and Write in the Multilingual Family*. Bristol: Multilingual Matters.

²⁶ Personal communication, 7 November 2011.

²⁷ Simpson, J. (2013) Identity alignment on an ESOL class blog. *International Journal of Applied Linguistics* 23 (2), 183–201.

²⁸ García, H. (1985) Family and offspring language maintenance and their effects of Chicano college students' confidence and grades. In E. García and R. Padilla (eds) *Advances in Bilingual Education Research* (pp. 226–43). Tucson, AZ: University of Arizona Press.

²⁹ Wang, X.-L. (2011) *Learning to Read and Write in the Multilingual Family*. Bristol: Multilingual Matters.

³⁰ Baker, C. (2011) *Foundations of Bilingual Education and Bilingualism*. Bristol: Multilingual Matters.

³¹ Wang, X.-L. (2008) *Growing Up With Three Languages: Birth to Eleven*. Bristol: Multilingual Matters.

³² Heritage language is a term that is often used to refer to languages from one's heritage other than the mainstream language used in a given social context. The alternative terms for heritage language are community language and home language.

³³ Gee, J.P. (2010) *An Introduction to Discourse Analysis: Theory and Method*. New York, NY: Routledge.

³⁴ Wang, X.-L. (2013) Multilingual family welfare. In T.K. Bhatia and W.C. Ritchie (eds) *The Handbook of Bilingualism and Multilingualism*. Boston: Wiley-Blackwell.

³⁵ The following chapter is the first to address multilingual family wellbeing: Wang, X.-L. (2013). Multilingual family welfare. In T.K. Bhatia and W.C. Ritchie (eds) *The Handbook of Bilingualism and Multilingualism*. Boston: Wiley-Blackwell.

[36] *Mr Bean* is a British television programme starring actor Rowan Atkinson. His dry humour is hilarious.
[37] Creole is a language that originated from a mixture of two or more languages. It is developed from a pidgin, a simplified version of a language. Creoles differ from pidgins because creoles have been nativised by children as their primary language, with the result that they have features of natural languages that are normally missing from pidgins, which are not anyone's first language.
[38] Sakamoto, M. (2000) Raising bilingual and trilingual children: Japanese immigrant parents' child-rearing experiences. Doctorate dissertation. University of Toronto.
[39] Bialystok, E. and Martin, M.M. (2004) Attention and inhibition in bilingual children: Evidence from the dimensional change card sort task. *Developmental Science* 7(3): 325–39.
[40] Gollan, T.H., Forster, K.I. and Frost, R. (1997) Translation priming with different scripts: Masked priming with cognates and noncognates in Hebrew–English bilinguals. *Journal of Experimental Psychology, Learning, Memory, & Cognition* 23, 1122–39.

2 Heritage-Language Maintenance and Multilingual Development in the Teenage Years

Shortly after his 16th birthday, while our family was in Switzerland for the summer vacation, Dominique declared that he was going to change his lifestyle and eat healthy food. During lunch, he asked his Swiss grandmother to serve him only carrots and water. He professed that he no longer had any desire for fruit juice, *pain au chocolat* (chocolate pastry) or *Rivella* (a milk-based soft drink), which he had been bingeing on each time we visited Switzerland.

This sort of teen exaggeration probably resonates with anyone who has raised or worked with teenagers. De Vries Guth and Pratt-Fartro[1] presented the following vivid descriptions about adolescents: 'Adolescents are a strange and wonderful mix of mature and child-like qualities, manifested in no particular order. They shift from serious, concerned citizens to teasing children with one comment and can be reduced to silence or tears with a look from a peer or teacher…' Indeed, the teenage years are full of contradictions and surprises.

The purpose of this chapter is to help you understand the physical, cognitive, social and identity changes associated with adolescence. Knowing the characteristics of adolescence will help you work with teens more effectively in their heritage-language maintenance and multilingual development. Moreover, this chapter discusses the major challenges associated with adolescent heritage-language maintenance. Finally, this chapter will provide many useful strategies for you to consider when working with your teenage children.

The Nature of Adolescence

The etymology of adolescence derives from the Latin word *adolescere,* which means growing up and near maturity. **Adolescence** is a transitional period from middle childhood to adulthood. Over a century ago, psychologist Stanley Granville Hall spread the term *adolescence* in his book *Adolescence: Its Psychology and Its Relations to Physiology, Anthropology, Sociology, Sex, Crime, Religion and Education.*[2] Hall famously used two words, *storm* and *stress,* to portray adolescents.

Adolescence has been typically regarded in Western culture as a period of troubled time with emotional upheaval and turmoil.[3] This view seems to reflect the opinions of many of the proverbial men and women on the street. For instance, I once asked the graduate students in my child and adolescent development class to survey people about the words that they would use to describe adolescents. Eighty-three percent of the people they interviewed associated the following negative words with adolescents: *sloppy, argumentative, moody, stubborn, trouble, confused, rebellious, disrespectful, disobedient, loud, obnoxious, stinking, complex, sensitive* and *lost*; and only 17% of those surveyed used positive words such as *caring, curious* and *expressive*.

The truth about adolescence is far different from the popular perception, and adolescents do possess many wonderful qualities. Teenage years are a unique time to explore, as well as to learn to negotiate many physical, cognitive, social and identity changes. Thus, adolescents may appear to be edgy, difficult and extreme. Even though teenagers may not elicit the cuddly feelings in us that they once did as two-year-olds, and their rolling eyes and rebellious tone (such as the insolent behaviour exhibited by Léandre described in the opening vignette in Chapter 1) may turn us away sometimes, and they sometimes may take extreme actions (like the example displayed by Dominique in the beginning of this chapter), adolescents are beguiling human beings who are often energetic, thoughtful, idealistic and gullible and who have a deep interest in what is fair and right. If we, as parents, are willing to understand their variability, enjoy the challenges and learn how to communicate with them, we will be successful in working with these demanding yet giving adolescents,[4] and they will grow into distinct individuals with much potential.

Adolescent Age Boundaries

Most people tend to associate adolescence with the teenage years (i.e. between the ages of 13 and 19). In fact, the adolescent age boundaries are never quite agreed upon among developmental psychologists and educators. Various adolescent age boundaries have been proposed, ranging from age 10 to age 25. In this book, I have decided to cover the adolescent period from age 12 to age 19 for three main reasons. First, my last book, *Growing Up With Three Languages: Birth to Eleven*, discussed the multilingual development of my two sons from birth to age 11. Thus, it is logical for this book to start with age 12. Second, in most countries, children enter middle school at around age 11 or 12. This is the time period when children are transitioning from middle childhood to adolescence. Third, I purposely use age 19 as a cutoff age for adolescence because this is the time when many young people are enrolled in college (which some countries call university) or have entered the workforce. Yet, they are still lingering at the borderline of adolescence and young adulthood. I would like to show how these young people's heritage languages fare when they are trying their initial independence and semi-independence. Hence, I will use the terms *teenagers* and *adolescents* interchangeably throughout the book, with an understanding that the age range I refer to is from 12 to 19.

Changes During Adolescence

Many changes occur during the teenage years. Physical changes tend to begin first, followed by social and identity changes. The adolescent period usually ends with the assumption of adult responsibility.

Physical changes

Many of teens' behaviours are connected to their neurological development status. The brain and neurological system are not fully developed during adolescence. For example, the two key systems involved in making sound decisions and controlling impulses, the limbic system and the frontal cortex of the brain, are not quite mature. The **limbic system** is responsible for emotions, reward-seeking, novelty, risk-taking and sensation-seeking behaviours; and the **frontal lobe** is responsible for judgement and decision making. The limbic system develops earlier than the frontal cortex. As the limbic system becomes mature, adolescents become more responsive to pleasure and emotional stimulation. As a result, adolescents need more intense emotional simulation than both children and adults; that perhaps explains why teens tend to take risks and seek thrills. Their frontal lobe is also not quite ready for thoughtful decision-making during the adolescent period.[5]

Other dramatic physical changes, such as **growth spurts** (a rapid increase in height and sometimes also in weight) and **puberty** (biological changes such as sexual maturity), also occur during adolescence. These physical changes are not single events but a series of synchronised and interconnected changes involving and affecting cognitive, emotional, social and other changes. For example, the adolescent growth spurt can cause sleeping issues (e.g. irregular sleeping patterns) and the hormone changes can trigger moodiness.

Cognitive changes

Adolescents also demonstrate increased ability in hypothetical (scientific) and logical thinking. They no longer require concrete objects or events as support for thought but can come up with new and more general logical rules through internal reflection.[6] Unlike children in the previous developmental stages (early childhood and middle childhood), adolescents can solve problems by beginning to think about possibilities and then proceeding to reality. In other words, they begin to reason more like scientists by devising ways to solve problems and by testing solutions systematically.[7]

Teenagers also begin to demonstrate formal **operational thought**, which is also known as **abstract reasoning**; that is, they can make logical inferences merely through verbal representations. For example, children in the earlier developmental stages would need to see the concrete relationship between A, B and C to be able to make the logical inference that if $A > B$ and $B > C$, then $A > C$. Adolescents, on the other hand, can reach the logical conclusion $A > C$ without having to rely on concrete steps.[8] However, adolescents' cognitive ability is not restricted to abstract reasoning abilities, and their developing power of thought opens up new cognitive horizons, which drives them to idealism and to think in more expansive and idealistic ways. Equipped with these newly attained intellectual abilities, adolescents may become more argumentative and engage in extended speculation about ideas by excising their new intellectual muscles.[9]

Social, emotional and identity changes

Physical and cognitive changes may make teens become more self-conscious and self-focusing with an exaggerated sense of personal uniqueness. They may believe that they are the centre of attention and that others are highly attentive to their behaviour and appearance. This phenomenon is called **adolescent egocentrism**. Adolescents are also sensitive to public criticism and are prone to taking risks.

Teens may also adopt a stance of rigid dogmatism. For example, one evening when I drove home with Léandre, I saw no one was behind our car, and therefore I did not use the right-turn signal when turning into our driveway. Léandre (16; 9; 11) criticised me for not following traffic rules. He lectured me for about five minutes, explaining why I should use my turn signals all the time.

Adolescents' nascent physical and cognitive changes and their inexperience with them may also make adolescents more anxious. Research indicates that there is a possible relationship between hormonal changes and emotional states. The hormonal changes can affect mood variability, and as a result, the adolescent emotional experience does differ in intensity, frequency and persistence from that of adults and younger children.[10]

Furthermore, adolescents are grappling with some common issues related to independence, such as changes in their relationship with parents, identity exploration, an increased need for more privacy, and idealisation of others. To adolescents, independence means that they are able to free themselves from their parents; however, by trying out their wings or experimenting with their freedom, teens also notice that they cannot completely detach themselves from their parents. Thus, they connect with their parents in a new and different way.

Finally, adolescents tend to idolise famous individuals. Crushes and hero-worship are two of the hallmarks of adolescence. For instance, in sixth grade, Dominique wore his hair exactly like the soccer star Cristiano Ronaldo, which demonstrates how teens can be easily influenced by famous individuals.

Teenagers and Their Unique Discourse Style

In addition to the various changes described above, teenagers also have their own distinct communication, or discourse, style. Their unique way of using language has been termed as 'teen dialect', 'teen language', 'teen speech', 'pubilect' and 'self-centred speech'. Some researchers believe that emotion is a significant factor in teen speech.[11] Adolescents use language as an outlet to project their feelings, opinions, frustrations and reactions. The emotive language function allows teens to capture the attention of those around them.[12] It is necessary for teens to use their style of discourse to make connections with their peers and solidify their identity through their special **registers** (communication style).

Teens' special way of speaking includes pronunciation and word usage that differs from those used by adults and children. For example, the typical words used by

English-speaking teens include 'like', 'groovy', 'da bomb', 'sick' and 'way cool'.[13] Even though they use this unique discourse style, most adolescents know how to adjust their discourse style to appease different audiences. You have probably noticed that they speak differently when they talk to their peers in comparison to how they talk to you and to their teachers.

Challenges in Maintaining Heritage Language During Adolescence

The many complex developmental changes that adolescents experience do pose great challenges for both parents and themselves in terms of heritage-language maintenance and multilingual attainment. Having gone through the multilingual childrearing process myself and having observed many cases in other families, I can attest to the fact that that behind every successful story about heritage-language achievement, there lies hard work, sacrifice, dedication and unwavering commitment on the part of both parents and teenage children.

In the following sections, I will *foreground* a few of the challenges that parents and teens are likely to face on the multilingual development journey. I italicised the word *foreground* because I believe that the challenges that both parents and adolescents frequently face in maintaining a heritage language in the home environment need to be brought to the forefront so that both parents and teens can work together to overcome them. Let me use the following two well-known images to illustrate why I want to *foreground* challenges in adolescent heritage-language and multilingual development. Please take a look at Figures 2.1 and 2.2.

Obviously, depending on what you want to focus on, you see different images. In Figure 2.1, you either see a vase or profiles of two human faces, and in Figure 2.2,

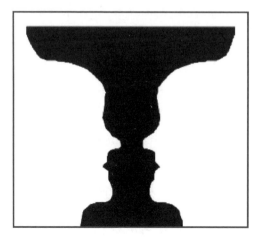

Figure 2.1 Robin Vase[14]

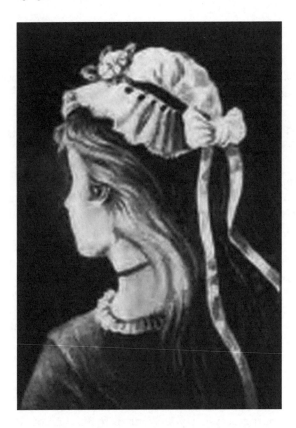

Figure 2.2 Young Woman vs. Mature Woman[15]

you either see a young woman or a mature woman. You see what you want to focus on (foreground). In other words, if we perceive something as the foreground, we see it clearly. Similarly, in adolescent heritage-language maintenance and multilingual development, if we foreground the challenges, we are likely to focus on and anticipate possible hurdles that may emerge on the adolescents' route to multilingualism, prepare to use effective strategies to optimise our teens' continued multilingual development, turn difficulties into teaching opportunities, and facilitate the overall growth and development of our multilingual adolescents. Below are some common challenges related to adolescent heritage-language maintenance and multilingual development.

Pressure to speak the mainstream language

Teenagers are most susceptible to peer pressure. If the majority of their peers are monolingual, multilingual adolescents may feel tremendous pressure to conform to the linguistic norm of speaking the mainstream language.[16] As you read in Chapter 1, Nikola complained to his mother that he felt embarrassed to speak his heritage languages, Croatian and Polish, when his friends were around and that his friends thought he sounded strange when he spoke his heritage languages to his parents. Likewise, Linjin's teenage daughter simply refused to speak her heritage Chinese. This is perhaps why many children of immigrants in the United States do not know their heritage language by the third generation.[17]

In addition, speaking a different language can cause unnecessary suspicion in social settings. In my previous book, *Growing Up With Three Languages: Birth to Eleven*, I mentioned that it was a challenge to converse in our heritage languages when others were around. In our case, the Chinese language seems to evoke more apprehensive reactions from people than French. Just recently on our vacation in Switzerland, I said something to Léandre during dinner in Chinese, and his great aunt thought we were talking about her. Indeed, using heritage language in a social setting sometimes does cause misunderstanding. More than once, people have asked us whether we were talking about them.

Inconsistency in belief systems

Parents from multilingual families are often from different linguistic and cultural backgrounds. Parents' childrearing beliefs and practices concerning teaching and learning may conflict with each other. In addition, parental beliefs may be different from that of the mainstream culture. These inconsistencies in belief systems may present themselves in how heritage language should be taught and learnt. JoAnn, who was originally from South Korea, wrote:[18]

> As a Korean, I believe in hard work in everything…Learning the Korean language is hard work. One needs to practice reading and writing everyday. That is why I help my daughter and son learn Korean and give them a lot of reading materials and language exercises sent by my Korean relatives. My husband is an American. He thinks I should not push too hard on our children…we sometimes argue about how to educate our children and how the Korean language should be taught…My children are teenagers now. They also tell me that I am too pushy…If I don't push, they are not going to learn the Korean language by themselves…

This kind of inconsistency in multilingual parenting beliefs affects how the heritage language is taught and, consequently, the multilingual attainment. I will further address this issue in Chapter 9.

Contrast of language teaching approaches

Teaching a heritage language in the home environment is not easy, and using effective strategies is essential for success. However, one may argue that our parents never formally taught us a language, and we just learnt it by talking to them. This is probably true in most cases, but with a condition; that is, besides our parents, we did have a larger linguistic supporting environment in which many other people helped us along the way. For example, our extended families, our teachers, our peers, the larger society and the media all supported our language development. In the case of Léandre and Dominique, their heritage French input was mainly from their father, and their heritage Chinese input was only from their mother. Without appropriate teaching strategies, it is unlikely that they could simply just 'get it', especially in terms of heritage-language reading and writing skills.

Moreover, even though many parents may be well versed in their heritage language, most of them are not taught how to teach that heritage language in the home environment. Parents often employ teaching methods by drawing on their own recollection of how they learnt as children.[19] In other words, parents often teach primarily in the same manner in which they were taught. As a result, when parents who are not educated in the same educational environment as their children (which is typical in multilingual families), the approaches that they take in heritage-language teaching may be in conflict with the methods with which children are familiar from their mainstream school. Thus, the methods used by parents may not be successful in engaging their children. A Chinese mother told me that she could not engage her 16-year-old son in reading and writing Chinese because he thought his mother's teaching was too rigid and boring. However, the mother maintained that this was the manner in which she had learnt to read and write back in China.[20]

Furthermore, to help maintain the family heritage language, many parents choose to send their children and adolescents to community heritage-language schools. There is no doubt that these community heritage-language schools are an important resource for helping heritage-language development, and many community heritage-language schools' contribution to promoting heritage language cannot be underestimated; however, the teaching style of some teachers (who are often parent volunteers) in these community language schools is often considerably different from the teaching style used in mainstream schools. Even though some teachers in community language schools may have received teaching training in their heritage countries, they are not familiar with the teaching style of their children's mainstream schools. In some cases, parents also have strong cultural beliefs about what learning should be. While some teachers in community language schools work hard to teach children and adolescents in the way that they believe to be effective for heritage-language learning, many children and adolescents are voicing their dissatisfaction. Such dissatisfaction may turn into objection during adolescence. Eventually, many teens may lose their motivation to continue with their heritage-language learning. The vivid account shown in Box 2.1, quoted from Xiao-lan Curdt-Christiansen's study, expresses the sentiment of a boy towards his Chinese heritage-language school in Montreal, and it also serves as a reminder for parents that something must be done to preserve children's desire to continue heritage-language learning.[21]

Léandre and Dominique shared the same reaction to their Chinese school. I remember that I used to have such a hard time getting them into the car for Chinese

Box 2.1 A Boy's Account of His Experience in Chinese School

I don't like the Chinese school, it's boring and the characters are too difficult to remember. Plus, there is no action in the class. I feel like sleeping. But my mom says I have to go. I like action. But in the Chinese school, we are not allowed to do anything. We are not allowed to talk or to write except dictations. So all the Chinese I have learnt I forget it all when I come home. In my French school, we are allowed to make up stories, we can talk about our stories in front of the whole class, and the teachers are nice.

school on Saturdays. Because of their unpleasant experience in the Chinese school (due to the rote learning, dull texts, repetition and the teacher's chastisement), they began to reject everything related to Chinese. At a certain point, they simply refused to go with me to any Chinese cultural events. In the end, I made a decision to stop enrolling them in a local Chinese language school because I feared that they would lose motivation to learn Chinese altogether if such a situation continued. In fact, the residual negative impact of their Chinese school experience could still be seen when Léandre was first in college. For example, during his freshman year of college, Léandre (18; 7; 5) told me that he did not want to ask for help in his statistics class from a teaching assistant who happened to be Chinese, for fear that he would act like his Chinese language school teachers (i.e. who would impart information repetitively) or nag like his Chinese mother (me).

Thus, the contrast in teaching styles may lead teens to be in favour of the teaching style of their mainstream teachers and to dislike the one used by their parents or teachers in community heritage-language schools. Unless community heritage-language schools and parents work together to negotiate and adjust the heritage-language teaching approaches, it will continue to be a challenge for the heritage-language schools to engage children and adolescents in heritage-language maintenance and multilingual development.

Time management in heritage-language learning and other activities

Heritage-language learning and development, especially heritage-language reading and writing development, requires time and energy. Heritage-language-speaking teens sometimes have to endure twice or more workload than monolingual teens in terms of language and literary learning. As a mother who was raising a bilingual child in Mitsuyo Sakamoto's study commented, 'having the child grow up to be bilingual is making a demand that far exceeds that expected of a child in a monolingual environment, requiring a bilingual child to manage twice the workload...'[22] Thus, balancing the time spent on heritage-language learning and other activities in adolescents' lives is a big struggle. Table 2.1 shows a typical day for Dominique when he was a junior in high school.

Table 2.1 A typical day for Dominique in his junior year of high school

6:00	Wake up and eat breakfast
6:45	Ride the school bus
7:30–14:15	Classes
14:30–15:00	Student governance meeting (Dominique was the junior class president) or other school activities
15:00–15:30	After-school fundraiser activities for the Math Honor Society
15:30–16:00	Varsity soccer practice/games or basketball coaching
16:00–17:00	Tutoring students who have learning needs or driver's education session and road practice
17:00–19:00	SAT[23] preparation class
19:00–midnight	Dinner and homework
Midnight or later, depending on the quantity of homework	Shower and sleep

Dominique obviously had a full plate during the week. It was indeed difficult for him to juggle between heritage-language learning (in particular, heritage-language reading and writing) and other activities. Without creative strategies and careful coordination of various activities, heritage-language learning is often unfeasible for many teens.

Lack of peer modelling

Teens who live in a typical language-learning environment are influenced by other peers around them and learn to use a different speech register when conversing with their peers. However, many heritage-language-speaking teens do not have peer heritage-language input, and thus they speak like their parents. For example, Philippe had his Swiss-German dialect input only from his parents. When he was a young man, he once had a conversation with some young people in Basel when he briefly enrolled for some courses at Basel University. They commented that he spoke like their grandparents. The challenge for heritage-language-speaking adolescents is that they often sound out of date when conversing with their contemporaries who live in the heritage-language-speaking environment.

Lack of societal and governmental support

Research has shown that the language choices and policies people make are largely influenced by social factors, and the consideration in promoting multilingualism and multilingual childrearing lies in the social settings and the available cultural mediating artefacts which parents can manipulate to achieve their goal.[24] It is unfortunate that in many developed countries, heritage language is often acquired and maintained in a very limited and restrained home environment without broader societal and governmental encouragement, recognition and support. This situation makes adolescent heritage-language development an even more challenging task. In my book *Growing Up With Three Languages: Birth to Eleven*, I expressed the sentiment that in many countries, the government and society at large had not really committed to providing resources for multilingual families to support their children's heritage languages. More than seven years have passed since my last book was published; the situation still has not really improved. The task for maintaining heritage languages largely rests on parents' shoulders.

It takes a community to raise multilingual children, teens included. Until governments in developed countries are committed to investing in multilingual education, parents will continue to be left alone to figure out ways to help their children and adolescents maintain a heritage language.

Language preference and bias

Scientific studies have long informed us that all human languages (including signed languages) and dialects are rule-governed communication systems. Therefore, all human communication systems deserve equal appreciation. Unfortunately, not all languages and dialects are embraced equally. In reality, some languages are valued more than others. My children's two heritage languages can be used as an example; their French has always been adored by neighbours, strangers, teachers and acquaintances, whereas their Chinese has been barely revered (except by Chinese speakers).

Adolescence is a period of conforming to other people's values. If an adolescent's heritage language is valued by the larger society and people around them, it is likely that they will be more motivated to maintain that language. Nikola's account of his friends' comments on his heritage languages (Croatian and Polish) discussed in Chapter 1 is an example of this phenomenon. Therefore, it is a real challenge for parents, especially immigrant parents, to battle against the language bias of the general public in the mainstream culture.

Proficiency gap in different languages

Another challenge during the adolescent period is the proficiency gap between teens' mainstream language and their heritage language. In the case of Léandre and Dominique, their two heritage languages were largely on a par with their mainstream language (English) when they entered kindergarten. To some extent, their two home languages were even stronger than their mainstream language. However, as soon as they entered school, beginning in kindergarten and first grade, their linguistic balance began to tilt. Their mainstream language, English, became stronger; and their home languages, French and Chinese, began to show signs of attrition. As they grew older and spent more time in school and with peers, their mainstream language topped their heritage language by far, especially in the aspect of reading and writing.

Moreover, the discrepancy between adolescents' heritage language and mainstream language widens also because of the settings in which their ambient languages are used. That is, before children enter school, their life experiences are generally quite similar. Therefore, the languages they use to communicate mainly revolve around their immediate environment: mostly toys, food and play. After children enter school, their experiences become more diverse as they move through grade levels. Consequently, the gap between their different languages broadens. It is likely that adolescents' heritage language is still limited to the home context, whereas their mainstream language is greatly expanded as they learn various academic subjects and socialise with peers. For instance, Dominique acquired a good amount of English vocabulary in his social-studies class to carry out a sophisticated conversation about Babylon in middle school, and he could do it moderately well in French because his father sometimes discussed it with him; however, he could only discuss the topic minimally in Chinese because I never discussed it with him. Unless proactive strategies are used, adolescents' heritage language and mainstream language proficiency levels will certainly be lopsided.

Furthermore, the properties of individual languages or the language particulars can also contribute to the proficiency gap in different languages and pose different types of acquisition difficulties for learners, thus influencing the course of language development.[25] For example, crosslinguistic findings have shown that Danish children's past-tense verb form attainment (inflectional past-tense morphology) is delayed relative to Icelandic, Norwegian and Swedish children due to the phonetic (sound) structure of the Danish language.[26] Additionally, different languages present children with different learning tasks. For instance, children who acquire Chinese will have to learn how to use classifiers (measuring words). The classifiers are used along with numbers to indicate the quantity of objects, such as *kuai* (块) in 'five *kuai* (块) of crackers' (five crackers) or classifiers can be used with demonstratives 'this' or 'that' to identify objects, such as *tou* (头) in 'this *tou* (头) cow' (this cow). Children who learn French have to learn gender difference in words such as *une table* (a table; feminine) and *un verre* (a glass; masculine).

To add to the complexity, the speed of children's literacy development in different languages can be also affected by the differences in **orthographic systems** (the writing systems). Research suggests that each writing system is based on a different set of symbolic relations and requires a different set of cognitive skills.[27] The world's writing systems can be roughly divided into alphabetic (such as English), **alphasyllabary** (such as Korean *hangul*), and nonalphabetic (such as Chinese). Alphabetic writing systems can be further divided into different scripts such as Roman scripts (e.g. Spanish), Semitic scripts (e.g. Hebrew), and Cyrillic scripts (e.g. Serbian). Overall, the alphabetic system tends to have more phonology (sound)-orthography (script) mapping than a nonalphabetic system. In other words, the alphabetic writing system is relatively more transparent than the nonalphabetic one. For instance, Finnish is a more transparent language than Chinese. Using the word 'cat' as an example, the sound [*kisa*] and the script *Kissa* in Finnish correspond closely to each other, whereas, the sound [*mao*] and the script 猫 in Chinese are not pellucid. Thus, it takes different information processing skills for children to learn these different orthographies.[28] Box 2.2 shows the degree of orthographic transparency of some languages.

Even within the alphabetic writing system, different languages vary in their degree of transparency. English, for instance, is known to be less transparent than Turkish, Czech, Welsh, French and German. Crosslinguistic studies have shown that English-speaking children consistently perform less well than those children from the relatively more transparent writing systems (such as Welsh and Turkish). Children learning relatively transparent writing systems not only appear to learn the basic phonological spelling more quickly but also demonstrate more advanced conventional spelling skills than those learning English.[29]

Box 2.2 Examples of Orthographic Transparency

(From most transparent to least transparent)

Korean Hangul
Serbian
Finnish
Turkish
↓
Italian
Spanish
Modern Greek
↓
German
Swedish
↓
French
Danish
↓
English
↓
Arabic
Hebrew
Aramaic
↓
Chinese

Such evidence has also been shown in children who simultaneously acquire three languages. For example, Léandre and Dominique, who simultaneously acquired French, Chinese and English from birth, tend to be more proficient in English and French reading and writing than Chinese partly because of the orthographic differences.

Lack of age-appropriate heritage-language reading materials

As hinted in the last section, literacy skills (e.g. reading and writing) may be the areas in which adolescents' heritage language tend to lag behind their mainstream language. To help their teens develop heritage-language literacy proficiency, many parents choose to introduce heritage-language reading materials to their children. However, because of the proficiency gap between adolescents' heritage language and their mainstream language, the reading materials chosen in their heritage language are often intended for younger children. For instance, at age 14 (14; 6; 1), Léandre was already reading Shakespeare and Dickens in his English literature class, but his reading materials in his Chinese language school were intended for younger children (see Box 2.3).

It was no wonder Léandre felt that his intelligence was being insulted, and he vehemently protested that he was offended to be asked to read materials for little babies (小宝宝). Indeed, one of the worst fears for teens is that they will be treated as

---

Box 2.3 Sample of Chinese Reading Material

(English Translation)

I Am Happier Than Before

A few years ago, father and mother sent me to school. I carried my school bag for the first time and entered school for the first time. I saw a huge playground, many classrooms, many classmates, and teachers. All these made me happy.

This year, I was promoted one more grade. I carried my school bag and went to school by myself. I also knew where to find my classroom. I saw the little tree had grown taller and my classmates and the teacher were having lovely conversations. All these made me happier than before.

(Original Chinese Text)

我比以前更快乐

几年前,爸爸妈妈送我去上学。我第一次背着书包,第一次走进学校。我看到了大操场,许多教室,和许多同学和老师。所有这些都让我高兴。

今年,我升了一级。我自己背着书包去上学。我知道在哪里可以找到我的教室。我看见小树长高,我的同学和老师都在谈话。所有这些让我比以前更快乐。

babies while they are striving to become adults. The reality was, however, that Léandre was not able to read the age-appropriate Chinese materials that his Chinese-speaking counterparts, who live in the Chinese-speaking environment, read. His chronological age did not match his Chinese reading proficiency.

Loss of interest in reading

Another area of challenge is that many adolescents (monolingual and multilingual alike) begin to lose interest in reading, particularly in classic literature, even though they were once avid readers as children. There may be many reasons for this, one of which is the nature of the reading materials. Young children often regard reading as a pleasurable activity because the books that they are reading are typically about children's lives, imaginary worlds or animals. As children advance through the grade levels, reading becomes **expository** (for information), and older children are increasingly asked to analyse texts they read. Léandre complained rightfully once to one of my colleagues, 'The extensive literary analysis in middle and high schools substantially lessened my motivation to read and read for pleasure.' Indeed, I could tell that his heritage-language reading was 'collateral damage' of his school English literature class. For a long time, he simply did not want to read any literature.

Time and effort may not result in expected outcomes

It is generally assumed that the time one spends doing something should be proportionally associated with the outcome; in other words, spending more time teaching and learning a language should result in higher achievement. However, heritage-language development may not necessarily happen in this way. Depending on the type of language and the context in which the language is learnt, as well as other factors, an adolescent's heritage languages may be acquired with different outcomes. For example, even though Léandre and Dominique spent more time studying Chinese and went to Chinese language school to learn how to read and write, in addition to their mother's unflagging effort, their Chinese reading and writing ability is not as proficient as their French, which they spent a lot less time learning. This can sometimes be frustrating and challenging for both parents and teens.

Strategies for Heritage-Language Maintenance and Multilingual Development During Adolescence

Given the various characteristics of adolescence and the many challenges involved in heritage-language maintenance and multilingual development, you may want to develop a thoughtful plan that includes strategies that are based on your specific family situation. In the remaining part of this chapter, I will share some strategies for you to consider.

Setting achievable goals and adjusting them when necessary

In order to better support adolescents' heritage-language maintenance and multilingual development during the adolescent period, it is important to set realistic and achievable goals based on your circumstance.

In our case, my husband and I revisited the multilingual development goals we had set when our kids were younger. At that time, our goal for Léandre and Dominique's multilingual development was to help them develop the four basic language skills in three of their ambient languages: listening, speaking, reading and writing.[30] The goals for our children during their teenage years were still, to a larger extent, the same as their early childhood and childhood. However, we did adjust the goals for their French and Chinese reading and writing. As I previously mentioned, both Dominique and Léandre had lots to do in their adolescent lives, and their daily schedules would not allow them to devote substantial amounts of time to their literacy attainment of both of their heritage languages. It would be unrealistic to expect them to achieve a heritage-language reading and writing proficiency of the same level as their counterparts who live in the Chinese- and French-speaking environments. We thought that as long as their heritage-language literacy foundations were built, they would be able to catch up when future opportunities arose. We did not give up on their heritage-language literacy development either. Instead, we employed alternative ways to help them develop their heritage-language literacy skills. For example, the teens took advantage of their high school's AP French classes to improve their French literacy, in addition to doing some focused French literacy activities (see Chapter 7 for details). It worked well, as both teens enjoyed the AP French class. Léandre even commented that he finally figured out many French verb conjugations that he knew how to say but did not know how to spell. For their Chinese literacy development, the goal was to continue to help them get a foundation in basic literacy. We focused on using daily conversation as our main vehicle for providing focused language and literacy teaching (this topic will be discussed further later in this chapter and in Chapter 7). By adjusting our goals for Léandre and Dominique's heritage-language literacy development, we all felt less stressed.

Determining the focus of multilingual development

By the time Léandre and Dominique were engaged in the process of applying for college in their senior year of high school, both kids contemplated attending universities outside the United States, in particular at French-speaking universities. As a family, we weighed the pros and cons of attending a French-speaking university. One of these pros was that their French (particularly their academic French) could improve drastically. However, one of the cons was that they would interrupt their continued English education in terms of their further English academic language development.

I have heard more than one multilingual person expresses the sentiment that he or she feels inadequate in more than one of his or her several languages with regard to reading and writing proficiency. Stavros is a case in point.[31] He came to the United States after he finished high school in Greece. Stavros lamented that his Greek was at the high-school level in terms of reading and writing. After spending 10 years in the United States, his English was on a par with his Greek; however, he always felt insecure (to use his exact words) in both languages in terms of writing. He wished that he could have finished university in Greece and then gone abroad. That way, he believed that he would have been strong in reading and writing in at least one language.

After many family discussions, we decided that it was better for Léandre and Dominique to attend college (university) in the United States to further develop their mainstream language: English. Even though both Léandre and Dominique were doing exceptionally well in oral and written English, they still needed to develop a solid academic English ability. Realistically, their English would have the best chance to develop as their most competent language in terms of speaking, listening, reading and writing. We believed that their heritage languages would benefit from having their mainstream language solidly developed.

Agency, empowerment, affect and motivation

In order to make heritage-language maintenance and multilingual development successful, we must take at least four factors into consideration: agency, empowerment, affect and motivation. First, adolescents must have **agency** (the capacity of individuals to act independently and to make their own free choices) in the decision-making process concerning matters related to their lives. Longing for independence is a healthy and typical desire for adolescents. When parents fail to grant their teens increasing decision-making opportunities, adolescents will become extremely peer-oriented and find their own solutions. I learnt this lesson from Léandre. During his college application process, a particular university admitted Léandre (17; 8; 10), and he and we, the parents, believed this university was not a good fit for him; however, because one of Léandre's good friends had decided to go there, Léandre insisted on visiting the university with his friend. I was concerned because the university was far from where we lived and Léandre had to miss school. I decided not to let Léandre go with his friend for the visit. Not giving Léandre the opportunity to make his decision and not including him in the decision-making process backfired. Léandre talked with his high-school counsellor, asking her to intervene in the situation. In the end, I gave in, but honestly, it was not pleasant for Léandre or me. This situation showed me that adolescents will not heed parental rules if they are not provided with opportunities to be involved in the decision-making process. When rules are too extreme, they may resist. Thus, negotiating limits is a better solution, and it is more productive if adolescents have a say in setting the limits or rules. For example, when Léandre wanted to come back at 2:00 am from his friend's house, I negotiated with him that he would come back at midnight with 20 minutes leeway. In this way, he felt that he had an opportunity to negotiate and tended to abide by the co-decision.

Agency is crucial in heritage-language learning as well. Negotiating between parents' demands and adolescents' emergent independence will work more effectively for adolescents' heritage-language maintenance. When adolescents feel that they can contribute to decision making regarding their own heritage-language learning, they will be more active in participating in the process. When Léandre and Dominique were younger, I basically made all of the decisions regarding their Chinese language learning. As time went on, I realised that the kids would not cooperate if they were told what to do and if I did not include their choices and decisions. We had lots of struggles in their early adolescent years. The successful scenarios often came from the situations when the teens were given a choice.

Second, adolescents must feel empowered in their heritage-language learning process. Because the heritage-language learning environment presents many limitations, it is likely that adolescents' heritage-language communication is not as proficient as their mainstream languages, and they may make mistakes as a result. However, they must feel empowered to continue with their multilingual development. Box 2.4 is an example of agency and empowerment.

This example shows that when I asked Léandre to use the new Chinese characters to make sentences, he did not want to complete the task. However, when he was given the choice to write them first instead of making sentences, he did it because it was also his choice. When showing him that these characters can be put together to make funny sentences (even nonsense sentences), he was more motivated because, as described in Chapter 1, Léandre is a humorous guy. He would not let a chance to make jokes pass by. When I told him that his sentences were not bad, he was even more empowered to go on. A few days later, on Mother's Day, I was pleasantly surprised to receive an e-mail from Léandre in Chinese. In this e-mail, he actually used the characters he had learnt a few days earlier.

Third, adolescents must develop a sufficiently affective bond to their heritage language and heritage culture to want to learn the heritage language. As indicated in my previous book, *Growing Up With Three Languages: Birth to Eleven*, Léandre and Dominique formed a close bond to one of their heritage countries, Switzerland (or specifically, the French-speaking part of Switzerland). Because of their frequent visits to and pleasant experiences in Switzerland, they were eager to speak and read French. However, they were ambivalent towards their other heritage country, the People's Republic of China. On one hand, they liked their Chinese maternal grandparents and they were very eager to talk to and visit them. They also enjoyed Chinese food delicacies and artefacts and were enthralled with the cultural relics. On the other hand, they disliked some things they experienced or observed. For instance, once on a flight back to New York from Shanghai after visiting their Chinese grandparents, Léandre had an empty seat next to him. He took advantage of it and used it to sleep. A Chinese man from the back of the plane came and pushed Léandre's legs away from the seat and occupied two seats for his own comfort. Although examples like this do not really represent China, Chinese culture or Chinese people,

Box 2.4 Examples of Agency and Empowerment

(Mother takes out ten cutout Chinese characters from a basket.)

Mother: Today, I want you to use these new words and phrases to make sentences. (今天我想让你们用这些新的字词造句。)

Léandre (12; 9; 11): [No response.]

Mother: Did you hear me? (你有没有听到?)

Léandre: I don't want to make sentences. I can learn to write them. (我不想造句, 我想学怎么写。)

Mother: That is fine. (可以。)

Léandre: [Writes the Chinese characters] I finished. (我写完了。)

Mother: Good. (好。) [Puts the Chinese characters together in a nonsense sentence on the dining table.]

Léandre: [Laughs and uses these characters to make funny and nonsense sentences.]

Mother: Do you really know how to use these words in a real sentence? (你真的知道怎么用这字造句?)

Léandre: Maybe. (可能。)

Mother: Show me how you do it. (那你造给我看看。)

Léandre: [Puts the characters to makes sentences.]

Mother: Not bad. Maybe you can write these sentences on a piece of paper? (不错。你能不能把这些句子写在纸上?)

Léandre: [Writes sentences.]

Léandre and Dominique did not develop a close **affective** (emotional) bond with the country as they did with Switzerland (more on this will be discussed in Chapter 8). Coupled with their negative impression of one of their Chinese schoolteachers, who again did not represent any other Chinese teachers, they were less eager to learn Chinese. As mentioned earlier, they even resented anything related to Chinese at a certain point. Fortunately, this changed in their later adolescent period when they became more mature. It seems that affective filters can affect a person's motivation and performance in learning and maintaining a heritage language; when individuals have a negative feeling towards a language, their feelings may block their ability to learn that language.[32]

Fourth, adolescents must be motivated to learn their heritage language. Not surprisingly, most adolescents are motivated to learn if they are interested in something or find personal relevance in something. Each time I saw an interesting book, I would suggest it to Léandre and Dominique and would encourage them to read the material. But, they rarely read what I recommended because the books were about topics that interested me, not them. However, if they found something interesting, they were unstoppable. One weekend, I paid Léandre (16; 6; 28) to proofread a book draft for me. I was waiting for him to send back his proof via e-mail, but it never came. I went upstairs and asked why he had not sent the proof. He said that he was fascinated by the paragraph I wrote about Genie, a 'wild child' who did not acquire a language because of abuse and neglect.[33] He found the case was so interesting that he went online and began to read the story and lost track of the time. This is a telling example of how interest can motivate and incentivise reading.

Fifth, relevance can make a difference in teens' motivation to learn. For example, Léandre (16; 4; 26) complained that that his father only wanted him to learn how to conjugate verbs, and he found the exercises boring. However, in his AP French class, and later in his French film class in college, he was asked to write in French. He finally realised the relevance of French verb conjugation to French writing and became eager to do French conjugation exercises.

Finally, adolescents' mindsets also influence whether or not they are motivated to continue their heritage-language development. The renowned psychologist Carol Dweck's motivation theory[34] indicates that there are two kinds of mindsets: the **growth mindset** (success is based on hard work, learning, training and persistence) and the **fixed mindset** (success is based on innate ability). When teens have a growth mindset, they are more likely to continue working hard despite setbacks in their heritage-language learning; and when they have a fixed mindset, they will attribute their setbacks to their innate ability and may stop learning. Because the progress of heritage-language learning is slow and the results may not be seen immediately, some teens may be discouraged and gradually form a fixed mindset. For instance, Dominique (13; 4; 7) complained that although he spent quite a few years in the Chinese language school, he still did not read and write Chinese well. One strategy that I have found most successful is to show my children their heritage-language achievements. After Dominique made the above comments, I played a word game with him (the game I invented by putting different Chinese characters in a basket and asking the children to select them and create sentences). After he completed the game, I said to Dominique, 'See, how many words you actually know?' Vitalising their heritage-language achievements (even the smallest achievements) can help teens see their potential to grow further in their heritage language(s) and boost their confidence.

Moreover, to cultivate a growth mindset, it is also important to emphasise effort over ability. Every teen learns differently, and as a result, some may learn faster than others. The amount of effort they put into their heritage-language learning needs to be emphasised. Both Léandre and Dominique are fast learners. Yet, both tend to profit from their wits rather than push themselves to their fullest potential. However, some areas in heritage-language development, such as writing, do require a substantial amount of work for teens to progress. Even established writers still put a lot of time and effort into their work. In my interactions with the teens, I have valued their efforts over their abilities.

Carrying on metacognitive conversation

As described earlier in this chapter, adolescents make significant improvement in their **cognition** (intellectual ability), and they can see the cause and effect relationship through their abstract thinking ability. Thus, carrying on metacognitive conversations will provide them with opportunities to reflect on their heritage-language learning process. **Metacognitive conversations** are in-depth, reflective conversations in which both parents and teens become aware of their own thinking. In doing so, parents can reflect on their own thinking and communicate that thinking to their children; and conversely, adolescents can make their thoughts known to their parents. In such metacognitive conversations, adolescents can come to see themselves as having the capacity to succeed in heritage-language learning, as well as having opportunities to discuss the difficulties they have had with their heritage-language learning. Parents can discuss their thinking on the setbacks and explain that struggle is a typical aspect of growth.

Using technology to aid heritage-language learning

When our kids were little, we used to carry trunks of books each time we came back from our heritage countries. Time flies and technology improves. Nowadays, thanks to advances in technology, teens have a lot more opportunities to learn their heritage language(s) by interacting with their heritage families and peers via digital means, such as Skype, Facebook, web chats and FaceTime. For instance, Léandre and Dominique are able to meet with their Chinese grandparents frequently via Skype and thus receive heritage-language and cultural support (see Box 2.5).

In this Skype conversation sample (unfortunately, the English translation does not do justice to the original Chinese version), Léandre and Dominique's Chinese grandfather passed a lot of Chinese language and cultural information to the teens. Linguistically, the grandfather taught the teens idioms 熙熙嚷嚷 (crowded and noisy; this Chinese idiom depicts the vivid image of crowded and noisy street and the beauty is lost English translation) and 烧香拜佛 (burning incense and praying; although the idiom was used by the grandfather literally here, I was later able to teach the children a different and related idiom, 临时抱佛脚: Do not prepare beforehand and only act when things are happening). The grandfather also taught the teens a vivid expression, 倒流的树影 (shadows backwards). Culturally, the grandfather taught the

> **Box 2.5 Example of Language and Cultural Support via Skype**
>
> (September 3, 2010; Skype conversation with Chinese grandparents)
>
> **(Translated Version)**
>
> Grandfather: When I was a young child (in Shanghai), my favourite thing was to take a rickshaw with my mother, whether we went to shopping in the main road (now called East Nanjing Road) or went to the Jingan Temple to burn incense and pray, or went to theater in Fuzhou Road. I sat in the rickshaw, watching the crowded and noisy street and looking at the shadows at both sides backwards. I was so happy.
>
> (Original Chinese Version)
>
> 我小时候在上海最喜欢跟我妈妈坐黄包车出去了。无论到大马路，现在叫南京东路买东西，还是到静安寺烧香拜佛，或者到福州路的共舞台看戏都要妈妈抱我坐黄包车去。我坐在车上，看着大街上熙熙嚷嚷的人群，望着两旁向后倒流的树影，心里开心极了。

teens the common transportation tool in old Shanghai 黄包车 (rickshaw). Ancestrally, the grandfather introduced to the teens their great-grandmother. Geographically (in Shanghai), the grandfather helped the kids link the places they visited in Shanghai and their functions in the past before the revolution in 1949 '大马路，现在叫南京东路买东西，还是到静安寺烧香拜佛，或者到福州路的共舞台看戏'(shopping in the main road, now called East Nanjing Road, or burning incense and praying at the Jingan Temple, or going to theater in Fuzhou Road). As you can see, communicative technology (such as Skype) can bring the heritage family together and provide heritage-language and cultural support.

Using intentional conversation

Given the time constraints in adolescents' lives, it is often unfeasible for them to spend increased time learning their heritage language(s). Thus, daily conversation can be a good context for heritage-language learning. Research conducted in the classroom setting has shown that well-planned teacher-student conversations (called instructional conversations) can help new-language learning students develop language and literacy skills.[35] In my personal experience of working with my own children, I also found that the instructional conversation method, which I have termed **intentional conversation**, is particularly useful for heritage-language learners like Léandre and Dominique. The basic steps of intentional conversation and examples are shown in Box 2.6.

The advantage of intentional conversation for heritage-language learning adolescents is that it is natural and spontaneous in parent–adolescent interaction; it is free from

Box 2.6 Steps and Examples of Intentional Conversation

Topic Focus: Parents selects a topic related to the heritage language (such as a specific grammatical structure) and develops a general plan on how to carry out the conversation around the topic to allow optimal exploration of the topic. For instance, Chinese measurement words or classifiers are an area of difficulty for Léandre and Dominique. I had a general plan to help them with some commonly used classifiers 块 (pieces), 杯 (cups) and 门 (number of classes). During one of their after-school snack times, I asked them how many 块 (pieces) of homemade cookies they wanted. After they told me the number of cookies they wanted, I asked them how many 杯 (cups) of fruit juice they wanted. During our conversation, I asked them how many 门 (numbers) of classes they took that day.

Activation and Use of Background and Relevant Schemata: Parents can either 'hook their children into' or provide their children with the pertinent background knowledge necessary for understanding a topic by weaving the information into the discussion. Using the above example again, after I deliberately used the classifiers in the context (块, 杯, 门), I asked Léandre and Dominique whether they noticed the differences in the classifiers I just used and asked them how these classifiers can be used in other contexts by recollecting their experiences.

Direct Teaching: When necessary, parents can provide direct teaching of a specific language feature in daily conversations. For example, I asked Léandre and Dominique whether they knew the kinds of classifiers to be used for speech (e.g. 一番话), essay (五篇文长) and forest (一片森林). I explicitly taught these classifiers by using different examples in the context. Because these classifiers are difficult, deliberate teaching in intentional conversation is necessary.

Promotion of More Complex Language and Expression: Parents can also elicit more extended child contributions by using a variety of elicitation techniques, such as invitations to expand and questions. For example, I invited Léandre and Dominique to use these newly introduced classifiers with different words and provided them with opportunities to ask questions. When they made mistakes, I gently probed them, asking 'What makes you think to use this particular classifier?'

Responsiveness to Children's Contributions: While sticking to the initial plan and maintaining the focus and coherence of the discussion on a topic, parents can also be responsive to their children's initiation and take advantage of opportunities to help their children learn. For instance, Léandre asked why it was illogical for him to use 匹 with horse and 头 with cow. I used this opportunity to discuss the possible reasons.

(Continued)

> **Challenging Atmosphere (but nonthreatening):** Parents can create a challenging atmosphere that is balanced by a positive and affective climate. Parents should act more like collaborators than evaluators, and children should be challenged to negotiate and construct the meaning of the topic under discussion.
>
> **Parent-Child Participation:** Parents should not hold the exclusive right to determine who talks; children should be encouraged to influence the selection of speaking turns.
>
> Modified from ERIC Clearinghouse on Languages and Linguistics, ED347850, Washington, DC, 1992.

the didactic nature of formal teaching, and it is relevant and meaningful. Thus, the intentional conversation method can activate adolescents' **schemata** (a mental framework or concept that helps organise and interpret information), promote complex language, create a nonthreatening environment, involve direct teaching and include parent responsiveness to teens' ideas. Consequently, it can help adolescents develop their heritage language(s).

Explicit teaching of the marked features in heritage languages

Because the heritage-language learning environment at home is different from the learning environment of the adolescents in the heritage-language countries, leaving heritage-language learning to the naturalistic setting is simply not enough. Therefore, explicit teaching in **marked** (difficult) areas of a heritage language is both necessary and effective. Using **pragmatics** (how language is used in a proper social context) as an example, explicit and **deductive teaching** (explaining rules first and followed by exercises) are more effective for pragmatic learning than implicit and **inductive teaching** (rules are inferred in the examples). Attention-drawing activities are more helpful for pragmatic learning than exposure alone. Research shows that learners who received pragmatic instruction outperformed those who did not.[36]

However, explicit teaching and deductive teaching do not really mean parent dominance; rather, they mean parental coaching. In other words, explicit teaching and deductive teaching suggest that parents purposefully make certain marked (difficult) heritage-language features more noticeable. Even though you, as an adult and a proficient heritage-language user, know what areas are important to pay attention to and draw your teens' attention to them, your role is to provide opportunities for them to explore, and you must coach them to get there. It is always important to remember that piquing teens' curiosity about their heritage language is fundamental.

Sowing the seeds

When interacting with adolescents, encountering resistance is typical. When forced to confront resistance, I thought about giving up many times. However, I noticed that when I kept on trying, I saw the results of my efforts later. Even though, at certain point, Léandre and Dominique resisted doing many things that I wanted them to continue to do, such as playing piano and attending Chinese school, I was pleasantly surprised that later on, some of the early resistance became acceptance and even aspiration. For example, Léandre unexpectedly told me one day (17; 4; 2) that he wanted to play piano again (the activity he and Dominique, like many other children, hated so much when they were younger). He printed the score *Rondo Alla Turca* by Mozart and began to practice it by himself. Similarly, he was suddenly interested in French writing. He (16; 3; 11) asked Philippe to say something in French so that he could write it down. Finally, out of the blue, Léandre (17; 3; 10) asked me why they did not go to Chinese school anymore. He said that he wanted to learn how to write Chinese well.

The metaphoric image I use to envisage my efforts as a parent is that of a gardener who sows seeds. Once seeds are sown, if the environment is supportive, the seeds will bud, even though there may be some bad weather during the growing process.

Effects of peers and idols

As mentioned earlier in this chapter, peer influence is essential in adolescent development. Research shows that having a peer group that values the heritage language is critical.[37] Peers can support and undermine heritage-language growth. If teens hang out with narrow-minded peers, such as the peers surrounding Nikola (in Chapter 1), they may not have the motivation to continue their heritage-language development. On the other hand, if teens are connecting with peers who are multilingual, they may be more motivated. In middle and high school, Léandre had a classmate, Joanna, who grew up in Geneva. They often discussed their experiences in French. This seemed to make Léandre feel that there were other teens who shared the similar linguistic experience. Léandre (15; 4; 26) commented that Joanna spoke more colloquially than him. Similarly, both Léandre and Dominique had e-mail exchanges and personal meetings with their Swiss friend David, who taught them many French words that were not used by their father, such as *stile* (style) and *nickel* (nice). Having a teen language teacher is a lot more effective than having a parent teacher.

In addition to peer influence, idols can also help teens in their heritage-language learning. The Swiss tennis player Roger Federer is multilingual. Dominique was impressed each time he saw Federer's interviews in different languages. The idol effect does help teens to have aspirations.

Avoiding information overload

Eager to help Léandre and Dominique learn how to read and write Chinese, I bombarded them with e-mails written in Chinese for a period of time. Because there was too much information in my e-mails, both of the boys stopped reading e-mails from me. I learnt that to work effectively with teens, it is better to avoid information overload. In other words, less is better than more; one e-mail message a day works better than 10 messages a day.

Working with teens: The bottom line

Adolescence is a fascinating and challenging period. Because of the many changes that happen in a relatively short period of time, adolescents may show anxiety and sometimes may seem to be difficult to work with. The good news is that the anxiety and conflicts sometimes exhibited during adolescence are transitory and relatively short term. These behaviours are neither inevitable nor normative. With maturity, most adolescents will become productive young adults.[38]

Although I have suggested some strategies for you to consider, I do believe that whatever works best for your adolescent children is the best method for them. Michael Riera, author of *Uncommon Sense for Parents with Teenagers*, had an interesting comment on the role of parents. He noted: 'During our child's early life, we are the manager. As the parent of an adolescent, it's time to shift our role, from manager to consultant. As a consultant, our job is a lot more hands off. He advised us that we need to back off on the "shoulds" and the "shouldn'ts" before we step over a cliff.'[39]

Indeed, if we try to 'manage' our adolescent children, they will most certainly go out of their way to defy us in order to make their *own* decisions. Riera reminded us that if we tell our teens 'Tonia is too wild, you shouldn't hang out with her,' we will be lucky if we ever see our children alone again. If we say, 'I saw you smoking and I'm very upset. You should quit,' be prepared to find cigarette butts from now until a very long 'then' from now. As a consultant (rather than a manager), our job involves more trust and 'back up' and less direct decision making. The bottom line is that adolescents must been seen as individuals who are able to make decisions with the support of parents and other adults.

Even though adolescents try to become independent, they still need our guidance. For example, the phenomenon of **invincibility** is common (i.e. things will happen to others, but not to me). While planning a family vacation, Léandre insisted on reserving hotels with no possibility of cancellation because he was sure that nothing would happen and we would be there. Our ferry from Jersey to Portsmouth was cancelled due to a small accident. Consequently, we had to make alternate hotel arrangements. This was a good opportunity for me to help him understand a Chinese saying: '不怕一万, 只怕万一' (always plan for the worst).

As we leave this chapter, I will highlight some good ideas proposed by Michael Riera with regard to working with adolescents:

- As a consultant, parents are still deeply involved. Make yourselves available for your children.
- Continue to provide the love, limits, structure, consequences and all that other good positive parenting 'stuff.'
- Don't feel abandoned by your adolescents. They are actually listening to you.
- During adolescence, communication is more important than ever. Here are a few ideas for maintaining (or gaining) communication flow:
    - Listen and know that you don't and won't have the answers to some of the things that are bothering your adolescent. This is the time for formulating new ideas and ideals, and your children may be paying more attention to the world than they ever have. Nobody has all the answers to the world's ills and injustices, but it's important to think about them, and to help your children develop critical thinking skills by talking and expressing opinions and feelings.
    - Focus on treating your teens with compassion, trying to understand the situation, and allowing (and encouraging) your teens to use their resourcefulness to negotiate difficult situations. Just yelling at them or condemning their behaviour will only distance you from them.
    - Do not criticise your teens directly. Tell a story about somebody you both know, or use a media example. Keeping the situation slightly removed will make it easier for your children to hear the message.

Summary of Key Points in Chapter 2

- Adolescence is a transitional period from childhood to adulthood.
- Adolescents experience many complex physical, cognitive, social, emotional and identity changes.
    - The two key systems involved in making sound decisions and controlling impulses, the limbic system and the frontal cortex of the brain, are not quite mature during adolescence.
    - Growth spurts and puberty affect changes in cognition, emotion, social and other dimensions of adolescents' development.
    - The development of scientific (hypothetic), logical and abstract thinking abilities opens up new cognitive horizons and drives adolescents to idealism and to think in more expansive and idealistic ways.
    - Adolescents become more self-conscious and self-focusing, with an exaggerated sense of personal uniqueness. They are sensitive to public criticism and prone to taking risks. Moreover, they may adopt a stance of rigid dogmatism. The hormonal changes may also affect mood variability. They are experimenting with their relationship with their parents and with their identity.

- Teenagers also have their own distinct communication or discourse style. They use their distinct communicative style as an outlet to project their feelings, opinions, frustrations and reactions.
- As a result of the many changes that occur during this period, adolescents face many challenges in heritage-language maintenance and multilingual development, such as:
  - Pressure to speak the mainstream language.
  - Inconsistency in parental cultural beliefs as well as in mainstream cultural ideology.
  - Contrast in language teaching approaches.
  - Time management in heritage-language learning and other activities.
  - Lack of peer modelling.
  - Lack of societal support.
  - Language preferences and biases.
  - Proficiency gap in different languages.
  - Lack of age-appropriate reading materials.
  - Loss of interest in reading.
  - Inconsistency of time invested in heritage-language learning and outcome.
- To support adolescent heritage-language maintenance and multilingual development, the following strategies may be considered.
  - Set up heritage-language development goals.
  - Determine the focus of heritage-language development.
  - Empower adolescents in their own heritage-language development by letting them be the part of the decision-making process.
  - Help them develop affective bonds with their heritage culture to motivate them to attain their heritage language.
  - Take advantage of their cognitive advancement and help them reflect on their heritage-language learning.
  - Use technology to help them attain and maintain their heritage language.
  - Use intentional conversation as an effective way to engage them in heritage-language learning.
  - Explicitly teach the difficult (marked) areas in their heritage language.
  - Sow the seeds for future success.
  - Use peers and idols for heritage-language aspiration and motivation.
  - Avoid information overload.
  - Change the parent's role from that of a manager to that of a consultant.

Recommended Readings

Adams, G.R. and Berzonsky, M.D. (eds) (2005) Blackwell Handbook of Adolescence. Malden, MA: Blackwell Publishing Ltd.

Kondo-Brown, K. (ed.) (2006), *Heritage Language Development*. Amsterdam, NL: John Benjamins.

Riera, M. (2012) *Uncommon Sense for Parents with Teenagers* (3rd edn). New York: Ten Speed Press.

Notes and References

1. De Vries Guth, N. and Pratt-Fartro, T. (2010) *Literacy Coaching to Build Adolescent Learning: Five Pillars of Practice*. Thousand Oaks, CA: Corwin.
2. Hall, S.G. (1904) *Adolescence: Its Psychology and Its Relations to Physiology, Anthropology, Sociology, Sex, Crime, Religion and Education*.
3. Rosenblum, G.D. and Lewis, M. (2003) Emotional development in adolescence. In G.R. Adams and M.D. Berzonsky (eds) *Blackwell Handbook of Adolescence* (pp. 269–89). Malden, MA: Blackwell Publishing.
4. De Vries Guth, N. and Pratt-Fartro, T. (2010) *Literacy Coaching to Build Adolescent Learning: Five Pillars of Practice*. Thousand Oaks, CA: Corwin.
5. Woolfolk, A. and Perry, N.E. (2014) *Child and Adolescent Development* (p. 468). Boston, MA: Person.
6. Berk, L.E. (2009) *Child Development*. Boston, MA: Pearson.
7. Santrock, J.W. (2007) *Adolescence*. Boston: McGraw Hill.
8. Santrock, J.W. (2007) *Adolescence*. Boston: McGraw Hill.
9. Owens, K.B. (2002) *Child and Adolescent Development: An Integrated Approach* (p. 532). Belmont, CA: Wadsworth/Thomson Learning.
10. Rosenblum, G.D. and Lewis, M. (2003) Emotional development in adolescence. In G.R. Adams and M.D. Berzonsky (eds) *Blackwell Handbook of Adolescence* (pp. 269–89). Malden, MA: Blackwell Publishing.
11. Nippold, M. (2000) Language development during the adolescent years: Aspects of pragmatics, syntax, and semantics. *Topics in Language Disorders* 20 (2), 15–28.
12. Telley, S.A. (2008) The Teenage Dialect. Unpublished MA Thesis. Indiana University.
13. Woolfolk, A. and Perry, N.E. (2014) *Child and Adolescent Development* (p. 469). Boston, MA: Person.
14. Image downloaded from https://www.google.com/webhp?sourceid=chrome-instant&ion=1&espv=2&ie=UTF8#q=image%20of%20background%20and%20foreground
15. Image downloaded from https://www.google.com/webhp?sourceid=chrome-instant&ion=1&espv=2&ie=UTF8#q=image+of+background+and+foreground+old+woman+and+young+woman
16. Caldas, S.J. (2006) *Raising Bilingual-Biliterate Children in Monolingual Cultures* (p. 107). Clevedon: Multilingual Matters
17. Portes, A. and Schauffler, R. (1994) Language and the second generation: Bilingualism yesterday and today. In R.G. Rumbaut and S. Pedrazgo (eds) *International Migration Review* 28, 640–61. New York: Wadsworth.
    Portes, A. and Schauffler, R. (1996) Language acquisition and loss among children of immigrants. In S. Pedraza and R.G. Rumbaut (eds) *Origins and Destinies: Immigration, Race, Ethnicity in America* (pp. 432–43). New York: Wadsworth.
18. E-mail communication on October 3, 2012.
19. Ran, A. (2000) Learning to read and write at home: The experience of Chinese families in Britain. In M. Martin-Jones and L. Jones (eds) *Multilingual Literacies: Reading and Writing Different Worlds* (pp. 71–90). Amsterdam: John Benjamins.
20. E-mail communication on July 23, 2013.
21. Curdt-Christiansen, X.-L. (2006) Teaching and learning Chinese: Heritage language classroom discourse in Montreal. *Language, Culture, and Curriculum* 19 (2), 189–207.
22. Sakamoto, M. (2006) Balancing L1 maintenance and L2 learning. In K. Kondo-Brown (ed.) *Heritage Language Development* (p. 47). Amsterdam, NL: John Benjamins.
23. SAT stands for Scholastic Aptitude Test. It is required for college application in the United States.
24. Sakamoto, M. (2006) Balancing L1 maintenance and L2 learning. In K. Kondo-Brown (ed.) *Heritage Language Development* (p. 53). Amsterdam, NL: John Benjamins.
25. Slobin, D.I. (1985) Crosslinguistic evidence for the language-making capacity. In D.I. Slobin (ed.) *The Crosslinguistic Study of Language Acquisition (Vol. 2): Theoretical Issues* (pp. 1157–256). Hillsdale, NJ: Lawrence Erlbaum.

[26] Bleses, D., Basboll, H. and Vach, W. (2011) Is Danish difficult to acquire? Evidence from Nordic past-tense studies. *Language and Cognitive Processes* 26 (8), 1193–231.
[27] Bialystok, E., Luk, G. and Kwan, E. (2005) Bilingualism, biliteracy, and learning to read: Interactions among languages and writing systems. *Scientific Studies of Reading* 9 (1), 43–61.
[28] Huang, H. and Hanley, R. (1994) Phonological awareness and visual skills in learning to read Chinese and English. *Cognition* 54, 73–98.
Wang, X.-L.(2011a) *Learning To Read and Write in the Multilingual Family*. Bristol: Multilingual Matters.
Wang, X.-L. (2011b) Teaching children to read and write in more than one orthography: Tips for parents. *Multilingual Living* 26 September 2011 issue.
[29] Caravolas, M. (2004) Spelling development in alphabetic writing systems: A cross-linguistic perspective. *European Psychologist* 9 (1), 3–14.
[30] Wang, X.-L. (2008) *Growing Up With Three Languages: Birth to Eleven* (p. 46). Bristol: Multilingual Matters.
[31] Personal communication on September 13, 2010.
[32] Brown, S. and Attardo, S. (2008) *Understanding Language Structure, Interaction, and Variation*. Michigan: The University of Michigan Press.
[33] Curtis, S. (1977) *Genie: A Psycholinguistic Study of a Modern-Day "Wild Child."* New York: Academic Press.
[34] Dweck, C.S. (2006) *Mindset: The New Psychology of Success*. New York: Random House.
[35] Cohen, A.D. and Horowitz, R. (2002) What should teachers know about bilingual learners and the reading process. In J.H. Sulli- van (ed.) *Literacy and the Second Language Learner* vol. 1. Greenwich, CT: Information Age.
[36] Soler, E.A. and Martínez-Flor, A. (2008) Pragmatics in foreign language contexts. In E.A. Soler and A. Martínez-Flor (eds) *Investigating Pragmatics in Foreign Language Learning, Teaching and Testing* (pp. 3–21). Bristol: Multilingual Matters.
[37] Li, G.-F. (2002) The role of parents in heritage language maintenance and development. In K. Kondo-Brown (ed.) *Heritage Language Development* (p. 47). Amsterdam, NL: John Benjamins.
[38] Adams, G.R. and Berzonsky, M.D. (2004) Introduction. In G.R. Adams and M. D Berzonsky (eds) *Blackwell Handbook of Adolescence* (p. xxv). Malden, MA: Blackwell Publishing.
[39] Riera, M. (2012) *Uncommon Sense for Parents with Teenagers* (3rd edn). New York: Ten Speed Press.

3 Multilingual Sound System Development During Adolescence

One summer a few years ago, in the French-speaking part of Switzerland, Léandre, Dominique, and their Swiss friend David were walking their grandmother's dog Kalina on a country road. When the dog saw a biker dashing by, she ran to him and pinched the biker's left leg, leaving tiny teeth marks. Enraged by what had just happened, the biker dismounted his bike and yelled at the teens and then asked, *'Où habitez-vous?'* (Where do you live?). Léandre replied, *'On habite à New York,'* (We live in New York) and made a sincere apology for the dog's mishap. Hearing Léandre's reply, the biker became even angrier. He shouted *'Menteur!'* (Liar!). Obviously, Léandre's native French accent made the biker believe that Léandre was trying to pull his leg and to dodge his responsibility by telling him that he lived far away (in New York). It was not until later, when the biker was in Léandre's grandmother's house, that he realised that Léandre was telling the truth. Before he left, having been given a case of local wine by Léandre's grandmother as a gesture of apology, he expressed his disbelief about the fact that Léandre grew up in *'les États-Unis'* (the United States) with such a *'parfait accent français'* (perfect French accent). This episode indicates that a person's accent influences the listener's judgement and perception about the speaker;[1] accent is the first thing people notice and, therefore, they use it to determine of the authenticity of a speaker's native-ness.

This chapter is about multilingual phonological (sound-system) development during adolescence. It begins with a brief overview of the general trend of adolescent phonological development. It then describes the specific features of Léandre and Dominique's heritage-language phonological development. The chapter concludes with some thoughts about and suggestions on how you can help your teens further develop their heritage-language phonological skills by drawing upon information from research and strategies that I have found to be successful with my children.

General Trend of Phonological Development During Adolescence

The development of the phonological system in a language is more than just the development of a repertoire of sounds. It is also the process of developing mental representations of the **phonemes** (the smallest meaningful sound unit) of a language and the knowledge of the rules of how sounds are combined in the language. Below are several areas in which teens make steady progress in their phonological system.

Increased refinement and control of sound system

Children typically master of all the sounds in a given language around age eight; however, it is not until late adolescence that the **phonetic inventory** (all the sounds in a language) is refined for both males and females.[2] From the ages of 11 to 12, adolescents are able to use **prosody** (such as stress, intonation, pitch, rate and rhythm) and emphasis to express their precise intent in communication, and from the ages of 16 to 18, they are able to use **vowel-shifting rules** (the rules that account for the vowel alternation such as *divine-divinity*, *sane-sanity* and *extreme-extremity*).[3] During the adolescent period, teens increasingly gain articulatory control of the sound system in their ambient language(s).

Increased gender differences

It is a known phenomenon that men and women tend to produce some phonemes, the smallest meaningful sound unit in a given language, differently. For example, in English, a gender difference in producing phonemes such as /f/, /θ/, /s/ and /ʃ/ have been observed with the increase of age. In Chinese, there is a distinguished male and female articulation style. Females are socialised to speak with a high pitch, as well as to pronounce certain palatal consonants as **dental sibilants** (sounded with a hissing effect), such as pronouncing /tx/, /tx'/ and /x/ as /ts/ /ts'/ and /s/. Females begin to use dentalised consonants during puberty and continue to do so until early adulthood. When a male violates such articulation conventions, he will be regarded as 娘娘腔 (speaking like a woman).[4]

Overall, research suggests that even though the gender differences in phonological production emerge early, usually around the age of six, they become more pronounced in late adolescence and young adulthood.[5]

Peer influence in accent change

Accent change is an interesting phenomenon during adolescence, as it is often a result of peer influence. Studies have shown that the maximum accent sensitivity to peer influence seems to be between ages 4 and 14.[6] Adolescents' accent changes may occur when moving to a new social circle. For instance, it has been reported in the literature that accent change was common among black adolescents of Caribbean descent who were born and lived in London. These native Londoners began to adopt the British-Jamaican accent to show their identity and affiliation when they were teenagers. Even some white teens who became friends with black teens adopted their friends' Jamaican pronunciation.[7] One interesting phenomenon I observed about Dominique is that when he turned 11, he was interested in the African-American English accent. He sometimes spoke with his friends in that accent, which was apparently regarded as cool among his peers. He also changed his cell-phone voice message to sound like an African American.

Once, when I tried to call him on his cell and heard the message, I thought I had dialled a wrong number.

Nonetheless, the peer influence on accent seems short-lived. At around age 14 or 15, most adolescents start to move away from the peer-group accent towards the more prestigious form of accent revered by the dominant culture, especially in formal situations.[8]

Increased phonological decoding ability

Perhaps the most important phonological achievement in adolescence is the development of the sophisticated phonological decoding ability. This attainment allows teens to decipher complex new words that they encounter. For example, in English, adolescents are able to decode the sound elements of complex multisyllable words such as *seismology, superconductivity, stockbrokerage* and *commodity*.

Heritage-language phonological development characteristics

Adolescents who are consistently exposed to more than one language from birth or at an early age are generally able to master the sound systems in their respective languages. Similarly, both Léandre and Dominique established stable phonetic representations for sounds in all of their three **first languages** (languages that are simultaneously acquired from birth) – French, Chinese and English – with native accents at adolescence. It is indeed an incredible phonological achievement; that is, they not only learnt to produce intelligible sounds in all their first languages and attain the different phonological variations (given such contrast phonological systems Chinese vs. French and English), but they also learnt to pronounce them according to the language-specific phonetic norms in the three speech communities.

However, because of the home environment in which they acquired and developed their two heritage languages (Chinese and French), as well as the language-specific features of these two languages, the two teens also exhibited some unique phonological characteristics that are different from their counterparts who grew up in a Chinese- or French-dominant environment. These differences are discussed below.

Prosody

Prosody features such as stress, intonation, pitch, rate, rhythm and tone are some of the first language properties children learn.[9] Children are sensitive to language-specific prosodic patterns early in life. It is well known that delays in exposure to the sound system of a language may result in a 'foreign' accent. In general, if adolescents are exposed to a language from birth or at an early age, they are usually able to acquire a native-like accent. However, because many heritage-language-speaking adolescents have limited input in their heritage language(s), some prosodic properties may not be well developed.

English prosodic interference on French

English stress can fall on any syllables, and sometimes changing stress may change the meaning of a word. For instance, if you place a stress on the first and last syllable of the words *record, object, suspect* and *content*, you will get different meanings. As a general rule, English bisyllabic nouns (e.g. record) are more likely to have initial syllable stress, and the bisyllabic verbs (e.g. record) are more likely to have final stress. French does not have word-level stress like English. Instead, it has a phrase-level accent in which lexical items (words) that have close semantic (meaning) or syntactic (sentence) relations are grouped together into a single phonological phrase with an accent in the final syllable.[10] In other words, in French, the stress tends to fall on the last syllable.

Influenced by the English stress pattern as a result of the dominant English input in his phonological development, Léandre occasionally put the stress of French words on the initial syllables rather than on the last ones; for example, he placed the emphasis on *'va'* in *'Va au lit'* (Go to bed) during early adolescence (between ages 12 and 13). This phenomenon gradually disappeared in mid to late adolescence. However, there is individual difference; Dominique did not show such a tendency at all in French.

Tone issue in Chinese

Chinese is a tonal language. Tones affect one's understanding of word meanings. For example, the same sound *ma* would result in different meanings depending on which tone is pronounced. When *ma* is pronounced with the first tone (high level) *mā*, it means *mother* (妈); when it is pronounced with the second tone (rising) *má*, it is a marker of *a question* (吗); when it is pronounced with the third tone (falling-rising) *mǎ*, it means *horse* (马); and when it is pronounced with the fourth tone (falling) *mà*, it means *scold* (骂).

Léandre and Dominique sometimes had tone issues in Chinese, both in production (speaking) and in comprehension (understanding). Overall, their mistakes made with the Chinese tones are about 2% in production and 1% in comprehension.[11] For instance, when I read a story called 懒猫 (Lazy Cat) to Léandre and Dominique, Léandre (14; 7; 21) misunderstood 神气 (energetic) for 生气 (angry). I discussed the tone change issues in my previous book *Growing Up with Three Languages: Birth to Eleven*. I stated there that both children were fine with the tones until English became more dominant when they went to English-dominant school. Studies have shown that English in particular seems to have an effect on Chinese tones.[12] However, the tone issue in Léandre and Dominique's Chinese showed improvement in later adolescent years (from ages 17 to 19) as a result of my intentional modelling and their increased exposure to Chinese, including Chinese media such as television.

Accent choice and adjustment

In every society, there tends to be an accent of privilege. As discussed before, at around age 14 or 15, most adolescents start to move towards the more prestigious form of accent. However, multilingual adolescents may form their own ideas about what accent to use, perhaps as a result of their constant interactions with different language speakers. For example, a study of Norwegian bilingual adolescents shows that these youngsters intentionally abandoned the native-speaker accent privilege (i.e. the formal school-associated British English accent or the media-influenced American English) and chose to use their own hybrid English accent.[13]

When Léandre and Dominique were younger, they tended to speak to every Chinese speaker with the same accent, which was closer to my accent. During their adolescent years, Léandre and Dominique gradually chose to speak Chinese with a neutral accent or their own accent in everyday communication; that is, their accent was neither mine nor the Putonghua[14] accent. Nonetheless, if they spoke to Chinese speakers whom they regarded as important, they tended to speak with a more Putonghua accent; in other words, they tended to make special efforts to articulate sounds with **retroflex** (sounds are articulated with the tip of the tongue curled upwards and back against or near the juncture of the hard and soft palates). After a Skype conversation with his Chinese grandparents, Léandre (15; 5; 24) told me that he purposely pronounced certain words such as 玩 (play) and 圈 (circle) in a 'super correct' way to impress his grandparents.

Similarly, my two sons also chose a neutral accent in French, as they neither had the Swiss-French accent (specifically the typical Neuchatel French accent), nor the typical Parisian French accent (which their father acquired as a child). Instead, they spoke with a 'plain' French accent. In other words, it is difficult to pinpoint what French accent they had.

As long as more than one accent or pronunciation is involved, people tend to make a decision about which one to use in context. Most frequently, they will choose an accent that helps them to fit in with the rest of the people around them. If you listen to former US President Bill Clinton carefully, you will notice that he sometimes speaks with a very strong southern American accent when he wants to show his southern roots. When he talks to New Yorkers, however, he speaks with a less southern accent. Likewise, three years ago I was in line to buy a tomato-mozzarella sandwich in a rest stop in the southern part of the United Kingdom, and everyone in front of me ordered it by saying 'tom*a*to' with the typical British English /a:/. When it was near my turn, I hesitated about whether I should pronounce *tomato* like everyone else in front of me or whether I should just pronounce the /a/ in the American way/ei/. In the end, I decided to say it like everyone else to avoid standing out. Similarly, when I buy my plants each spring in a local plant market, I always purposefully pronounce the *a* in *pl*a*nts* with a typical American /æ/ to show my localness, although I normally choose to use a quite neutral pronunciation of the sound /a/; that is, I use a pronunciation that is between the American /æ/ and British /a/.

Phonological translation

Research shows that phonological abilities appear to be especially acute in multilingual speakers, even at a very young age. Multilinguals may have more of an advantage in phonological translation than their monolingual counterparts. **Phonological translation** is the ability to hear a word in one language and to render that word, not its meaning but its phonological form, in the other language. For example, a Spanish speaker pronounces the name *Fernando* with the Spanish pronunciation, and when an English speaker hears the name, he repeats it in English pronunciation. This phonological translation requires a mapping of sounds between the two languages.[15] In multilinguals' daily environment, it is common for them to use phonological translation for names and linguistic borrowings (words borrowed from one language to the other). Thus, multilinguals are not only capable of making their phonological translation freely but are also capable of choosing whether to use it or not.[16]

Switching between languages requires multilinguals to use the phonological translation mapping of phonemic units of one language onto the phonemic units of the other. Because Léandre and Dominique acquired three languages simultaneously from birth, they automatically use phonological translation when articulating a person's name, pronouns, places, food and brands based on language-specific conventions of a particular language. For instance, when saying the names *Rousseau* and *Charlesmanie*, Léandre and Dominique consistently pronounce them in French, English and Chinese according to the pronunciation conventions of the respective languages, whereas people like me, who acquired other languages later in life, often do not have this ability (at least, not without conscious effort). I often tend to pronounce names, places and brands in the language that I first learnt. For example, I tend to pronounce *Rousseau*, *Charlesmanie* and *Hermès* in English with French pronunciation convention instead of using their English pronunciations. I often find that I have to correct my pronunciations of these names when speaking to English or Chinese speakers.

Positive and negative transfer in phonological skills

According to the **Unified Competition Theory** proposed by psycholinguist Brian MacWhinney,[17] multilinguals are sensitive to phonological properties that are common across languages. When phonological knowledge is transferred accurately from one language to the other, it is called **positive transfer;** and when the phonological knowledge is not transferred accurately from one language to the other, resulting in mistakes, it is called **negative transfer** or **phonological interference**. Research has shown that children and adolescents who are exposed to more than one language at home tend to show more advanced phonological skills (such as consonant accuracy, consistency and a fewer number of error patterns) than those children who are only exposed to one language.[18]

Proportionally speaking, Léandre and Dominique demonstrated more positive phonological skill transfers (98% for Léandre and 96% for Dominique) than negative transfers (2% percent for Léandre and 4% percent for Dominique).[19]

Phonological awareness and knowledge across languages

As mentioned earlier, the development of the phonological system in a language is more than just the development of a repertoire of sounds. It is also the process of developing mental representations of the phonemes in a language and the knowledge of the rules regarding how sounds are combined and represented in the language.

Native speakers, including native-speaking young children, develop **phonotactic knowledge** (knowing the constraints of the sequencing of sounds and the phonological rules) in their native languages. A well-known classic study by renowned psycholinguist Jean Berko Gleason[20] suggests that by age four, young children intuitively understand the phonological rules in English by applying English phonological rules to made-up words, such as pronouncing s in plural form *wugs* as /z/ instead of /s/ and the past tense of *rick* as *rickt* /t/ instead of /d/. Adolescents who are exposed to more than one language early in life also develop phonotactic knowledge in their ambient languages. For instance, Polish-English-speaking adolescents know that /zl/ is a permissible combination of sounds in Polish but not in English.

Léandre and Dominique continuously demonstrated remarkable phonological awareness, knowledge and progress across multiple phonologies in their early teen years. They increasingly verbalised their phonological awareness and knowledge after the age of 11. For example, each time we drove by the French town *Besançon*, they would tell me that 'ç' (cedilla) should be pronounced as /s/. On a trip with his Chinese grandfather to the ancient town *Qibao* (七宝) near the city of Shanghai, Léandre (17; 11; 22) came up with many theories about the road signs and shop names outside the window of the tea house where he was having a snack. He commented on the words and analysed their connections; for example, he suggested that the characters 魚 and 泗 must have something to do with water. Moreover, Léandre and Dominique not only demonstrated phonological awareness and knowledge in their heritage languages but also extended their phonological awareness to the other languages. Box 3.1 shows some examples.

Moreover, as a result of being exposed to more than one language from birth, Léandre and Dominique have developed a better intuition about the pronunciation of words in other alphabetic languages. For example, when we drove out of a garage in Aachen (Germany), we saw the word *Uitrit* (*Exit* in Dutch). Léandre (18; 11; 14) was able to pronounce it correctly in a way that sounded like Dutch.

Furthermore, Léandre and Dominique were always curious about any new languages they encountered, and they spontaneously researched information about them. Once during breakfast in a hotel in Cardiff (Wales, the United Kingdom), my colleague and I learnt from the lady who served us that in Welsh, /dd/ is pronounced as /th/. When Léandre (16; 0; 10) joined us later in the dining room, I told him about this. He said that he had already checked online and showed me all the rules for Welsh pronunciations.

> **Box 3.1 Examples of Phonological Awareness and Knowledge**
>
> Léandre (17; 11; 24)
>
> On the way back to Basel (Switzerland) from Freiburg (Germany), Léandre saw a German road sign that read *'Éqisheim.'* He commented that it was strange to see an accent aigu (´) on a German word. As we drove further in Alsace (France), we saw a sign for *BÂLE* (Switzerland). Léandre explained to me that the accent circumflex (^) means old 's' like in the word *même*.
>
> Dominique (13; 0; 24)
>
> While driving around Loch Ness in Scotland, Dominique saw Scottish words, such as *loch* (lake) and *onich* (place), on the road signs. He could guess the meanings of these words based on his linguistic inklings.
>
> Léandre (17; 10; 24)
>
> When Léandre saw a street sign in Basel with ß (esszet), he commented that ß means double *ss*.
>
> Léandre (15; 3; 4) and Dominique (13; 4; 8)
>
> While the family was watching the movie *The Kite Runner*, Léandre and Dominique could name the language that the characters were speaking (*Pashto*). They went on to discuss the relationship between *Pashto* and *Persian* (*Farci*).

Sound play and accent imitation

As a result of their early exposure to three languages, Léandre and Dominique developed exceptional awareness, knowledge and sensitivity of sounds in different languages. In fact, since early childhood, part of their play and leisure had included imitating others' accents. During our long road trips each summer, Léandre and Dominique would entertain themselves and us by mimicking different accents based on different situations. For example, while waiting for food to arrive in a Portuguese restaurant in Jersey (a UK Channel Island), Dominique (17; 0; 11) pretended to be a World Cup announcer/commentator commenting on soccer games in Spanish. His imitation was vivid and sounded just like the one I heard a few days before on TV. Also, on the way to Aachen, Léandre (18; 11; 12) shifted accents by impersonating a car salesperson from the southern part of the United States. A few minutes later, he pretended to report the news as a television anchor in Russian, American and British accents. It was quite entertaining and amusing. On a trip to Scotland, I bought a book on the history of Scotland for Léandre and Dominique. In the car, Léandre (14; 11; 16) began to read it in Scottish accent. It was amazing that he sounded like a real Scot after just a few days in Scotland.

Also, the teens were sensitive to the sounds of a new language, even when they didn't know it. For example, Léandre (16; 5; 4) and Dominique (14; 6; 8) pretended to speak Japanese to each other by making up words. Even though what they said made no sense, the accent, intonation and rhythm sounded just like the father-son conversation of our Japanese neighbours who had dinner with us a few days previously. Most impressively (as I mentioned in Chapter 1), after studying German for only about five or six months, Léandre (18; 8; 27) sounded like a real German in his college class recording, and our native-German-speaking neighbour praised his accent. Likewise, when Léandre came home for spring break, our German neighbour invited us over for lunch. She was visibly impressed with Léandre's German accent.

During each Skype conversation with their Chinese grandparents, the teens would learn a few words and phrases in Shanghai dialect. Their grandparents were pleasantly surprised that both Léandre and Dominique could imitate the Shanghai dialect pronunciation very well.

Also, Léandre and Dominique often played with or joked about the sounds of different languages. For example, when I commented in a restaurant that the dish was too 油腻 (greasy), which sounded like 有你 (have you), Léandre (18; 11; 27) joked 'you mean 有我' (have me). Dominique (15; 3; 19) imitated his soccer mate Filipe in the way he would speak in Portuguese to his mother. Even though most of the words were made up, he definitely sounded Portuguese. Once Dominique imitated our neighbour Teresa's Portuguese accent in English so vividly (15; 10, 7) that for a moment I thought Teresa was at our door.

Dominique became interested in African-American rapping when he was about 11 years old. From ages 13 to 17, he wrote many raps and often performed them at his high school. If you listened to his recordings, you would be convinced that he was African American. He was also interested in Verlan, a form of French slang that consists of playing around with syllables. Dominique was (and still is) very knowledgeable about Verlan rules, and he (17; 0; 4) showed me some Verlan words such as *pécho* (*chopper*), *chémar* (*marcher*), *bégère* (*gerbep*), *teubet* (*bête*), *meut* (*femme*) and *beur* (*arabe*). Dominique was also a fan of Grand Corps Malade (the stage name of Fabien Marsaud, the French slam artist), and he could recite many of his texts.

Accent sensitivity and bias

As mentioned in my previous book *Growing Up With Three Languages: Birth to Eleven*, both Léandre and Dominique were sensitive to people's accents and liked to make extensive comments about them. This phenomenon continued during the adolescent period. Once, we stopped for lunch in south of France, and during the lunch, Dominique (16; 0; 0) kept eavesdropping on the conversations of diners around us and commenting on the southern accent of these people.

Because Léandre and Dominique were exposed to multiple languages from birth, one would expect that they would be more flexible and accepting of different accents and different ways of speaking. On the contrary, they are actually quite biased about how sounds in their respective languages should be pronounced. They clearly demonstrated an accent preference from early childhood to adolescence. For example, Dominique ordered a hot cider in a café called *Unisex* in Paris. The manual was printed in English. After taking the order, the waiter confirmed with Dominique, *'Vous avez commandé un* outsider,' which he intended to mean 'You ordered a hot cider.' Dominique (14; 0; 3) immediately corrected him and said it *'Je voudrais* **hot cider***!'* pronouncing hot cider in an authentic American English way. Similarly, Léandre (15; 10; 10) commented that he was bothered by the way his high school AP French teacher (who is an American) pronounced *'Je ne sais pas'* (I don't know). He said that native French speakers never separate every word when saying this sentence. During his freshman year of college, Léandre also demonstrated bias towards two of his German professors. He said that the nonnative German professor was *barbante* (boring) because she spoke German with an accent, and the native German-speaking professor was enthusiastic because he was accent-free. I also noticed that in middle and high school, both Dominique and Léandre spoke highly about their Spanish teachers when they were native speakers, and they tended to be very critical of their teachers who were not native Spanish speakers. Research indicates that like monolinguals, multilinguals at various ages also tend to show preference for native-accented speakers.[21] Although multilinguals may have cognitive flexibility (see Chapter 1), they may not have accent flexibility.

Language-specific phonological phenomena

Léandre and Dominique demonstrated some language-specific phonological phenomena during adolescence. Below are some specific areas that are important to note.

Chinese heteronyms or heterophones

Heteronyms or **heterophones** are words that are spelt the same but have different pronunciations and meanings, such as *row* (propel with oars) and *row* (argument). Léandre and Dominique sometimes had difficulty with the pronunciation of some Chinese heteronyms, such as the word 和. When 和 is combined with 你和我 (you <u>and</u> me), it means *and,* which is pronounced as /hé/. When it is combined with 和面 (<u>mix</u> flour), it means *mix* and is pronounced as /huò/. The same is true with the word 落. When 落 is combined with 落枕, it means *stiff neck* and pronounced as /lào/. When it is combined with 落后, it means *fall behind* and is pronounced as /luò/. The issue for both the boys was with the pronunciation rather than the meaning. In fact, heteronyms are often a common issue for many mature Chinese speakers. Only people who are well versed in the Chinese language, such as Chinese teachers and television or radio announcers, can pronounce heteronyms correctly.

Chinese homophones

Homophones are words that sound alike, and may be spelt alike or differently, but have different meanings such as *bear* (animal) and *bear* (tolerate) and *mean* (unkind) and *mean* (average) in English. Both Léandre and Dominique had some homophone issues in Chinese. For example, I asked Léandre to finish the green tea I bought from Hangzhou (China). I said that was too 珍贵 (precious) because I made a special trip to the village in Hangzhou to buy the tea. Léandre (17; 2; 29) thought that I said 真贵 (expensive), because both 珍 and 真 are pronounced the same as /zhēn/.

In general, Léandre and Dominique did not have issues with homophones in spoken French. However, they had some issues in the early and mid-adolescent period when spelling some French homophones. For example, *sang* (blood), *cent* (a hundred), *sent* (feel) and *sans* (without). In spoken French, these words sound alike, yet they are spelt differently and have different meanings.

French /b/ and /p/ distinction

During the early adolescent period, Léandre sometimes had a slight /b/ and /p/ distinction issue in French. For example, when he said '*C'est bon* (This is good),' it sounded like '*C'est pont* (This is bridge).' This could be the result of a negative phonological transfer from English to French. However, with constant reminders, Léandre corrected this problem towards late adolescence. There is an individual difference with sound distinction as well, as Dominique did not exhibit this issue at all.

Superb Chinese pinyin (phonetic) abilities

Pinyin is the phonetic system for transcribing the pronunciations of Chinese characters into the Latin alphabet. For example, the Chinese word 中 (middle) is transcribed as *zhong* in pinyin. In Chinese school, Léandre and Dominique learnt the pinyin system to help them pronounce Chinese characters. Because pinyin is the Latin alphabet, both Léandre and Dominique had a great advantage in mastering it because they had knowledge of French and English. In fact, their pinyin ability surpassed mine. I still have to ask them for help each time I struggle to spell some Chinese words when using the alphabetic computer keyboard.

Gendered prosody

Since I am the major Chinese language input for Léandre and Dominique, during early childhood, middle childhood and early adolescence, both kids had a tendency to have slight feminine prosodic patterns in their Chinese communication, specifically regarding intonation and rhythm. As time went on and when they had more exposure to male adult input via conversations with their Chinese uncle, grandfather and other male Chinese-speaking adults, they gradually attained the masculine prosody.

Strategies for Supporting Heritage-Language Phonological Development

In any spoken language, meaning is expressed though sounds. A clear and accurate articulation of sounds in a language is particularly important in intelligibility and communication. Inaccurate pronunciation can cause phonological interference[22] and can affect listeners' understanding; consequently, it can lead to loss of meaning in communication. Some languages may contain the same sounds but use them differently when conveying meaning. For example, the sound /p/ in English can take two different forms depending on where it is in a word. The /p/ in the word *pill* is an aspirated /pʰ/(when it is produced, it is accompanied with a burst of air coming out of the mouth) and the /p/ in the word *spill* is an unaspirated /p/ (which does not have a burst of air when it is produced). English native speakers automatically use /p/ and /pʰ/ correctly. There is never a case in which two words differ only in the use of /p/ or /pʰ/, because aspiration is never the basis for a contrast between two words in English. Thai also has an aspirated /pʰ/ and unaspirated /p/; however, these two sounds change the meaning of words. The aspirated/pʰaa/means *to split* and the unaspirated /paa/ means *forest*.[23] Thus, helping your teens further develop a clear articulation and phonological knowledge in their heritage language(s) should be one of your priorities in supporting their heritage-language development.

Moreover, because heritage languages are often learnt in the home environment, some phonological processing skills may need to be taught explicitly. Below are some thoughts and suggestions for you to consider.

Acoustic modelling

Research suggests that pronunciation can improve with more exposure to acoustic modelling, even for older language learners.[24] Contrary to conventional perception, adults and adolescents actually have a better ability to imitate accents than young children.[25] Thus, even though the period in which children are sensitive to accent may decrease as they grow older, continuing to provide your teens with a good heritage-language acoustic model is still important. A study indicates, for example, that older native speakers of a stress language, such as Spanish, can learn some aspects of the English stress system successfully, even though early learners tend to be more successful.[26]

To promote your teens' phonological development, you may want to draw their attention to pronunciation. You can help your children by guiding them to listen carefully to the way you, other native speakers and native-language television anchors pronounce words. You can intentionally segment words and show your teens how sounds are articulated. By doing so, you are helping others to understand their speech and thus facilitate better communication and social relationships.

Media exposure

Even though research suggests that young children do not learn a language via watching television, adolescents and adults can be influenced by media exposure. A study of Norwegian multilingual adolescents suggests that media does have an impact on accent.[27] I actually know a law professor who learnt English by watching American films in Vienna as a young man.

Reading to teens

Being read to is often regarded as an activity for young children. However, teens also enjoy being read to.[28] Because the heritage-language environment (with limited input that often comes only from parents) is different from the typical language environment (with ample multiple input from many people), additional phonological input is necessary. When choosing texts to read to teens, you can select materials that interest them or allow them to choose what materials to read. Before reading, you may want to rehearse and try to emphasise the phonological areas that you want to model in your heritage language, such as proper stress, intonation, rhythm, rate and other language-specific phonological features. Mealtimes are often a good time to do this activity because eating is usually an enjoyable event, and associating reading with something enjoyable may result in positive acceptability.

Spelling and sound representation

To help auditory discrimination and increase phonological representation awareness, you can use spelling as a springboard to help your teens understand visually how sounds are represented. For example, up until age 15 (15; 7; 6), Léandre did not know how to represent the sounds of *'il y a'* based on its pronunciation until he learnt how to spell it. Thus trying auditory discrimination activities with your children will be helpful. For instance, Philippe played French songs by Georges Brassens and asked Léandre and Dominique to listen to them while he pointed out those difficult words. He then asked the boys to spell them. Making sounds visual will help teens develop not only their abilities in heritage-language representation but also their spelling abilities in general.

Another way to help draw teens' attention from sounds to spelling is to use a direct **Multisensory Structured Learning (MSL) approach**. MSL utilises several sensory channels simultaneously and synthesises stimuli coming from these channels. In other words, while learning how to spell words, teens integrate visual, auditory, kinesthetic and tactile stimuli. This multisensory training helps teens learn how to spell words by hearing, seeing and pronouncing them; tracing them on various surfaces such as paper and sand; and writing them. The underlying idea is that the more perceptual channels that are open, the greater the possibility of forming associations between the graphic (visual) and phonetic (auditory) aspects.[29]

Exposure to native speakers

Frequent travel to heritage countries or heritage-language-speaking regions is another very effective way to expose your teens to the native-language speaking environment. When Léandre and Dominique spent two or three months in French-speaking or Chinese-speaking environments, we observed a great change in their phonological advancement each time.

When travelling to a native-speaking environment is not possible, other opportunities to talk with native speakers are also helpful. For example, encouraging your teens to volunteer in your heritage community and to converse with family and native speakers though Skype and FaceTime are valuable means of providing extra opportunities to speak with native speakers. Studies have confirmed that when adolescents are emerged in more multiplex native-speaking networks, they tend to have higher native-accent ratings.[30]

Explicit teaching of phonological process skills

Because the environment in which heritage-language speakers acquire their languages with limited input, explicit teaching of phonological skills is important. Research has confirmed the important role that phonological processing skills play in the reading and writing development of children and adolescents' language development. [31] Below are a couple of strategies for you to consider.

Teaching auditory discrimination explicitly

Earlier, I mentioned that Philippe used French songs to teach Léandre and Dominique auditory discrimination. In fact, explicit teaching of auditory discrimination within a minimal pair has shown to be successful in helping children and adolescents who are learning English as a new language.[32] **Minimal pairs** or **contrasting phonemes** are pairs of words in a given language that differ in only one phonological element and have distinct meanings, such as *bad-bed*, *let-lit, pan-pen, pat-bat, pin-bin* and *rot-lot*. I found that explicitly teaching auditory discrimination of minimal pairs is also helpful for heritage-language learners. You can intentionally help your teens discriminate between sounds, while making them aware of the meaning changes that occur as a result of phoneme variation. For example, by changing the vowel in the word *b<u>a</u>nd* to *b<u>e</u>nd*, the meaning is altered. I have intentionally pointed out the minimal pairs in Chinese such as *b<u>i</u>àn* (变—change) and *p<u>i</u>àn* (骗—cheat), *b<u>à</u>n* (半—half) and *p<u>à</u>n* (盼—hope) in my daily conversations with the teens. This seems to be more effective during adolescence than when they were younger. Similarly, Philippe also tried to draw attention to the French minimal pairs such as *f<u>ê</u>te-b<u>ê</u>te* (celebration-beast) and *l<u>i</u>n-v<u>i</u>n* (linen-wine) in his daily conversations with the kids to help teach them auditory discrimination.

Teaching difficult sounds explicitly

It is particularly important to pay attention to and teach difficult sounds in a heritage language. The difficult sounds in a language are called **marked sounds**. The same sound in different languages may not be acquired at the same rate. One can look to the English and Arabic/z/ sound as an example. In early language acquisition, English-speaking children master the sound at around age four, whereas Arabic-speaking children do not mater this sound until after age six. Researchers have explained that in English, /z/ has **higher functional load**[33] (the importance of a phoneme in the phonemic inventory of the language); for example, /z/ is used for pluralisation (van_s and dog_s). In Arabic, however, it has a low functional load.

Moreover, some sounds such as /m/ exist in 97% of world languages, whereas /r/ only exists in 5% of world languages.[34] Therefore, you may want to focus on teaching sounds that are more marked (difficult) in your heritage language(s).

Relationship between phonological development and lexical development

There is certainly a relationship between phonological development and lexical development; however, the debate among language researchers is whether phonological development influences lexical development or vice versa. In studies of young children, some researchers found that words that conform to a child's phonology are more readily learnt than words that do not. Moreover, children's phonological skills are linked to their vocabulary size. Children with larger phonetic inventories tend to have larger vocabularies. However, other researchers have argued that vocabulary growth is a major factor that pushes children towards a phonological analysis of their language and the presentation of a phonological system. Although there is no conclusion on this issue and debate is likely to continue, it is clear that there is a connection between phonology and lexicon.

Thus, it is important to deliberately focus on heritage-language phonological analysis when you interact with your teens by helping them become conscious of the sound structures. If you make this exercise a routine, you will help your teens achieve vocabulary advancement.

Useful measure of phonological progress

To monitor your teens' phonological progress and understand how to provide support for them, you may want to try the **nonword repetition** (NWR) task. Although this task is often used for young children, it is also useful for heritage-language-learning teens. The NWR task requires repeating novel phonological forms such as *woogalamic* or *noitauf*.[35] It mimics one of the most basic and important language-learning mechanisms: the immediate repetition of unfamiliar words. A language speaker's NWR is especially important because the skills used in repeating nonwords play an important role in learning new words and **morphemes** (the smallest meaningful unit, such as *s* in *works*). Numerous studies show that performance in NWR tasks can predict children's vocabulary development and syntactic (sentence) development, albeit to a lesser degree.[36] Compared to traditional language measures, such as standardised language tests, NWR relies less on a child's prior knowledge of events, vocabulary or language structures. In a NWR task, a child repeats increasingly longer nonwords comprised of syllables that conform to the **phonotactic constraints** (rules governing possible sound sequence) of a particular language. Immediate recall of meaningless phonological sequences depends heavily on a speaker's ability to perceive, store, recall and accurately reproduce strings of phonological sequences.

Multilingual children and adolescents may rely on similar language-learning mechanisms to mediate the NWR tasks. For example, more exposure to Spanish may increase abilities to repeat longer nonwords. This knowledge may shift across levels of multilingualism. Past research shows that NWR performance was similar across English and Spanish, with differences in performance patterns based on accuracy. NWR performance in both English and Spanish was also significantly correlated to cumulative language experience. Furthermore, there were significant correlations between NWR and **morphosyntax** (**morph** is the short form of morphology, which means the internal structural of words such as *s* in *works*; and **syntax** means sentences) in both English and Spanish, and there were no correlations with semantics (meaning). Children learning languages in which multisyllable words are frequent, such as Portuguese and Greek, appear to be better at producing longer nonwords (up to five- and six-syllable nonwords, respectively). Because longer words are more frequent in Spanish than English, children exposed to Spanish are also able to produce longer nonwords.[37]

Summary of Key Points in Chapter 3

- During adolescence, teens have generally mastered the sound system in their environmental language, as evidenced by their increased refinement and control of their phonological inventory.
- There are increased gender differences in articulation.
- Teens' accents may change as a result of peer influence. However, at around age 14 or 15, most adolescents start to move away from the peer-group accent towards the more prestigious form of accent.
- The most significant phonological achievement during adolescence is teens' phonological decoding abilities, which help them to decipher complex new words.
- The dominant language of multilingual adolescents may impact their prosodic patterns, such as stress and tone in their heritage language(s).
- Multilingual adolescents may also choose to have their own accent and abandon the native-accent privilege.
- Multilingual adolescents have better phonological translation abilities.

- For the most part, multilingual adolescents tend to have more positive phonological transfers than negative ones.
- Multilingual adolescents develop advanced phonological awareness and knowledge in some areas, such as their advanced phonotactic knowledge and accent imitation.
- Multilingual adolescents are sensitive to accents and may have accent bias.
- There may be some language-specific phonological phenomena with multilingual adolescents.
- To help heritage-language-speaking teens further develop their heritage-language phonological awareness and skills, you may want to try the following strategies:
  - Provide acoustic modelling via media exposure, rehearsed reading, spelling activities and exposure to native speakers.
  - Expose your teens to media technology.
  - Read to your teens.
  - Conduct spelling and sound representation exercises.
  - Expose them to heritage-language native speakers.
  - Explicitly teach phonological awareness such as minimal pair distinction and difficult sounds.
- Moreover, when you interact with your teens, focusing on heritage-language phonological analysis will help them become conscious about the heritage-language sound structures and promote heritage-language vocabulary development.
- Finally, you can use nonword response as a way to help you understand your teens' current phonological ability and provide necessary support to their heritage-language development.

Recommended Readings

Souza, A.L., Byers-Heinlein, K. and Poulin-Dubois, D. (2013) Bilingual and monolingual children prefer native-accented speakers. *Frontiers in Psychology* 4, 1–6.

Notes and References

[1] Souza, A.L., Byers-Heinlein, K. and Poulin-Dubois, D. (2013) Bilingual and monolingual children prefer native-accented speakers. *Frontiers in Psychology* 4, 1–6.
[2] Smith, A. and Goffman, L. (2004) Interaction of motor and language factors in the development of speech. In B. Maasen, R. Kent, H. Peters, P. van Lieshout and W. Hulstijn (eds) *Speech Motor Control in Normal and Disordered Speech* (pp. 227–52). Oxford: Oxford University Press.
[3] Pence, K.L. and Justice, L.M. (2008) *Language Development from Theory to Practice.* Upper Saddle River, NJ: Pearson.
  Krohn, R. (1970) The vowel shift rule in English. *Working Papers in Linguistics* 2 (9), 141–54.
[4] Erway, C.C. Downloaded on 31 August 2014 from http://chris.erway.org/portfolio/cce3_ling101_final_chinese_gender_diff.pdf
[5] Owens, R.E. (2012) *Language Development: An Introduction.* Boston: Pearson.
[6] Hoff, E. (2009) *Language Development.* Belmont, CA: Wadsworth.
[7] Hewitt, R. (1982) *White Talk Black Talk: Inter-racial Friendship and Communication amongst Adolescents.* Cambridge: Cambridge University Press.

[8] Hoff, E. (2009) *Language Development* (p. 332). Belmont, CA: Wadsworth.
[9] Guion, S. (2005) Knowledge of English stress patterns in early and late Korean-English bilinguals. *Studies in Second Language Acquisition* 27 (4), 503–33.
[10] Di Cristo, A. (1998) Intonation in French. In D. Hirst and A. Di Cristo (eds) *Intonation Systems: A Survey of Twenty Languages* (pp. 195–218). New York: Cambridge University Press.
[11] Data were calculated based on 28 hours of video-recorded tapes over 7 years (from ages 12 to 19; 4 hours each year with 2 hours for the birthdays and 2 hours for Christmas).
[12] Wang, X.-L. (2008) *Growing Up With Three Languages: Birth to Eleven*. Bristol: Multilingual Matters.
[13] Rindal, U. (2010) Constructing identity with L2: Pronunciation and attitudes among Norwegian learners of English. *Journal of Sociolinguistics* 14 (2), 240–61.
[14] Putonghua is the official language of the People›s Republic of China, which uses Beijing pronunciation as the basis of the standard pronunciation.
[15] Oller, D.K. and Cobo-Lewis, A.B. (2002) The ability of bilingual and monolingual children to perform phonological translation. In D.K. Oller and R.E. Eliers (eds) *Language and Literacy in Bilingual Children* (p. 256). Clevedon: Multilingual Matters.
[16] Oller, D.K. and Cobo-Lewis, A.B. (2002) The ability of bilingual and monolingual children to perform phonological translation. In D.K. Oller and R.E. Eliers (eds) *Language and Literacy in Bilingual Children* (p. 258). Clevedon: Multilingual Matters.
[17] MacWhinney, B. (2005) A unified model of language acquisition. In J. Kroll and A.M.B. De Groot (eds) *Handbook of Bilingualism: Psycholinguistic Approaches* (pp. 49–67). Oxford: Oxford University Press.
[18] Grech, H. and Dodd, B. (2008) Phonological acquisition in Malta: A bilingual learning context. *International Journal of Bilingualism* 12, 155–71.
[19] Data were calculated based on 28 hours of video recorded tapes over 7 years (from ages 12 to 19; 4 hours each year with 2 hours for birthdays and 2 hours for Christmas). A corpus of 52 phonological transfers were identified for Léandre, among which 51 (98%) were positive phonological transfers and 1 (2%) was a negative transfer. A corpus of 69 phonological transfers were identified for Dominique, among which 66 (96%) were positive transfers and 3 (4%) were negative transfers.
[20] Gleason, J.B. (1958) The child's learning of English morphology. *Word* 14, 150–77.
[21] Cohen, E. and Haun, D. (2013) The development of tag-based cooperation via a socially acquired trait. *Evolution and Human Behavior* 34, 230–35.
Lev-Ari, S. and Keysar, B. (2010) Why don't we believe non-native speakers? The influence of accent on credibility. *Journal of Experimental Social Psychology* 46, 1093–6.
Souza, A.L., Byers-Heinlein, K. and Poulin-Dubois, D. (2013) Bilingual and monolingual children prefer native-accented speakers. *Frontiers in Psychology* 4, 1-6.
[22] James, C., Scholfield, P., Garrett, P. and Griffiths, Y. (1993) Welsh bilinguals' English spelling: An error analysis. *Journal of Multilingual and Multicultural Development* 14 (4), 287–306.
[23] Hoff, E. (2009) *Language Development*. Belmont, CA: Wadsworth.
[24] Snow, C. and Hoefnagel-Höhle, M. (1978) The critical period for language acquisition: Evidence from second language learning. *Child Development* 49, 114–18.
[25] Snow, C. and Hoefnagel-Höhle, M. (1977) Age differences in the pronunciation of foreign sounds. *Language and Speech* 20, 357–65.
Snow, C. and Hoefnagel-Höhle, M. (1978) The critical period for language acquisition: Evidence from second language learning. *Child Development* 49, 114–18.
[26] Guion, S. (2005) Knowledge of English stress patterns in early and late Korean-English bilinguals. *Studies in Second Language Acquisition* 27 (4), 503–33.
[27] Rindal, U. (2010) Constructing identity with L2: Pronunciation and attitudes among Norwegian learners of English. *Journal of Sociolinguistics* 14 (2), 240–61.
[28] Zehr, M. (2010) Reading aloud to teens gains favor among teachers. *Education Week* 29 (16), 12–13.
[29] Ideas based on Nijakowska, J. (2008) An experiment with direct multisensory instruction in teaching word reading and spelling to Polish dyslexic learners of English. In J. Komos and E.H. Kontra (eds)

Language Learners With Special Needs: An International Perspective (pp. 130–57). Bristol: Multilingual Matters.

[30] Polat, N. (2011) Nature and content of L2 socialization patterns and attainment of a Turkish accent by Kurds. *Critical Inquiry in Language Studies* 8 (3), 261–88.

[31] Stackhouse, J. and Wells, B. (1997) *Children's Speech and Literacy Difficulties: A Psycholinguistic Framework.* San Diego: Singular Publishing Group Inc.

[32] Seeff-Gabriel, B. (2003) Phonological processing: A platform for assisting second-language learners with English spelling. *Child Language Teaching and Therapy* 291–310.

Van Borsel, J. and Demeulenaere, H. (1998) The minimal pair technique and the remediation of spelling problems. *Clinical Linguistics and Phonetics* 12, 379–87.

[33] Ingram, D. (1989) *First Language Acquisition: Method, Description, and Explanation.* Cambridge: Cambridge University Press.

[34] Hoff, E. (2009) *Language Development.* Belmont, CA: Wadsworth.

[35] Archibald, L.M.D. (2008) The promise of nonword repetition as a clinical tool. *Canadian Journal of Speech-Language Pathology and Audiology* 32 (1), 21–8.

[36] Archibald, L.M.D. (2008) The promise of nonword repetition as a clinical tool. *Canadian Journal of Speech-Language Pathology and Audiology* 32 (1), 21–8.

[37] Summers, C., Bohman, T.M., Gillam, R.B., Penã, E.D. and Bedore, L.M. (2010) Bilingual performance on nonword repetition in Spanish and English. *International Journal of Language Communication Disorders* 45 (4), 480–93.

4 Multilingual Word and Meaning Development During Adolescence

Once during breakfast, Philippe asked me whether I wanted some raisins. Having already had a lot of them in my homemade granola, I declined his offer. A few minutes later, when I saw that he brought some washed grapes to the table, I told him that I also would like to have some. Philippe was a little annoyed and said that I just told him that I didn't want any and that he had only washed enough for himself. It turned out that neither of us was really at fault in this miscommunication; we had both stated our intentions clearly. The only issue here was Philippe's misuse of the French word *raisin* (grape) in the English context (in French, *raisin* is *grape* and *raisins secs* is *raisins*).

This anecdote shows that in everyday communication, lexicon (word) errors are more detrimental in understanding meaning than grammatical or syntactic (sentence) errors. In other words, listeners tend to consider lexicon errors to be more disruptive than grammatical or syntactic errors.[1] Grammatical or syntactic errors could be generally understood by listeners in the context (e.g. 'Can you tell me where *is* the restroom?'), whereas lexicon errors may interfere with meaning comprehension, and misused words will lead to a misunderstanding of the speaker's intended meaning (e.g. Philippe's misuse of the French word *raisin* for *grape* in the English context).

This chapter is about the lexical and semantic (word and meaning) development of multilingual adolescents. It begins with a description of the general trend of adolescent vocabulary development. It then focuses on Léandre and Dominique's heritage-language vocabulary development. Finally, it introduces some practical strategies and useful measurements to support teens' heritage-language lexical and semantic development.

General Characteristics of Lexical-Semantic Accomplishments during Adolescence

Adolescents generally make steady progress in their overall vocabulary development in their ambient language(s). Several changes warrant special mention.

Changes in vocabulary quantity

It has been estimated that by the end of high school, an adolescent will know between 40,000[2] and 60,000[3] different words altogether. This means that they usually add thousands of new words per year to their vocabulary repertoires.

The quantitative change of adolescent vocabulary growth can be attributed to many factors, such as the enlargement of their social circles, the improvement of their cognitive ability, the development of their reading and writing abilities and the enrichment of their vocabulary input (e.g. teacher lectures, news broadcasts and exposure to the internet). Moreover, the development of an organised semantic (meaning) network in which related words become more closely associated may also contribute to the increase in adolescent vocabulary size. Furthermore, adolescents' understanding of word components (or the morphological process) may also be responsible for adolescent vocabulary expansion. For example, when adolescents have an understanding of word roots (e.g. *work*), inflected words (e.g. *work<u>s</u>* and *work<u>ing</u>*), derived words (e.g. *work<u>er</u>*), and compound words (e.g. *<u>workman</u>*), they tend to learn words more efficiently.

However, studies show that deviational word knowledge develops later than compound word knowledge. **Deviational words** are words that are formed by adding a prefix (e.g. adding *un-* to *happy* becomes *<u>un</u>happy*) or suffix (e.g. adding *–ness* to *slow* becomes *slow<u>ness</u>*). **Compound words** are words that are formed by adding two or more words together (e.g. *grapefruit* and *schoolteacher*). Even 16-year-olds may not demonstrate full productive control of derivational words.[4] Like children, adolescents may still learn words from **incidental exposure** (i.e. they learn the new meaning of words in context by looking for cues and drawing from background knowledge).

Changes in vocabulary quality

The quality of vocabulary development also progressively improves during adolescence. While being exposed to school subject areas and reading, adolescents increasingly use longer, rarer, more specialised, more abstract and more complex words, especially in formal writing. The quality change in adolescents' vocabulary development can been observed in their increased **lexical diversity** (use of different types of words), **lexical density** (use of a variety of lexical items such as nouns, verbs, adjectives and adverbs) and **lexical complexity** (use of multisyllabic words).

Changes in vocabulary use

In addition to the improvement in lexical quantity and quality, teens also make a gradual progress in their use of words. Even though young children may already use some words, they may not completely understand the function of these words until adolescence. For example, young children may use the words *because* and *before*. However, they are only understood as intrasentential (within sentence) connectives until early adolescence. Moreover, young children may use the words such as *cold*, *bright*, *sweet* and *crooked* based on their physical meanings, while their psychological meanings are not understood until early adolescence.[5]

Even though vocabulary use qualitatively improves during adolescence, teens may still have partial knowledge about word meanings and sometimes still make mistakes when using unfamiliar and new words. For example, some researchers[6] reported that adolescents still have trouble grasping the meaning of English words when using the words *meticulous*, *relegate* and *redress* accurately, as shown in the following examples:

> I was *meticulous* about falling off the cliff.
> I *relegated* my pen pal's letter to her house.
> The *redress* for getting well when you're sick is to stay in bed.

Improvement in lexical and semantic ambiguity

Teens also make great progress in understanding ambiguous words, such as **homophones** (words that sound alike and may be spelt alike, e.g. *bear* vs. *bear*; or that may be spelt differently, e.g. *bear* vs. *bare hands*), **homographs** (words that are spelt the same and may sound alike, e.g. *row a boat* vs. *row of homes*; or may sound different from each other, e.g. *record player* vs. *record a speech*), and **homonyms** (words that are spelt and pronounced in the same way but are different in meaning, e.g. *brown bear* vs. *bear weight*). The ability to understand word ambiguity not only enables teens to understand humour and jokes that take advantage of lexical and semantic ambiguity but also enables them to make jokes by applying lexical and semantic ambiguity. This is a major lexicon achievement of adolescents.

Heritage-Language Lexical and Semantic Development Characteristics

Heritage-language-speaking adolescents also show the general development trajectory in their mainstream language as described above. However, their heritage-language learning environment is significantly different from the environment of their counterparts who live in the heritage-language-speaking environment. In the heritage-language learning environment, the language input is mainly from parents, often from only one parent; and is learnt mostly in the home setting. In contrast, those who are living in the heritage-language dominant environment have a wider input from many agents, such as parents, teachers, peers and other adults, in addition to formal school education. As a result, the heritage-language lexical and semantic development of multilingual adolescents is likely to be lopsided, with a stronger mainstream-language vocabulary than the heritage-language vocabulary, and it tends to result in different developmental characteristics.

In the discussion below, I will first address the challenges that parents face when providing the heritage-language vocabulary input, and I will then discuss the unique heritage-language developmental phenomena as a result of the input.

Challenges in parental input

Parents, who are usually the major heritage-language models for their children, may experience tremendous challenges when their own native language goes through attrition as a result of living in a different language environment. Using myself as an example, I have lived in the United States for 30 years. Even though I try to go back to my country of origin every year, my own Chinese lexicon is not on a par with other parents who have been living in the Chinese linguistic environment undisrupted. Thus, my Chinese vocabulary attrition as well as my infrequent contact with the Chinese linguistic environment affected the model that I provided for my two children. For example, I did not know many terms related to internet search engines, such as 百度. Below are a few of the commonly observed challenges.

Limitation in active vocabulary use

Because of detachment from the native-speaking environment, parents often have trouble using heritage-language vocabulary in **online production** (immediate and on-the-spot communicative situations), which is the nature of everyday communication. It sometimes takes a while to recall an adequate word. By the time a word is recalled, the uncertainty and hesitation in word searching may result in communication breakdown. For example, once I was negotiating with Léandre about when he should return home from his friend's house. I tried to use the words 底线 (the bottom line) and 纠结 (entangle). Because these words were no longer included in my active vocabulary, I had to stop talking and search for them in my memory. By the time I could recall the words, Léandre was in another room, and I had lost the opportunity to have a successful negotiation with him. This example indicates the importance of immediate vocabulary accessibility in communication flow.

Lack of up-to-date vocabulary

Because some parents live outside of their heritage-language environment, their vocabulary may be out of date. For example, once at Pudong Airport in Shanghai, I saw a woman abandoning her cart in the middle of a busy corridor without putting it back in the cart rack. I commented to Léandre (17; 11; 17) in Chinese that this type of behaviour was 小农意识 (peasant mentality). Léandre immediately criticised me, saying I had insulted peasants. I tried to explain that this was merely an expression that I used as a child in China to describe people who only thought about their own individual interests and failed to consider others' interests or the larger picture. In retrospect, my use of the phrase 小农意识 (peasant mentality) does sound rather derogatory and out of date. I checked with some of my Chinese colleagues at a conference in China, who told me that it is no longer politically correct to use this phrase. The proper way to express this sentiment would be to say 不文明行为, which means 'uncivilised behaviour.' This example does show that when discussing situations like this in Chinese, I did have trouble using more updated vocabulary, and many times I sounded ancient or out of date, to say the least.

Generation gap in vocabulary use

Another issue that Philippe and I ran into when providing lexicon input for our sons in our heritage languages was that there was a generation gap in our vocabulary use due to our lifestyle change and age differences. For instance, when the boiler in our place was under repair, Philippe joked that we would need to wear nightcaps. Dominique (16; 7; 0) thought Philippe was talking about an alcoholic beverage called a 'nightcap.' Indeed, in Dominique's lifetime, there has always been heating, and he has not needed to wear a nightcap to bed.

Unique heritage-language lexical and semantic phenomena

Discrepancy in crosslinguistic synonyms

Much of multilingual learning involves learning to understand different words from different languages that share the same meaning. Since early on in life, multilingual children will have been used to hearing the same thing referred to in more than one way (**crosslinguistic synonyms**) such as *cup*, *tasse* and 杯子 in English, French and Chinese, respectively. Even though young multilingual children understand the crosslinguistic synonyms, they may initially attribute different meanings to them. For instance, a child may think that the Dutch word *fles* (bottle) means the bottle he drinks his milk out of, which his mother usually fixes; and when he hears English *bottle*, he may believe that it only refers to the kind of bottle that contains his favourite juice, which his father usually gives to him.[7]

By the time multilingual children enter the adolescent period, they may vary greatly in their production of crosslinguistic synonyms. Due to the language acquisition environmental differences in their society's dominant language and their heritage language(s), multilingual adolescents tend to have a lexicon discrepancy or gap in their various languages. For example, Léandre and Dominique acquired more vocabulary in their mainstream language, English, than in their other two heritage languages (French and Chinese) during adolescence. Moreover, they also tended to have more heritage-language **receptive lexicon** (vocabulary that one can understand but not necessarily use in communication) than their **expressive lexicon** (vocabulary that one can use in communication) and had less literate and academic lexicon in their heritage languages. Such a lexicon gap in different languages is typical and most multilinguals do not produce a similar set of words (crosslinguistic synonyms) in their respective languages, even though some multilinguals do.

There may be different reasons for the vocabulary discrepancy in multilinguals' respective languages. One major reason is because of their different environmental input (e.g. teacher language input vs. parental language input) and another one is their different interactive contexts (such as school and peers vs. home). Moreover, the lexicon gap also depends on how close their various languages are to one another. For example, Spanish and Catalan are closely related. Therefore, children and adolescents who acquire these two languages will tend to have a large set of **cognates** (words in different languages that share the same etymology; they tend to have similar form and meaning, but not always pronunciation: e.g. *activate* in English and *activer* in French). However, children and adolescents who are acquiring Chinese and Spanish will have no cognates to share. In Léandre and Dominique's case, French and English are closer to each other, and thus, the boys were able to benefit from the cognates. I noticed that the two teens (especially Dominique) used lots of words in English that are considered to be academic vocabulary in writing. These words often may not appear in monolingual English adolescents' typical lexicon. I believe that Léandre and Dominique simply profited from French cognates. But, neither of the teens' Chinese lexicons benefited from their French or English and vice versa; because Chinese is a logographic language, it does not share cognates with an alphabetic language such as French and English.

Another cause of Léandre and Dominique's lexicon gap is word learning in different contexts. For example, both Léandre and Dominique knew a lot of words related to mathematics in English and few words related to mathematics in Chinese; Léandre knew more French words related to trains (because one of his hobbies is Mäklin trains) than both Chinese and English words, and both teens knew more words used to describe a variety of dumplings in Chinese than in French. This vocabulary imbalance is called **distributed characteristic of multilingual word learning**,[8] and it is a characteristic of multilingual development due to varying amounts of exposure to different languages.

False cognates
   False cognates, sometimes referred to as **false friends**, are words in different languages that have overlapping orthographic (spelling) or phonological (sound) properties but have little or no semantic (meaning) overlap.[9] In other words, false cognates are pairs of words in different languages that look or sound similar but differ significantly in meaning. Examples are the English word *embarrassed* and the Spanish word *embarazada (pregnant)* and the English word *library* and the French word *librairie (bookstore)*. Multilinguals sometimes use false friends in their communication. Although this is a common phenomenon among multilinguals, Léandre and Dominique typically did not use false friends in their different languages. There are a couple of explanations for this. First, it is possible that they were acquiring English and French simultaneously from birth, and their lexicon production in the two languages is clearly separated. Second, Chinese is a logographic language; thus, it is impossible for them to have false friends with either English or French because both of them are alphabetic languages.

Lexical and semantic inaccuracy

Because heritage-language speakers tend to have less input models than their counterparts who live in the heritage-language environment, they may have issues with heritage-language lexical and semantic accuracy in communication. For instance, when we were driving to Edinburgh, Léandre (14; 11; 15) said, '苏格兰人不喜欢英国人' (the Scottish do not like the British). I asked him why, and he said it was because they 打架 (fight between people) instead of 打仗 (war between two groups). Likewise, when I asked Dominique '你为什么在 Ossining 足球队? Marco 为什么不在你的足球队'? (Why are you on the Ossining Soccer Team? Why isn't Marco on your team?), he (15; 10; 15) said, '他比我年轻' (He is junior-er than me) instead of '他比我小' (He is younger than me). At Dominique's age, 小 is more appropriate than 年轻. These examples show that multilingual children and adolescents sometimes may not use heritage-language vocabulary accurately in communication.

Lack of tier-three words

Literacy experts have categorised words into three tiers[10] in terms of level of difficulty. **Tier-one words** are the basic and frequent words that rarely require purposeful instruction because they are embedded in the everyday environment (e.g. *clock* and *walk*). **Tier-two words** also appear frequently (e.g. *coincidence*, *absurd*, *industrious* and *fortunate*). Mastering tier-two words can have a powerful impact on children's reading and writing development because of the large role these words play in a language user's repertoire. Therefore, instructions directed towards tier-two words can be most useful. **Tier-three words** are not frequently used or are limited to a specific domain, and they are quite technical and sophisticated (e.g. *isotope* and *lathe*). They often need special exposure or teaching.

Both Léandre and Dominique tended to lack tier-three vocabulary in their heritage languages. This was to be expected because they were not educated in their heritage languages and were rarely exposed to domain-specific or technical terms in their heritage languages. For example, Léandre (17; 1; 28) did not know the word *dégommer* (beat someone at a war game) when his French-speaking friend David used it for the first time. Their lack of tier-three words was more pronounced in Chinese than French, because I almost never used tier-three Chinese words with them.

Crosslinguistic lexical mixing or loan blending

Because multilingual adolescents are exposed to their mainstream language under a more full-acquisition condition (i.e. they receive more adult and peer input and read and write in school) than their heritage language(s) (which often have limited input in the home environment), they tend to be on a more solid footing in their mainstream-language vocabulary than their heritage language(s). As a result, they tend to have advanced adolescent cognitive abilities but less advanced vocabulary in their heritage language(s). For example, Léandre (15; 9; 23) could not express the idea of 幽默感 (a sense of humour) when making a comment in Chinese, and he had to borrow the expression from English. This phenomenon is called **lexical mix** or **loan blending**.

Although mixing or loan blending can be a result of insufficient vocabulary in a heritage language, multilingual speakers can also use it intentionally to emphasise what they want to say. For instance, when I reminded Léandre to bring extra batteries to his SAT exams, Léandre (17; 1; 15) was annoyed and told me, '妈妈，我知道了。我已经跟你说了un million 次了我会带电池 (Mother, I know. I have told you a million times that I will bring the batteries).' In this case, I knew that Léandre could have said '一万次' instead of 'un million.' However, by blending the French words, he expressed how he felt about his mother's constant nagging more clearly. It is interesting to note that he mixed French with Chinese, which he rarely did (he tended to mix English with Chinese) to show that his father, to whom he spoke French, did not usually nag. Clever indeed!

Furthermore, there tends to be a different reaction from people with regard to loan blending. For instance, when an English speaker blends French words in his or her speech, it is often perceived as prestigious or educated, whereas if a speaker blends words from South-American Spanish, it is not considered favourable. Research has corroborated this bias. A study in a Danish school has shown that the blending of English, French and German is privileged and the blend of Arabic languages is not privileged.[11]

Lexical innovation

Besides borrowing words from other languages to fill in the vocabulary gap in communication, multilinguals sometimes also invent words to compensate for their vocabulary insufficiency. For instance, when Léandre and Dominique did not have enough vocabulary in their heritage languages, especially in Chinese (as I mentioned elsewhere,[12] French does not allow much invention), they invented words. For example, Léandre (16; 1; 29) told me '妈妈，那个饭的水跑出来了' (Mom, the water is running out of the rice cooker), instead of '水浦出来了' (the water is coming out of the rice cooker). Similarly, Léandre (14; 3; 5) said 'cafards 的鸡蛋' (cockroaches' chicken eggs), instead of '蟑螂的卵'(cockroaches' eggs). Although these lexical inventions are not authentic, they are creative and contextually understandable. By using lexical invention, heritage-language learning children and adolescents are able to carry out coherent conversations in their heritage language without communication breakdowns caused by a vocabulary shortage.

Literal understanding of Chinese word meaning

Because of linguistic input limitations, Léandre and Dominique sometimes interpret some Chinese words in their literal meanings instead of their intended meanings. For instance, when I told Léandre that he was '不听话' (does not listen to what I said or obey; the literal meaning is *do not hear*), Léandre (14; 1; 28) answered, '听到了' (I heard). Both Léandre and Dominique had a tendency to interpret Chinese words based on their literate meaning; this is a particularly prominent phenomenon during early and middle adolescence. With constant explanation, they began to do well in late adolescence.

Chinese semantic overextension

When young children acquire a language, they often use **overextension** (extending the meaning of a word). Adolescent heritage-language speakers sometimes also overextend word meaning in their heritage language(s) for lack of vocabulary availability. For example, I once asked Dominique how to get to a restaurant for his soccer team celebration dinner. Dominique (13; 4; 4) said, '去次教练告诉' (Past time, my coach told me) instead of '上次教练告诉我' (Last time, my coach told me). Even though this is not correct, one can trace the origin of it; that is, Dominique overextended from 去年 (last year) to 去次 (last time).

Family lexicon

Because several languages are frequently used in our family, Philippe and I have shared a set of words over the years that are used regularly in our family communication. For example, we use the Chinese words 大便 (bowel movement) and 小便 (urination) and the French words *poussette* (stroller), *chariot* (cart) and *pain perdu* (French toast).

As is common with linguistic input, both Léandre and Dominique use these mixed words in our family communication as well. However, they have never used them outside of the family environment or in a non-French-speaking environment.

Lexicon fixture in Chinese

As I reported in my last book, *Growing Up With Three Languages: Birth to Eleven*, Léandre and Dominique tended to misuse the Chinese words 穿 (wear clothes) and 戴 (wear gloves and or glasses). Both continued to use 穿 instead of 戴 in their speech production in addition to other words such as using 旧 (used) for 老 (old) and 脏 (dirty). For example, while travelling in Paris, Léandre did not bring enough socks. He (18; 11; 26) said to me, '我要穿我的旧的袜子' (I want to wear my old socks) instead of '我要穿我脏的袜子' (I want to wear my dirty socks). Both Léandre and Dominique seemed to have a lexical fixture in some Chinese words even in late adolescence, though they did not have difficulties comprehending these words. It seems that once a habit is formed in using the wrong words, it is hard to change. However, both teens did not have this lexical fixture issue in French.

Semantic interference

The two teens also showed semantic interference in their various languages. For instance, Léandre and Dominique often made mistakes in Chinese, such as using '你不认识我' (You don't recognise me) for '你不知道我' (You don't know me). When we discussed this, Léandre (18; 10; 12) reflected that this could be the interference from French 'Tu ne me connaîs pas' (You don't know me). Most notably, the teens tended to have proportionally more English interference in their heritage languages as a result of the dominant language exposure. Box 4.1 lists some examples.

Multilingual Word and Meaning Development During Adolescence 83

> **Box 4.1 Examples of Dominant Language Interference on Heritage Languages**
>
> **Example 1:**
> Dominique (13; 4; 17) said, 'Quand une personne a *leur* téléphone…' instead of 'Quand une personne a *son* téléphone …' (when a person has his telephone…).
>
> **Example 2:**
> Léandre (14; 10; 15) directly used the English phrase *make a face* for French *fair un visage* instead of *fair des grimaces* (make a face).
>
> **Example 3:**
> Dominique (13; 2; 8) saw that our neighbour took her sister somewhere, and he said, 'Teresa 拿她的妹妹' instead of '带她妹妹去.' This is a direct influence from the English *took*.
>
> **Example 4:**
> Also, when we came back from our annual trip abroad, we filled our refrigerator. Léandre (18; 0; 6) directly used the English word for French, 'Le réfrigérateur est stoki' (the refrigerator is stocked) instead of 'Le réfrigérateur est complète.'
>
> **Example 5:**
> Léandre (18; 6; 15) used *sans doute* (probably) to replace *sans aucun doute* (no doubt).
>
> **Example 6:**
> Léandre (16; 0; 19) used *numéro* (number) in places where he needed to use *chiffre* (number 0–9 or amount). This is an English influence.

Life experience and vocabulary

Vocabulary is linked to life experience. If a person does not have opportunities to experience something, it is likely the person will not have the words to describe that experience. For example, Léandre (17; 10; 23) did not know how to say 'well done' in French when he ordered a beef steak in Nîmes, France, because I don't eat meat and we don't cook meat at home. He turned to Philippe for help to communicate what he wanted to the waiter. Another example of interest is the word *clothespin*. Once there was an article in the *New York Times* magazine[13] about who invented the clothespin. In this article, a seven-year-old boy asked his father 'What is a clothespin?' In developed countries, most people don't use clothespins any more. So, I showed a clothespin to Léandre (16; 9; 5) and asked him what he would call it. He did not know the word in Chinese. I then asked him whether he knew it in English, and he said, *'clothes* something.' He then said that he knew how to say it in French, *pince à linge*. The reason he knew the word in French was that each summer in Switzerland, we often dried our clothes in the sun using *pinces à linge*. Indeed, vocabulary is closely linked to experiences.

Special things for a special language

Multilinguals sometimes have some special concepts or words 'reserved' only for a specific language. Often, these words are not shared with other languages. For example, I asked Léandre (15; 7; 27) what he was doing while waiting for me to pick him up from one of his examinations. He said that he was *petrir 我的橡皮* (kneading his eraser). He said he did not really know how to say this word exactly in other languages.

Errors in the French words de, à, dans, tes and des

Up until mid-adolescence, Dominique and Léandre still had some issues using the French words *de, à, dans* and *tes*. Dominique (13; 3; 25), for example, said, *'voler quelque chose de quelqu'un'* instead of *'voler quelque chose à quelqu'un'* (to steal something from someone). Léandre (15; 3; 16) used *'dans la gym'* instead of *'à la gym'* (in the gym). Léandre (15; 10; 26) commented that Dominique wore his pyjamas to the mall. He used *'tes pyjamas'* instead of *'ton pyjamas'* (your pyjamas). When eating Sardinian parchment crackers, Dominique (16; 6; 28) commented that the crackers were *'La vrai choses'* (the real thing) instead of *'des vrai choses.'*

Heritage-language vocabulary stabilisation

Fossilisation has been discussed in literature as a language phenomenon in which a new-language learner or second-language learner reaches a plateau and does not make any progress. In this case, the language learner's **interlanguage** (their own version of a target language) continues to exist regardless of further exposure to the target language. Because it is difficult to determine when the language learning process has ceased, this phenomenon is now often referred to as **stabilisation**. Some believe that there is no solid research evidence at the moment to support the idea of fossilisation, and stabilisation[14] is a better concept for the phenomenon.

Although little is mentioned in the literature about whether or not the heritage-language stabilisation phenomenon also exists, I have observed stabilisation in Léandre and Dominique's Chinese. Between the ages of 14 and 17, their Chinese vocabulary went through a stabilisation phase. Over these three years, the boys' vocabulary did not increase significantly.[15] However, their French vocabulary increased. There are several explanations for this. First, both Léandre and Dominique stopped going to the Chinese school during these years. Second, the conversation between them and me was reduced due to their busy extracurricular activities. Third, they spent significantly less time in China than they did in the French-speaking environment.

Cognate transfer

Earlier in the chapter, I mentioned cognate transfer. As noted, crosslinguistic cognates are words that share form and meaning in two languages (e.g. the English *helicopter* and the Spanish *helicóptero*). Research has consistently demonstrated a performance speed and/or accuracy advantage for processing cognates versus noncognates in older multilinguals. Studies have shown that older multilinguals are faster and more accurate in processing both written and spoken cognates as compared to noncognates of comparable length, difficulty or frequency. However, it is important to note that not all adolescents demonstrate this cognate advantage.[16]

Intuition about word components

When a person has a good lexical knowledge in a language, he or she can instinctively segment a word into meaningful parts. This is called **morphological analysis**. For instance, in Dover (the United Kingdom), while waiting for the ferry to Calais (France), Philippe wanted to type in the hotel address in Aachen (Germany). I tried to read the road name *Adenauerallee* to him. At first glance, the word looked like a difficult long word, and I had a hard time segmenting it. I showed the word to Léandre (18; 11; 17), and he looked at it and segmented it immediately because he knew that the last part of the word meant *allee* (avenue) and the first part is a surname. Léandre had a good lexical knowledge, perhaps as a result of being exposed to different languages early in life. Such knowledge seems to be transferable (in this case, to German).

In sum, heritage-language-speaking adolescents have their own unique lexical and semantic development characteristics. Despite the input limitations, they are able to use various strategies such as loan blending, cognate transfer, lexicon innovation and overextension to compensate for their lexicon limitation.

Strategies for Supporting Heritage-Language Lexical and Semantic Development

Vocabulary is the building block for a language. It is basic to listening, speaking, reading, writing, and language use in general. It has been estimated that about 70%–80% of our comprehension is based on vocabulary.[17] For example, in the sentence, 'The futility of winning the jackpot has been demonstrated by scientists,'[18] the word *futility* is central to understanding the meaning of the whole sentence. Having a rich vocabulary can help teens form better concepts and make their learning in many areas easier. A rich vocabulary can also enhance thinking and communication and allow teens to communicate in precise, powerful, persuasive and interesting ways. Further, a rich vocabulary can promote reading fluency (as it accounts for 70% of fluency) and improve the speed of reading.[19] Taken together, vocabulary knowledge is the primary indicator of a language proficiency level.[20]

Therefore, the most important part of helping multilingual adolescents develop a rich vocabulary is to help them build heritage-language mental lexicon. **Mental lexicon** is the mental storage of words that can be activated by a language user. In other words, mental lexicon is an individual's knowledge of words in a given language and the ability to process these words in comprehension (understanding) or production (use). For example, Jim was writing a speech to thank Martha for her donation to the school library. He searched his metal lexicon for a right word to describe Martha's contribution. He retrieved several words for consideration: *generous, philanthropic, unselfish, giving, magnanimous, ungrudging, altruistic* and *benevolent*. In the end, he decided that the word *generous* was the best word for him to use. Similarly, when Jim's 12-year-old son Marcus came across the new word *malevolent* in a book, he searched in his mental lexicon for other words he knew in order to decipher the meaning, such as *mean, malicious* and *vindictive*.

Mental lexicon, particularly the productive mental lexicon in young children, has been shown to predict later reading ability and comprehension.[21] During adolescence, mental lexicon continues to be important for effective communication and academic learning. Language experts have suggested that older children and adolescents develop their mental lexicon through three primary approaches: **direct teaching** (being directly taught the meaning of words), **contextual abstraction** (learning words by using context clues to determine the meaning of unfamiliar words), and **morphological analysis** (analysing the components of words and using that information to infer the meaning of the entire word; e.g. learning the word *talkativeness* by analysing the parts *talkative-* and *-ness*).[22]

In my own interactions with my two multilingual adolescents in the family context, I have come to realise that these three approaches are equally applicable in heritage-language vocabulary attainment. However, the order of the three components may need to be adjusted; that is, it should be changed so that contextual abstraction comes first, followed by direct teaching and then by morphological analysis. In the school context, a subject content area teacher may teach some new words before students are asked to read the materials. For example, a social studies teacher may first define the meaning of the words *tyranny* and *revolution* before exposing students to the readings and lectures. Conversely, in the everyday home context, new words first appear often in the communicative context and parents can then go on to teach these words explicitly, including through morphological analysis.

I advocate using the aforementioned three approaches for new vocabulary learning in heritage languages because as children become older, the common practice in the home context is often to teach words through oral communication. While oral communication is still useful for heritage-language vocabulary learning, it is not enough for adolescents to develop more advanced heritage-language vocabulary. As adolescents go to school and make great progress in their societal dominant language (in Léandre and Dominique's case, they developed far more vocabulary in

English than in their other two heritage languages), they should pay equal attention to their heritage language. Their heritage language needs a big boost so that they could catch up with their mainstream-language vocabulary and move forward. Below I will suggest some concrete ideas in these three areas for you to consider.

Contextual abstraction

Researchers have long found that young children acquire a large amount of vocabulary in a short period of time due to their **fast-mapping cognitive ability**[23] (the mental process whereby a new concept is learnt based only on a single or limited exposure to given information.) Some researchers think fast-mapping is particularly important for language acquisition. Like young children, adolescents also often use fast-mapping in new word learning; that is, they make a guess about a word's meaning based on the available knowledge they accumulate and contextual clues surrounding a new word they encounter for the first time. However, compared with children, adolescents are more sophisticated in using contextual abstraction (context clues) to guess word meanings. Parents' deliberate efforts in helping adolescents develop the contextual abstraction have been shown to be an effective way for adolescents to increase the breadth and depth of their word knowledge.[24]

An adolescent's initial exposure to a new word is through several contextual channels: spoken communication, multimedia (e.g. news reports and films) and reading (books, the internet, Twitter and magazines). Thus, you may want to encourage your teens to use contextual clues presented in these channels when encountering new words in their heritage language(s).

Specific strategies include exposing your teens to these channels and increasing the frequent opportunities for new word exposure with immediate contextual guidance. For instance, I often turned on Chinese news channels while Léandre and Dominique were around. When detecting words that were new to them, I asked them to tell me the meanings by encouraging them to guess. Also, I frequently use the everyday context to help the teens learn new words. Box 4.2 shows more examples.

Thus, using the context to help teens extract meaning is an effective way to help them learn new words. I have noticed that there is no need to fear that your teens cannot understand you when you use new words. Even if in the very beginning they do not, if you keep on talking in your heritage language and paraphrase what you say, your teens will understand the words from the context.

Direct Teaching

Because of the nature of heritage-language learning, directly teaching the word meaning may be extremely important, since many heritage-language-speaking teens will not have opportunities to be taught their heritage language(s) in school as they

Box 4.2 Examples of Teaching Vocabulary in the Everyday Context

Example 1:

Dominique (12; 8; 26) kicked the soccer ball against a stonewall in our neighbourhood. A woman shouted at him. Dominique told me about it and used the English word *bitch* to describe her. I told him that there was no need to get upset with 这种泼妇 (this kind of shrew). In the context, Dominique could guess the meaning of 泼妇 (shrew), which he had never heard before in Chinese.

Example 2:

Dominique was reading about *karma* online. We then carried out a lively discussion about it. I deliberately used 因果报应 (what goes around comes around) several times in the conversation, and he could infer the meaning from the context.

Example 3:

At the breakfast table, Dominique (13; 5; 22) wanted me to give him the arts section of the *New York Times*, but he did not know how to say 文艺版 (arts section). I handed the arts section to him and said, 'Here is the 文艺版 (arts section).' I then purposely asked him whether he also wanted to have 新文版 (the news section) and 体育版 (the sports section). In the context, he could guess the meanings of these words. I then continued to ask him which section was his favourite, 新文版 (the news section), 体育版 (the sports section) or 文艺版 (the arts section) in order to reinforce the new words in the context.

Example 4:

I called Dominique for dinner. He replied that he did not feel like eating because he just had diarrhoea. I told Léandre (15; 3; 4) that Dominique did not want to eat because he had a special situation (他有特殊情况). In the context, Léandre understood the new words he had not known before.

Example 5:

Dominique (14; 1; 3) had a new laptop; I used it to check e-mail in a hotel in Tier (Germany). He complained that I had made scratches on his new laptop because I dropped it in Mons (Belgium). He said that it was not in perfect condition anymore. He did not know how to say 'perfect condition' in Chinese. Below is a conversation I had with Dominique and Léandre:

Mother: Why is it not in perfect condition? (为什么不完美？)

Dominique: Because there are scratches. (因为有印子。)

(Continued)

Mother:	Show me where it is not perfect. (你给我看哪里<u>不完美</u>？)
Mother:	(to Léandre): Léandre, can you tell where it is not perfect? (理昂，你看哪里<u>不完美</u>？)
Léandre:	What is 不完美? (什么是不完美？)
Mother:	不完美 means imperfection. (不完美就是有缺限。)
Léandre:	I don't see the imperfection. (我看不到哪里不完美。)

do in their societal mainstream language. Research shows that explicit teaching of vocabulary is an effective means of building a stock of known words,[25] and it is the best way for building vocabulary[26] or mental lexicon. Below are some ideas you may want to try in the home context.

Teaching rare words

Vocabulary is related to life. Chances are that we gain vocabulary through our experiences. However, our lives are also limited, and we cannot experience everything. Thus, to help heritage-language-learning teens gain rare vocabulary, we must find various opportunities to teach those words in the context. The first and most relevant way to directly teach heritage-language vocabulary is to use activities in which teens are already engaged. For example, Léandre (15; 5; 12) was playing a war videogame called *Uncharted*. This was a very good opportunity for me to teach him Chinese vocabulary related to war. As much as I felt uncomfortable teaching him vocabulary related to war, I decided to use this opportunity to help him gain the kind of vocabulary that it is necessary to know in order to have a basic understanding of war-related topics in Chinese. I watched him playing and made comments such as 'This solder used a <u>grenade</u>, gun and <u>bayonet</u> to eliminate his enemies' (这个士兵用<u>手榴弹</u>, 抢和<u>刺刀</u>消灭他的敌人).

Frequency of exposure to words has been shown to help adolescents as well as children obtain the knowledge of words.[27] Reading in the heritage language (both reading to teens and teens reading independently) and talking about words that appear in texts is a good way to expose teens to new and rare words. For instance, Philippe identified some words in the book *La Nuit*[28] (The Night) that Léandre was reading and asked him whether or not knew these words. If you can make this kind of activity as a routine, your children will have a better chance to learn more rare words that are not used in everyday communication.

Teaching words in the everyday context

Teaching words in the everyday context is an effective way for teens to increase their heritage-language vocabulary. For example, when Philippe walked Léandre and Dominique to the school bus stop each morning, he would usually give them a French word to rhyme. This is a fun way to learn words. Also, using meals and snack times to teach heritage-language vocabulary is a realistic approach to accommodating teens' busy schedules. I used to cut Chinese words into small pieces and then asked Léandre and Dominique to guess their meanings and then put them together into a sentence. Similarly, when I made cookies for the teens for a snack, I put new words related to cookies in a basket. The children were asked to pick words from the basket, guess their meanings, put these words on the table and make sentences. Both teens enjoyed these kinds of puzzle games (拼字游戏). Even though Dominique (13; 6; 23) commented 'This is a trap to make us learn Chinese,' he still enjoyed the experience.

Moreover, capitalising on naturally occurring events to teach new words is also effective. For instance, Dominique wanted to drink sparkling water (气水). Knowing this, I would create opportunities to expose him to words that were related to 气水. Below is an example:

Mother: What do you want to drink? (你想喝什么？)

Dominique: I want sparkling water. (我想喝 sparkling water.)

Mother: You want to drink 气水. You want the kind of water that has bubbles (你想喝气水。有气泡的水。)

Dominique: Yes. (是的。)

Mother: [Poured the water into a cup.] You see the bubbles are moving up. (你看气泡往上冒。)

In this conversation, I introduced several new words for Dominique: 气水 (sparkling water), 气泡 (bubble), 往上 (going up), 冒 (erupt). Teaching new vocabulary in such a manner is natural and more motivating

Philippe used a different method to teach the boys French vocabulary. He would let the teens listen to French songs (such as songs by George Brassens and Maurice Chevalier) and would ask them whether they understood certain words in the lyrics. If not, he would explain them to the teens. Dominique (15; 5; 1) began to listen to music by George Brassens himself and imitated him. This is an excellent way to learn French vocabulary.

Teaching vocabulary through expanding life experience

One efficient way to help adolescents continue to build their heritage-language vocabulary is to expand their life experience; richer life experience creates opportunities for wider vocabulary acquisition. For instance, visiting different places and engaging in different activities (e.g. community service and sports) can help increase chances for adolescents to hear different words used and to use different words to describe their experiences. A variety of life experiences will help them develop a larger mental lexicon.

Table 4.1 Mean number of new words acquired at the end of each summer

	French new words	Chinese new words
Léandre	338	267
Dominique	350	224

I am always amazed by the fact that each time Léandre and Dominique visited their heritage countries or travelled in the summer, there was a surge in their heritage-language vocabulary. This is because both Philippe and I had opportunities to supply them with French and Chinese words to describe their experiences, which we would not otherwise use in our daily contexts in the United States. Table 4.1 shows the average number of new words the boys gained in Chinese and French at the end of each summer vacation (over about two or three months) between ages 12 and 19.[29]

Teaching secondary word meaning

Words often have primary or common meanings and secondary meanings. For example, the word *bank* has at least two meanings: the place where money is kept (dominant meaning) and the edge of a river (secondary meaning). Research suggests that difficulties in understanding the secondary meanings of **polysemous words** (words that have multiple meanings) may persist well into adolescence.[30] Heritage-language-learning adolescents are likely to have trouble mastering the secondary meaning of words. Thus, teaching secondary word meaning is important in overall heritage-language lexicon development.

Léandre and Dominique acquired many words that are common and concrete in their everyday context. Yet, the secondary meanings of these words are less common and more abstract, and, as such, they appear in readings and are used in more sophisticated writings. Therefore, the teens sometimes lacked opportunities to learn the secondary meanings of these words. To help them learn the secondary meaning of words, Philippe, for example, tried to use jokes from *Le Chat* and other comic books to teach the secondary meanings of French words. It was quite an effective way to get the two boys attend to the secondary meanings of many words while getting a laugh from them.

Teaching literate lexicon

Although every word in a language is important, some words, such as literate lexicon, may be more crucial for more advanced development in reading and writing. **Literate lexicon** means words used in more advanced reading materials, such as abstract nouns (*freedom* and *challenge*), mental state verbs (*assume* and *explain*) and derivatives (*relationship* and *respectful*). Understanding literacy lexicon requires the ability to use contextual abstraction to infer the meaning of new words from the linguistic cues that accompany them. Heritage-language-learning adolescents may lag behind 'native' speakers in their heritage-language literate lexicon. One of the

> **Box 4.3 Important Literate Lexicons to Teach**
>
> **Polysemous words**: Words that have more than one meaning; often the secondary meanings bear little or no relationship to their primary meanings (e.g. *bank* and *bank*).
>
> **Double-function words**: Words that have both a physical meaning (literal) and a psychological (nonliteral) meaning (e.g. *cold* temperature and *cold* person).
>
> **Adverbs of likelihood and magnitude**: Adverbs that express likelihood (e.g. *possibly, probably* and *definitely*) and adverbs that describe magnitude (e.g. *slightly, somewhat, rather* and *extremely*).
>
> **Abstract nouns**: Words that refer to intangible concepts, mental states or emotions (e.g. *challenge, decision* and *enjoyment*).
>
> **Metalinguistic and metacognitive verbs**: Metalinguistic verbs refer to the action of speaking (e.g. *predict* and *interpret*) and metacognitive verbs refer to acts of thinking (*hypothesise* and *conclude*).
>
> **Factive and nonfactive verbs**: **Factive verbs** are verbs that presuppose the truth (e.g. *notice* and *see*) and **nonfactive verbs** are verbs that are uncertain about the truth (e.g. *guess* and *believe*).
>
> Modified from Nippold, M.A. (2007) *Later Language Development: School-Age Children, Adolescents, and Young Adults* (pp. 36–46). Austin, TX: Pro-ed.

reasons for this may be that parents rarely need to use literate lexicon to describe abstract concepts, such as *possibility* or *probability*, in the everyday home context. Therefore, it is necessary to provide explicit support in this area.

One way to support literate lexicon is to select some unfamiliar and difficult words in a heritage-language text that are important for comprehending a topic and help your teens to study these words. Box 4.3 suggests some important literate lexicon categories that you may want to consider when selecting words from texts to help your teens develop literate lexicon abilities in their heritage language(s). You can first ask your teens to guess what the difficult words mean and to explain why they define them as such. You can then guide them by looking for cues in the text.

Another way of teaching literate lexicon is to use words in daily conversations and help teens notice their uses. For instance, I purposely used the following Chinese words in my daily conversations with Léandre and Dominique in their early teen years: 可能 (probably), 也许 (perhaps), 大该 (in general), 差不多 (almost), 轻微 (slightly), 严重 (severely), 注意到 (noticed) and 我相信 (believe). By doing so, I have helped them to notice these words in their readings.

Teaching tier-two and tier-three words

As discussed earlier, tier-two and tier-three words usually need direct instruction. One simple way to determine tier-two and tier-three words in your heritage language is to sample a text to which you want to introduce your teens. This will be easier for you to do online. Calculate how frequently these words are used. Normally, tier-one words appear most frequently, tier-two words appear moderately frequently and tier-three words appear least frequently. Once you have the calculation, you can identify and decide what tier-two and tier-three words to teach. Because teens are often occupied with other activities, you can incorporate teaching these words in your daily conversations. Box 4.4 is an example.

In this example (Box 4.4), tier-two and tier-three words were taught in the daily context by linking them to the current event. Generally, words such as 岩浆 (magma), 岩石 (igneous rock), 地壳 (crust) and 熔融 (molten) were not the kinds of words I would use in my everyday conversations with the boys. However, because this particular conversation was carried out naturally, it did not appear to be 'teaching' but talking. I found that activities like this are very effective in introducing heritage-language tier-two and tier-three words in the home context.

Teaching word definitions

To help teens develop accurate and complete word definitions in their heritage language(s), you can work on enhancing their understanding of word meanings by identifying words that they have problems defining and making a list of them. Once the list is made, you will need to provide ample opportunities for adolescents to work with these words by engaging them in activities such as

---

Box 4.4 Example of Teaching Tier-Two and Tier-Three Words in an Everyday Context

Mother: Today I read in the newspaper about the volcano explosion in Italy. (今天我在报纸上看到在意大利有火山爆发)

Léandre: Really? (真的？)

Mother: When a volcano explodes, there is a lot of magma. (火山爆发时有好多的岩浆喷出来)

Léandre: What is magma? (什么时岩浆？)

Mother: Magma is molten material beneath or within the earth's crust. It then forms igneous rock (岩浆是地壳内或地壳下的熔融材料。岩浆冷却以后就形成了岩石。)

…

looking up the definition in the dictionary, reading texts that expose them to the variety of word meanings, reproducing words and generating word meanings. By doing so, teens will have a better grasp of the word definitions in their heritage language(s).

Teaching word relations

To be competent with heritage-language words, teens need to know more about the words than just their definitions. It is also necessary for them to know how words are related. There are several areas in which you may want to provide support.

First, you can help teens generate multiple meanings for words that often have more than one meaning by discussing them and asking questions. For example, 'Tell me what *run* means when you are talking about a race and what *run* means when you are talking about an election?' You can also help them compare and contrast word meanings to choose the best words to express their ideas.

Second, being limited in their heritage-language vocabulary, many teens may tend to use the same words repeatedly. You can help them substitute words with the same or similar meanings; in other words, help them develop a list of synonyms.

Finally, help your teens develop self-questioning abilities and encourage them to determine whether multiple meanings of a word need to be invoked to understand a word, an occurrence of **figurative language** (e.g. metaphors and jokes).

Teaching emotion and emotion-laden words

Research suggests that **emotion words** (words that directly refer to particular affective states, such as *scared* and *anxious*; or processes, such as *worry*) and **emotion-laden words** (words that do not refer to emotions directly but instead express emotion, such as *loser*; or elicit emotions from the interlocutors, such as *malignancy*) are represented, processed and recalled differently from concrete words (e.g. *cup* and *chair*) and **abstract words** (e.g. *myth* and *emancipation*).[31]

Depending on the heritage-language socialisation context, your teens may be hindered by their limited emotion and emotion-laden words in their heritage language(s), especially when they need to express anger and frustration.[32] Many emotion and emotion-laden words in the heritage language may not trigger teens' personal and affective associations or sensory representations; thus, they may have difficulty using vocabulary to express emotion.

Literature reports that individuals who are learning a new language tend to experience different processes in their emotion lexicon development (see Box 4.5). Heritage-language-learning teens may show the same tendency.

However, the processes described in Box 4.5 need to be looked at with caution, as multilingual expert Aneta Pavlenko[33] reminded us when she noted the following:

- The processes are based on older heritage-language speakers.
- None of the seven processes account for the whole emotion domain in the multilingual lexicon. Rather, they depend on an individual's personal history

Box 4.5 Multilingual Conceptual Processes in Emotional Lexicon

Coexistence: Categorise emotion-eliciting situations in each of their languages similar to monolingual speakers of the respective languages.

Dominant language conceptual transfer: Heritage-language learners rely on the dominant-language concept of emotions and have not internalised the representations of emotions in the heritage language (often teens who have not had an opportunity to be socialised into the heritage-language community. This reliance may result in positive transfer in the case of identical concepts in the dominant language and heritage language, and it may also cause negative transfer in the case of partially overlapping concepts in the dominant language and the heritage language or language–specific concepts).

Internalisation of new concepts: Heritage-language speakers are socialised into the heritage-language community and use the emotional words in the right context. However, heritage-language socialisation may not guarantee internalisation. Internalisation does not always happen. Heritage-language learners may be aware of the core meaning but do not appeal to the words. This may be because they have not yet formed a unified conceptual category that allows them to identify this emotion and to use the words accurately.

Conceptual restructuring: Previous existing dominant language-based concept has been modified but does not fully approximate the heritage language (initiated but not completed).

Conceptual convergence: Heritage-language learners create a concept or a category distinct from monolinguals of respective languages.

Conceptual shift: Heritage-language learners have resided in the heritage-language context, and their representations of partial concepts have shifted in the direction of heritage language-based concepts (as opposed to restructuring, where the shift has been initiated but not completed).

Conceptual attrition: As a result of living in the heritage-language environment, heritage-language learners have ceased to rely on particular conceptual categories to interpret their experiences. While it does not imply that they no longer recognise the categories, it means that the categories have ceased to be central in their interpretation of the world around them. Conceptual attrition may be further accompanied by attrition of emotion vocabulary and difficulties with expressing one's emotions in one's native language.

Modified from Pavlenko, A. (2008) Emotion and emotion-laden words in the bilingual lexicon. *Bilingualism: Language and Cognition* 11, 147–64.

and on the relationship between the concepts in question. Some conceptual representations may display evidence of restructuring and others may be evidence of attrition.
- The process is dynamic and not static. The conceptual configurations may change when heritage-language speakers' experiences and speaking contexts change.
- These processes are context-dependent; different aspects and dimensions are activated in different settings and in different languages.

Because teens have a need to express their emotions, it is an optimal time for you to help them develop emotion and emotion-laden words in your heritage language(s). The best way to do it is to observe your teens and listen to them carefully. You can seize opportunities to supply them with the vocabulary to talk about their emotion and emotion-related matters. Box 4.6 is an example.

As shown in Box 4.6, in the conversation, I taught Dominique the emotion and emotion-laden words 不安 (uneasy), 焦虑 (worried), 惊恐 (panic) and 恶毒 (vicious) so that he could learn to use these words to discuss his emotions.

Teaching words digitally

Teaching and learning new words via multimodality, especially by combining visual and verbal modes, can help retain new words in heritage language. Teens usually enjoy the digital creation of new words. For instance, Wordle (www.wordle.net) is a website for generating **word clouds** (a cluster of words) from text that you provide. The clouds show words that appear more frequently in the text you provide. You can change your clouds with different fonts, layouts and colour schemes. You can print them out or save them to the Wordle gallery. You can also generate your own word clouds quickly and easily. Teens usually enjoy using the web program to have fun with words because it is an engaging way to make word choice posters. For example, it can be used to create a visual list of synonyms for your teens. While it cannot be used for logographic languages such as Chinese, this web program has the capacity to accommodate most of the alphabetic languages. There are other websites such as www.animoto.com and www.glogster.com that

---

Box 4.6 Examples of Teaching Emotion and Emotion-Laden Words in the Daily Context

[Dominique talked about the rumour he read regarding the issue of 'the end of the world' in 2012.]

Mother: I understand that when we hear this kind of thing, we feel <u>uneasy</u>, <u>panicked</u> and <u>worried</u>. But these are rumors. People who spread these kinds of rumors are <u>vicious</u>. (我很理解为什么我们听到这样的消息，我们会感到<u>不安</u>。我们会<u>焦虑</u>, 我们会<u>惊恐</u>, 恐具。可是撒布这些摇言的人也很<u>恶毒</u>).

can also be used to inspire your teens to create visual representations of words with graphs and illustrations.

Creating awareness of cognates

Earlier in the chapter, I discussed the advantage of cognates. Research shows that training cognate awareness and using cognate pairs as target items are useful ways to improve children's skills in all of their languages concurrently.[34] You may want to spend some time making a list of cognates in your teens' heritage language(s) and their dominant language (given they are alphabetic languages). You can keep the list nearby and refer to it when you have conversations with your teens. By making your teens become aware of the cognates, you can help them learn their heritage-language vocabulary more efficiently. In fact, because Philippe did this cognate comparison between English and French frequently, Léandre and Dominique not only benefited from the vocabulary learning in French; it also improved their English.

Moreover, it is also important to draw your teens' attention to false cognates (or false friends). In speaking, false friends are usually not a problem, but in reading and writing, they may be. The words *die* and *bad* in English and German are examples in point. In German, *die* means the article *the,* such as *die Frau* (the woman); and *bad* means *bath*, such as the places *Bad Kreuznach* and *Bad Belligen* in Germany. Consciously pointing out false cognates to your children will help them see the differences between words.

Modelling in context

Modelling vocabulary use and filling in the word gaps in the context are also very important in exposing teens to heritage-language lexicon. Box 4.7 shows an example of how I deliberately modelled Chinese vocabulary use by supplying Chinese words that Léandre did not know.

Notice how in this conversation, I deliberately supplied the word 细节 (detail) and modelled how it could be used in the context several times. This kind of intentional teaching is natural and effective in vocabulary learning.

Box 4.7 Modelling Vocabulary Use by Filling in the Vocabulary Gap

After watching the movie *The Kite Runner,*

Léandre (15; 3; 4): This film omitted *many details*. (这步电影漏掉 *many details*).

Mother: You are right. This film omitted *many details*. Can you tell me again what *details* this film omitted? Does the book have this *detail*? Are these omitted *details* important? (对，这步电影漏掉许多细节。 你再说说这步电影漏掉什么细节。书里有这个细节？这些漏掉的细节重要吗？)

Explaining word meanings in the heritage language

Sometimes it is easier to explain word meanings to teens in their dominant language. Although it is perhaps unavoidable to use mainstream language to explain heritage-language word meanings occasionally, my experience with my children shows that trying to explain word meanings in the heritage language tends to be more effective in teaching new heritage-language vocabulary. Box 4.8 are two examples.

As you can see, in the first example, I did not have to use a single English word to explain the meaning of 消化. I simply paraphrase it in Chinese. This is a useful way not only to teach teens the target word 消化 (digestion), but also to introduce other new vocabulary words. In my example, several other new words, including 儒动 (a literate use of the word *move*) and 过程 (process), were introduced as well. Similarly, in the second example, I could have said that 元旦 is New Year's Day. Instead, I used the opportunity to expand the explanation by talking about 圣诞节 (Christmas) and 圣诞节前夜 (Christmas Eve).

Using targeted reading to increase heritage-language vocabulary

During early childhood and middle childhood, spoken language serves as the primary source of input for learning new words; however, when children reach late

---

Box 4.8 Example of Explaining Word Meaning in Heritage Language

Example 1:
(I invited Dominique (13; 2; 15) to take a stroll with me after dinner.)

Mother: Strolling after meals can help 消化 (digestion). (饭后散步可以帮助消化。)

Dominique: What does 消化 mean? (消化是什么意思？)

Mother: After you take in food, it moves in your intestines. The process is called 消化 (digestion). (你吃过饭以后，食物在你的肠胃里儒动，这个过程就叫消化)

Example 2:
[I just bought a form to make dumplings.]

Mother: I could use this new form to make dumplings on 元旦 (New Year's Day). (我在元旦的时候可以用刚买的模子做饺子。)

Léandre (12; 4; 16): What is 元旦? (什么是 元旦？)

Mother: Today is Christmas Eve and tomorrow is Christmas. Calculate how many days to the New Year. 元旦 is New Year's Day. (今天是圣诞节前夜, 明天是圣诞节。你算算过几天是新年。元旦就是新年。)

middle childhood (around 9 or 10 years of age), written language becomes a significant, additional source of word learning.[35] However, in the heritage-language environment, teens continue to receive vocabulary input from the spoken channel. Therefore, it is important to used targeted readings to help their heritage-language vocabulary development. In fact, advanced heritage-language vocabulary development depends critically on the type of readings that teens are asked to read.

Research indicates that reading a combination of **expository** (explaining and informing) and **narrative** (describing) texts can help adolescents gain more vocabulary than reading only an expository or narrative text. Moreover, those who read a text with text-target word ratios of less than or equal to 2% did not learn significantly more vocabulary than those who read a text with a ratio of 2% to 5%.[36] Thus, when you select texts for your teens, you may want to consider texts that contain the target word that are between 2% and 5%. It is usually easier to copy the text to the computer programs, such as the word document, and let the program identify and count the ratio for you.

Using humour to teach vocabulary

Using humour to teach vocabulary is an attractive way to make teens pay attention to words. Because of their English influence, Léandre and Dominique sometimes transferred English words into French. Instead of correcting them all the time, Philippe used humour to make the teens pay attention to those transferred errors. For example, once we bought a particular kind of chocolate mixed with wasabi. While tasting it, Dominique said 'tester' instead of *goûter* (taste). Philippe joked with Dominique (15; 11; 20) by pronouncing the wrong word 'tester' in a strange way, 'Tu veux t-e-s-t-er le chocolat au wasabi. On t-e-s-t-e le chocolat.' Dominique immediately realised his mistake and corrected himself with the right word, *goûter*.

Teaching culture-specific vocabulary

Because teens like Léandre and Dominique do not live in their heritage countries, they often do not have experiences with many things in the culture, and therefore they may not have some cultural-specific vocabulary. Intentional teaching becomes very important for them to attain these words. For instance, 烧饼 (a special kind of steamed bread) and 油条 (a fried dough stick) are commonly served at Chinese breakfast. Thus, knowing these words is an important part of knowing Chinese culture. However, we did not eat them for breakfast in our family. As a result, Léandre and Dominique did not know the words. I made an effort to ask their Chinese grandparents to buy these foods for Léandre and Dominique when they were in Shanghai and introduced the words to them in the context.

Using media to teach vocabulary

Using heritage-language media (e.g. television programmes) as a source of vocabulary exposure can be effective in terms of expanding heritage-language vocabulary.

For instance, Léandre (17; 11; 29) learnt words such as 溜达 (stroll) by watching the Chinese television programme 快乐驿站 (*Happy Relay*). I never used 溜达 to describe stroll in my interactions with him, but the television programme provided him with a good opportunity to hear and learn a different way of saying 'stroll.'

Teaching vocabulary through observing gestures

Gestures are part of human communication. When words are not available, gestures can reveal what a speaker wants to say. Thus, learning to observe your teens' gestures may help you supply appropriate heritage-language words. Below is an example:

Mother: Léandre, why did you buy a large sized T-shirt? (理昂, 你为什么买大的T恤衫？)

Léandre (17; 8; 5): I couldn't find a small-size T-shirt. It doesn't matter, it will [moving two hands to each other]. (他们没有小的。不要紧, 洗过以后会 [moving two hands to each other].)

Mother: It will shrink. (会缩水。)

My experience suggests that observing gesture use and using it as a base to supply heritage-language words can help teens learn vocabulary in context without interrupting the flow of conversation.

Explicitly teaching word formation rules

There are some general rules for word formation in every language. Teaching teens heritage-language formation rules can help them master the general rules and learn their heritage language well. For example, *-ment* is a general French adverb ending. Understanding this rule can help heritage-French-speaking children learn words effectively. Philippe explicitly showed Léandre and Dominique the rule using words such as *prudement* (cautiously). I also showed Léandre and Dominique some Chinese word formation rules, such as that the radical 扌 is often associated with words that have something to do with hands, including 打 (hit), 抱 (hold), 提 (lift). Explicit explanation of the word formation rules in the situational appropriate context can help teens learn heritage-language vocabulary faster.

Morphological analysis

Although some multilingual children, such as Léandre and Dominique, spontaneously engage in morphological analysis of words (see the examples I used earlier in the chapter), not all teens will do that automatically. Thus, it is essential to engage teens in deliberate morphological analysis to learn new words. Morphological analysis of words includes the process that takes place when encountering new words or unfamiliar words (such as *seabound, talkativeness* and *serviced*). Teens are encouraged to analyse the components of these words such as the root words (*sea, bound, talk* and *service*), inflectional morphemes (*-ed*) and derivational morphemes (*-ive, -ness*). With this analysis, they can then use the information to infer the meaning of the entire word. Research suggests that this strategy (morphological analysis) is a major contributor to vocabulary development.[37]

Therefore, in your everyday interactions with your teens, you can deliberately introduce new words to them in your heritage language and encourage them to analyse the components of words. In alphabetical languages, you can help them look at the root words and to add prefixes and suffixes to change the meaning. In logographic languages such as Chinese, you can help teens analyse the radicals of words and their relations to other words, such as the example I just demonstrated in the previous section: The radical 扌 is often associated with words that have something to do with hands: 打 (hit), 抱 (hold) and 提 (lift).

Be aware of the masking phenomenon

One important area that you may want to pay attention to is the **masking phenomenon** in heritage-language vocabulary development; that is, it appears sometimes that teens know some words in heritage languages, yet they actually either do not know or only have partial knowledge about the vocabulary. The best way to avoid the masking phenomenon is to ask and confirm that adolescents fully understand the words. For instance, Philippe made sure that Dominique (15; 1; 2) understood the word *bourre* when his Swiss friend David said, 'Je suis à la bourre (I am in a hurry).'

Useful measures to monitor adolescent lexical development

If you can use standardised tests to measure your teens' heritage-language lexicon development, you can always try; however, chances are that your teens may not cooperate. In addition, standardised lexicon test results may not be accurate, especially in the heritage-learning environment. It has been shown that the nature of the task may influence the language produced by children and adolescents. Therefore, the topic, the task and the listener should be considered as critical criteria in assessing adolescents' word production.[38] Thus, an authentic and natural way of measuring teens' vocabulary development is to measure what they can produce in a real communication situation by asking them to narrate an event. You can video- or audio-record the narrative and the measure the lexical diversity (use of more different types of words); density (use of more different lexical items the proportions of lexical items such as nouns, verbs, adjectives and adverbs[39]); and complexity (use of more polysyllabic words). Alternatively, you can record some language samples in different contexts (e.g. everyday dinner conversation, peer conversation or explaining things) and then measure the lexical diversity, density and complexity. You can compare the three areas over time (e.g. in January and in June) and see whether your teens have made any progress and determine what areas that they need more support.

Taken together, it is important to note before I end the chapter that word learning continues well beyond adolescence. Studies show that words may be learnt throughout a person's lifetime through active reading.[40]

Summary of Key Points in Chapter 4

- During adolescence, teens demonstrate progress in vocabulary quantity, quality and use. Moreover, they also show improvement in lexical and semantic ambiguity, such as homophones (words that sound alike and may be spelt alike), homographs (words that are spelt the same and may sound alike), and homonyms (words that are spelt and pronounced in the same way but are different in meaning).
- The heritage-language vocabulary input may be affected by parents' own heritage-language attrition as demonstrated in their limitations in terms of active vocabulary use, the lack of up-to-date words and the generational gap in lexicon use.
- As a result, teens' heritage language vocabulary may show the following characteristics:
    - Discrepancy in crosslinguistic synonyms.
    - False cognates.
    - Lexical and semantic inaccuracy.
    - Lack of tier-three words.
    - Loan blending.
    - Lexicon innovation.
    - Literal understanding of word meaning.
    - Meaning overextension.
    - Use of family lexicon.
    - Lexicon fixture.
    - Lexicon interference.
    - Vocabulary limitation .
    - Language-specific errors.
    - Vocabulary stabilisation.
    - Cognate transfer.
    - Intuition about word components.
- To help teens develop heritage-language vocabulary development and build mental lexicon, parents many want to try the following strategies:
    - Use contextual abstraction.
    - Practice direct teaching such as teaching words in the context, expanding life experience, and teaching rare words, secondary word meaning, literate lexicon,

    tier-two and -three words, word definition, word relations, emotion and emotion-laden words and digital words.
    - Moreover, direct teaching can be realised through making adolescents conscious of cognates and false friends, modelling word use, explaining word meaning, using targeted heritage-language reading to help increase heritage-language vocabulary, using media and humour to teach vocabulary and teaching vocabulary through observing gesture use.
    - Encourage morphological analysis.
    - Avoid masking phenomenon in vocabulary comprehension.
- To help you monitor your teens' heritage-language vocabulary development, parents may want to try to use natural narrative as a base to monitor the lexical diversity, lexical density and lexical complexity development.

Recommended Readings

Biemiller, A. (2006) Vocabulary development and instruction: A prerequisite for school learning. In D.K. Dickinson and S.B. Neuman (eds) *Handbook for Early Literacy Research* (pp. 41–51). New York: Guilford Press.

Notes and References

[1] Gass, M. and Selinker, L. (2001) *Second Language Acquisition. An Introductory Course.* Mahwah, NJ: Lawrence Erlbaum.
[2] Nippold, M.A. (2007) *Later Language Development: School-Age Children, Adolescents, and Young Adults.* Austin, TX: Pro-ed.
[3] Pence, K.L. and Justice, L.M. (2008) *Language Development from Theory to Practice.* Upper Saddle River, NJ: Pearson.
[4] Berwing, B. and Baker, W.J. (1986) Assessing morphological development. In P. Fletcher and M. Garman (eds) *Language Acquisition* (pp. 326–38). Cambridge: Cambridge University Press.
[5] Nippold, M.A. (2007) *Later Language Development: School-Age Children, Adolescents, and Young Adults* (p. 28). Austin, TX: Pro-ed.
[6] Miller, G.A. and Gildea, P.M. (1987) *How Children Learn Words.* Scientific America 257, 94–9.
[7] De Houwer, A. (2009) *An Introduction to Bilingual Development.* Bristol: Multilingual Matters.
[8] Oller, D.K. (2005) The distributed characteristic in bilingual learning. In J. Cohen, K.T. McAlister, K. Rolstad and J. MacSwan (eds) *Proceedings of the 4th International Symposium on Bilingualism* (pp. 1744–9). Somerville, MA: Cascadilla Press.
[9] Janik, V. and Kolokonte, M. (2015) False cognates: The effect of mismatch in morphological complexity on a backward lexical translation task. *Second Language Research* 31 (2), 137–56.
[10] Beck, I.L., McKeown, M.G. and Kucan, L. (2002) *Bring Words to Life: Robust Vocabulary Instruction.* New York: Guilford Press.
[11] Jørgensen, J.N. (2005) Plurilingual conversations among bilingual adolescents. *Journal of Pragmatics* 37 (3), 391–402.
[12] Wang, X.-L. (2008) *Growing Up With Three Languages: Birth to Eleven.* Bristol: Multilingual Matters.
[13] *New York Times* magazine (12 May 2012).
[14] Long, M.H. (2003) Stabilization and fossilization in interlanguage development. In C. J. Doughty and M.H. Long (eds) *The Handbook of Second Language Acquisition* (pp. 487–535). Oxford: Blackwell.

[15] This was calculated based on six videotapes of their naturalistic conversation in summer vacations in three years from ages 14 to 16 (2 hours each year).

[16] Kelley, A. and Kohnert, K. (2012) Is there a cognate advantage for typically developing Spanish-speaking English-language learners? *Language, Speech, and Hearing Services in Schools* 43, 191–204.

[17] Nagy, W.E. and Scott, J.A. (2000) Vocabulary processes. In M.L. Kamil, P.B. Mosenthal and R. Barr (eds) *Handbook of Reading Research* (Vol. 2, pp. 269–84). Mahwah. NJ: Erlbaum.

[18] The sentence is modified from an article in the *New York Times Science Times*, 27 May 2014, by John Tierney.

[19] The example and ideas are inspired by Bromley, K. (2014) Active engagement with words. In K.A. Hinchman and H.K. Sheridan-Thomas (eds) *Best Practices in Adolescent Literacy Instruction* (pp. 120–36). New York: The Guilford Press.

[20] Cummins, J. (2000) *Language, Power and Pedagogy: Bilingual Children in the Crossfire*. Clevedon: Multilingual Matters.

[21] Lugo-Neris, M.J., Jackson, W.C. and Goldstein, H. (2010) Facilitating vocabulary acquisition of young English language learners. *Language, Speech, and Hearing Services in Schools* 41, 314–27.

[22] Nippold, M.A. (2007) *Later Language Development: School-Age Children, Adolescents, and Young Adults* (pp. 29–35). Austin, TX: Pro-ed.

[23] Spiegel, C. and Halberda, J. (2010) Rapid fast-mapping abilities in 2-year-olds. *Journal of Experimental Child Psychology* 132–40.

[24] Nagy, W.E. and Herman, P.A. (1987) Learning word meanings from context during normal reading. *American Educational Research Journal* 24 (2), 237–70.

[25] Pressley, M., Levin, J.R. and McDaniel, M.A. (1987) Remembering versus inferring what a word means: Mnemonic and contextual approaches. In M.G. McKeown and M.E. Curtis (eds) *The Nature of Vocabulary Acquisition* (pp. 107–28). Cambridge, MA: MIT Press.

[26] Biemiller, A. (2006) Vocabulary development and instruction: A prerequisite for school learning. In D.K. Dickinson and S.B. Neuman (eds) *Handbook for Early Literacy Research* (pp. 41–51) New York: Guilford Press.

[27] Nippold, M.A. (2007) *Later Language Development: School-Age Children, Adolescents, and Young Adults*. Austin, TX: Pro-ed.

[28] Wiesel, E. (2013) *La Nuit*. New York, NY: Hill and Wang.

[29] Data were calculated based on 14 hours of video-recorded tapes in 7 years (from ages 12 to 19; 2 hours each year from the natural conversation at birthday meals).

[30] Durkin, K., Crowther, R. and Shire, B. (1986) Children's processing of polysemous vocabulary in school. In K. Durkin (ed.) *Language Development in the School Years* (pp. 77–94). Cambridge, MA: Brookline.

[31] Altarriba, J. and Basnight-Brown, D.M. (2011) The acquisition of concrete, abstract, and emotion words in a second language. *International Journal of Bilingualism* 16 (4), 446–52.

[32] Pavlenko, A. (2008) Emotion and emotion-laden words in the bilingual lexicon. *Bilingualism: Language and Cognition* 11, 147–64.

[33] Pavlenko, A. (2008) Emotion and emotion-laden words in the bilingual lexicon. *Bilingualism: Language and Cognition* 11, 147–64.

[34] Kelley, A. and Kohnert, K. (2012) Is there a cognate advantage for typically developing Spanish-speaking English-language learners? *Language, Speech, and Hearing Services in Schools* 43, 191–204.

[35] Nippold, M.A. (2007) *Later Language Development: School-Age Children, Adolescents, and Young Adults* (p. 26). Austin, TX: Pro-ed.

[36] Huang, S., Willson, V. and Eslami, Z. (2012) The effects of task involvement load on L2 incidental vocabulary learning: A meta-analytic study. *Modern Language Journal* 96 (4), 544–57.

[37] Nippold, M.A. (2007) *Later Language Development: School-Age Children, Adolescents, and Young Adults* (pp. 32–3). Austin, TX: Pro-ed.

[38] Cazden, C.B. (1970) The neglected situation in child language research and education. In F. Williams (ed.) *Language and Poverty* (pp. 81–101). Chicago: Markham.
[39] Johansson, V. (2008) Lexical diversity and lexical density in speech and writing: A developmental perspective. *Working Papers* (Lund University) 53: 61–79.
[40] Nippold, M.A. (2007) *Later Language Development: School-Age Children, Adolescents, and Young Adults*. Austin, TX: Pro-ed.

5 Multilingual Word- and Sentence-Structure Development During Adolescence

On the way back from school, Léandre (12; 1; 25) told Philippe, 'Il alairait malade' (he looked sick), talking about about his friend Galo. In this botched French sentence, Léandre made an interesting mistake. He constructed an imperfect French grammatical form based on what he took to be a simple verb instead of an expression. In other words, instead of conjugating *avoir l'air* and saying, 'Il *avait* l'air,' he attached the imperfect ending *–ait* to *a l'air* or *alair-*, in his mind, the root of an invented verb *alairer*. Although Léandre made a mistake here, the form he invented is ingenious.

This chapter is about adolescents' development of the structure of words and sentences. It begins with an overview of the general morphological (word structure) and syntactic (word order or sentence) accomplishments during adolescence. It then focuses on Léandre and Dominique's heritage-language morphological and syntactic (often termed **morphosyntactic** in research literature) development characteristics. It concludes with some practical strategies and useful morphosyntactic measures to help you with your teens' heritage-language morphosyntactic advancement.

Overview of Morphosyntactic Achievements During Adolescence

In the last chapter, the importance of adolescent vocabulary development was discussed. To be a competent language user, it is also crucial to develop knowledge about how words are constructed and related to each other in a sentence. For instance, knowing the word *house* is important, and it is also important to know how the word can be combined with other words to create new meaning (such as *housekeeper*) and how the word *house* is related to other words in a sentence (such as *'The house that is under construction is paid for using the money saved for community development'*). During adolescence, language users make several remarkable advancements in the areas of morphology and syntax.

Improvement in morphology

There are three general types of word (morphological) constructions in world languages: inflection, derivation and compounding.[1] **Inflectional morphemes** observed in alphabetic languages, such as English, are word endings that indicate case, verb tense, gender or syntax. For instance, adding –*ing* to the root word *work* indicates present progressive (e.g. She is *working*); adding -*s* to the root word *book* indicates plural form (He bought two *books*); adding –*s* to the root word *work* indicates third person singular (Susan *works* in a bank); and adding apostrophe '*s* to the root *student* indicates possessiveness (The custodian installed a towel rack in the *student's* room). As shown, inflectional morphemes show syntactic or semantic relations between different words without altering the meaning of the root word.

Derivational morphology observed in alphabetic languages is a more complex system. A single root word or root form can be used to generate a large number of derived forms through the addition of a prefix or a suffix. For example, the root word *construct* in English can generate words like *construction, destruction, structure, reconstruct* and *indestructible*.[2] Deviational morphology differs from inflectional morphology in a number of ways. First, deviational morphology often changes the functions of the root words. For instance, when the suffix –*ness* is added to the word *eager* (adjective), the word becomes a noun (eagerness). Second, deviational morphology also changes the meaning of the root words. For example, when the prefix *mis*- is added to the root word *inform*, the meaning changes (*misinform*). Third, deviational morphology may also change the pronunciation (phonetic structure) of the root words; for example, *reception* is pronounced significantly differently from its root word *receive*.[3]

Compounding morphemes are combinations of two or more root words that generate new meanings (e.g. *classroom*). Compounding morphemes are observed in both alphabetic and logographic languages, such as 教室 (class-room) in Chinese.

Improvement in deviational morphology in alphabetic language

In alphabetic languages, inflectional morphemes are mastered earlier (e.g. usually by the age of six or seven in English) and deviational morphemes usually take longer to develop. Sometimes the process can continue well into adolescence and young adulthood.[4]

Box 5.1 shows that there is a progression in the development of deviational morphology in English. Studies indicate that older children and adolescents perform better than younger students in their deviational morphology.[5] However, older children, including adolescents, do not always perform with complete accuracy, especially in production.[6] Nevertheless, they do improve over time.[7]

It has been suggested that the largest increase in deviational morphological skills occurs between ages 9 and 14.[8] The gradual improvement in the deviational

> **Box 5.1 Developmental Trend in Deviational Morphology in English**
>
> **Stage 1**: Develop an awareness of the root form and its meaning within the derived form
> **Stage 2**: Increase awareness of the meaning and syntactic purpose contributed by the suffix
> **Stage 3**: Become aware of the various constraints on attaching particular suffixes to particular root words or forms
>
> Modified from Nippold, M.A. (2007) *Later Language Development: School-Age Children, Adolescents, and Young Adults* (p. 66). Austin, TX: Pro-ed.

morphology development of older children and adolescents is largely a result of the development in three areas: spoken language abilities, metalinguistic skills (e.g. awareness of the rules of the word structure) and exposure to the morphologically complex words in written language via reading and writing (especially through spelling).[9] As their social circle enlarges and school subject-related conversation (such as teacher language use in lectures) deepens, teens are exposed to more complex word usage. This definitely helps their deviational morphology development. Moreover, reading materials such as textbooks for older children and adolescents include more complex words. For example, in eighth grade English social-studies textbooks, students are exposed to words such as *interchangeable parts, monotheism, polytheism, reincarnation, sharecropping* and *subcontinent*.[10] Derivational phonology is also associated with increased accuracy in spelling as children and adolescents move up through grades, even though accuracy in spelling derived forms tends to lag behind the knowledge of the derived forms.[11] Furthermore, when encountering new words, older children and adolescents tend to employ the morphological decomposition strategy (i.e. to analyse components of words, such as talk-ative-ness) to decipher their meanings.

Morphological differences between alphabetic and orthographic languages

Important differences exist between alphabetic and orthographic languages in terms of word construction. In English (an alphabetic language), inflections and derivations are the main word formation methods. However, in Chinese (an orthographic language), more than 75% of words are formed through compounding.[12] The salience of morphological features appears to influence the development of specific morphological skills. In a comparative study of English and Chinese children, researchers observed that Taiwanese children had more advanced compound awareness than American children, whereas American children had more advanced derivational awareness than their Taiwanese counterparts,[13] which demonstrates the effects of language features on adolescents' morphological development.

Although compounding is more prominent in Chinese, Chinese and English are rather similar in terms of rules for the formation and meaning of compound morphology. For example, in English, the word *classroom* refers to a room where a class takes place. In Chinese, 教室 (*teach-room*) is formed comparably. In general, Chinese compounds tend to be relatively **transparent**; that is, the meaning of the compound is predictable from the meaning of the constituent morphemes. For example, the Chinese word for birthday, 生日, is a combination of the symbols that represent the words *birth* and *day*. English has many transparent compounds, but it also has **opaque compounds**, in which the meaning of the compound is not closely related to one or both constituent morphemes, such as in the word *jailbird*.[14] As a general trend, transparent compound words tend to be mastered faster than opaque compound words.

Increase in complex sentence use

By age five, most children are able to use complex sentences in conversations. Each of their **utterances** (the smallest meaning unit such as 'I am hungry') has at least 6.0 morphemes (the mean length of an utterance) on average.[15] Despite the impressive accomplishments of a typical five-year-old child, research suggests that syntax continues to develop beyond adolescence into early adulthood (20–29 years) and remains stable into middle age (40-49 years).[16]

One of the major linguistic achievements during adolescence is teens' ability to understand and use more complex sentence structure. Across the board, adolescents' sentence complexity increases considerably over the years. This is evidenced by the fact that the sentences that adolescents produce become increasingly longer with more words, embedded phrases and clauses as they get older. Most notably, by the end of high school (grade 12), adolescents' average number of words per sentence in writing is about 13.27, which surpasses the average number of words per sentence in speaking (11.70) for the first time in their lives. Further, even though adolescents use simple sentences when they talk to their friends and use telegraphic phrases when composing text messages, they produce cohesively linked complex sentences when writing persuasive essays on controversial topics or explaining the rules of a game to adults[17], because this type of writing requires longer sentences that contain greater amounts of subordination and stronger linkages between sentences.[18]

Increase in sentence length and clause density

Two important markers of later syntactic advancement are shown in sentence length and clausal density. In early childhood, the sentence length is conventionally measured by using **mean length of utterance** (MLU). MLU is the average number of words used in utterances. Beyond the preschool years, MLU is considered by many researchers to be less accurate in measuring syntactic complexity. Thus, a different unit called the *terminable unit* or *T-unit* is often used to measure the syntactic development.

A T-unit consists of one main clause plus any subordinate clause that is attached to or embedded in it (e.g. *'I visited the Metropolitan Museum while I was visiting my aunt in New York,'* and *'The book that is on the shelf is the gift given by his grandfather.'*). The T-unit has been shown to be a more sensitive index of syntactic growth for older children and adolescents than MLU. Additionally, the T-unit is often used to measure syntactic complexity in writing. The *communication unit* (C-unit) is often used instead of the T-unit to measure growth in syntax in speaking. The T-unit and C-unit are identical, with the exception that a C-unit includes incomplete sentences when answering questions (e.g. when answering the question *'How long have you lived in New York?'* the answer *'for 16 years'* is a C-unit.).[19] More information about T-units and C-units will be presented at the end of this chapter. A steady increase in adolescents' syntactic complexity can be observed in their increased use of C-units. At grade 6 (about 11 years old), adolescents' C-unit is about 9.04, by grade 9 (about 14 years old) it is about 10.05, and by grade 12 (about 17 years old) it is 13.27.[20]

Clausal density[21] (also called the subordination index) is the average number of clauses (main and subordinate clauses) per T-unit. A subordinate clause (also called a dependent clause) begins with a **subordinate conjunction** (e.g. *after, before* and *while*) or a **relative pronoun** (e.g. *that, which* and *who*). A subordinate clause cannot stand alone as a sentence because it does not provide a complete thought, such as *after his boss left*. It needs a main clause to complete an idea, such as in the sentence *'After his boss left, John was able to make a quick phone call.'* Clause density also increases gradually during the adolescent years. It has been reported that clause density for adolescents in grade 8 (about 13 years of age) is 1.39, and for adolescents in grade 11 (about 16 years of age) is 1.52.[22]

Increase in complex sentences in the expository genre

Sentence complexity is often determined by the genre of a text. It has been observed that the number of words used in the **expository writing genre** (texts that explain and convey information) is more than in the **narrative discourse genre** (descriptive texts).[23] Crosslinguistic studies[24] that involved a comparison of narrative and expository discourses in seven different languages (Dutch, English, French, Hebrew, Icelandic, Spanish and Swedish) found that all types of subordinate clauses (such as relative, adverbial and nominal) occurred more often in expository discourse than in narrative discourse across languages. These studies also show that the use of subordinate clauses suggested an age-related increase in both genres. The production of **relative clauses** (a clause starts with relative pronouns such as *that, which* and *who*) was particularly sensitive to the effects of age and genre; adults used this type of clause far more often than did children, and both groups used them more frequently in expository discourse.[25]

One word of caution: despite a general trend towards greater syntactic complexity across the board during adolescence, there are wide individual differences. Some teens may use more elaborate syntax and others may speak quite simply.

> **Box 5.2 Examples of Advanced Syntactic Structure**
>
> | Noun phrase expansion | Examples |
> |---|---|
> | Appositives[26] | Margret, the corporate attorney, bought a town house. |
> | Elaborated subjects | Dogs such as collies, Cocker Spaniels, and Golden Retrievers were at the show. |
> | Postmodification via prepositional phrase | They knew the Italian cyclist in the lead pack would win the race. |
> | Postmodification via nonfinite verbs | The next runner to compete would anchor the relay. |
> | **Verb phrase expansion** | |
> | Modal auxiliary verb | We should have gone skating. |
> | The perfect aspect | She had been working all day. |
> | The passive voice | The house was carefully designed by a famous architect. |
>
> Modified from Nippold, M.A. (2007) *Later Language Development: School-Age Children, Adolescents, and Young Adults* (p. 265). Austin: Pro-ed.

Increase in the use of sophisticated syntactic structure

Another area of adolescents' syntactic progress is the emergence of sophisticated syntactic structures. These structures are not frequently used in everyday conversation or written communication but are more essential in more advanced levels of writing. Box 5.2 shows some examples of these more advanced syntactic structures.

Improvement in conjunction sentence structure

Adolescents also improve gradually in their use of **subordinate** (e.g. *after* and *before*), **coordinate** (*or* and *so*) and **correlative** (*either...or...*) conjunction sentence structures. Box 5.3 lists examples of the conjunctive links that are used to connect sentences. These conjunctions, in particular the correlative conjunction, are not often used in speech but instead are often used in the writing modality to indicate the sophistication of an individual's language ability. In addition, understanding these conjunctions is essential for academic reading and writing. A reader needs to be clear about the meaning of conjunctions in text comprehension or problem solving in a particular subject area. The conjunctions *although* and *but* are the most challenging to acquire, and it has been found that only 68% of teens can correctly comprehend them by 11 and 12 years of age (roughly by grade six).[27] With consistent exposure to subject-related readings, adolescents' understanding of these conjunctions improves as they progress through the grades. By the time they are in college, almost all adolescents can use conjunctions correctly. Adolescents also

> **Box 5.3 Examples of Subordinating, Coordinating, and Correlative Conjunctive Links**
>
> **Subordinating conjunctive links**
>
> After
> Although
> As
> As if
> Because
> Before
> Even if
> For
> If
> Since
> Unless
> Until
> Whatever
> When
> Whenever
> Whereas
> While
>
> **Coordinating conjunctive links**
>
> And
> But
> Nor
> Or
> So
> Yet
>
> **Correlative conjunctive links**
>
> Both...and
> Either...or
> Neither...nor
> Not only...but also
>
> Modified from Nippold, M.A. (2007), *Later Language Development: School-Age Children, Adolescents, and Young Adults* (p. 266). Austin: Pro-ed.

improve in their use of conjunctions such as *even though* and *because* when they move up through the grades.

Improvement in adverbial conjuncts and adverbial disjuncts

Moreover, adolescents also make progress in **adverbial conjuncts** like *moreover, however, accordingly, hence, similarly, consequently, therefore* and *furthermore*; and **adverbial disjuncts** like *in my opinion, to be honest, frankly* and *perhaps*. These linguistic devices make written discourse more cohesive. They frequently appear in more advanced contexts such as textbooks, essays, lectures and debates. The ability to both use and produce these linguistic devices is particularly important for adolescents' academic success. Adolescents do not usually use these adverbial conjuncts in their spontaneous conversations. Even if they do, they tend to use the more common ones such as *then, so* and *though*. Although adolescents tend to perform better than elementary children when asked to choose correct adverbial conjuncts in experimental studies, they still do not fully use these conjuncts correctly.[28]

However, adolescents are found to use more adverbial conjuncts when they are engaged in persuasive writing in which they need to make their points clear through analysing, discussing and convincing. At age seven, the mean use of adverbial conjuncts in English, for example, is 0.77, which is a significant increase from 0.33 at age 11.[29]

Increase in passive sentence use

In some non-Indo-European languages such as Inukititut and Zulu, passive forms tend to be acquired and developed early.[30] However, passive forms in languages such as English take a relatively long time to develop. For instance, passive sentences, especially the **instrumental nonreversible passives** in English (e.g. *The opinion that was held by the majority is also shared by the minister*) begin to appear frequently between the ages of 11 to 13. In general, adolescents continue to make gradual progress in passive forms in all languages, especially in their writing.

Characteristics of Heritage-Language Morphosyntactic Development During Adolescence

As demonstrated in previous chapters, multilingual children and adolescents tend to transfer their phonological and lexical knowledge and skills to their various languages (often from the more proficient one to the less proficient one). However, syntax seems to be an area that tends to be language-independent; that is, transfers of sentence structures do not occur as frequently as in phonology and lexicon.[31]

Research suggests that the morphosyntactic development order of multilingual children and adolescents is similar to that of their monolingual counterparts. In other words, the morphosyntactic development order trend develops based on universal morphosyntactic principles (see Box 5.4).

> **Box 5.4 Morpheme Acquisition Order in English**
> - Pronoun case (he/him)
> - Articles
> - Copula (be)
> - Progressive (-ing)
> - Plural (-s)
> - Auxiliary (be+V+-ing)
> - Regular past
> - Irregular past
> - Plural (-es)
> - Possessive ('s)
> - Third person singular (-s)
>
> Modified from Brown, S. and Attardo, S. (2008) *Understanding Language Structure, Interaction, and Variation* (p. 220). Ann Arbor: University of Michigan Press.

Nevertheless, because of the uniqueness of the heritage-language development environment, heritage-language-speaking adolescents inevitably also develop their unique morphosyntactic characteristics in their respective languages. In some languages, the use of morphology to pack complex meanings into a single word is much more elaborate than in English. For instance, in West Greenlandic, *tusaanngitsuusaartuaannarsiinnaanngivipputit* is a single word meaning '*You simply cannot pretend not to be hearing all the time.*' While English compounds of a verb and its object (like *scarecrow*) are rather rare, this constitutes a basic and quite general pattern in French and other Romance languages. English and German tend to have the head, when there is one, on the right, such as in the word *doll__house__*; while Italian and other romance languages more often have the head on the left, such as in the word *__caffe__latte* (coffee with milk). Most English compounds consist of two elements, though one of these may itself be a compound, as in *grade schoolteacher*. Other languages have compounds that consist of more components, which lead to complex morphological structures, such as *lebensversicherungsgesellschaftsangestellter* (life-insurance-company-staff) in German and 亭台楼阁 (pavilions-terraces-upper-stories-raised-alcoves)[32] in Chinese.

Language-specific morphosyntactic characteristics

Depending on adolescents' heritage-language background, morphology in different languages may pose different challenges. Using English tenses as an example, when expressing time in English, one uses inflectional morphology. Adding suffixes, such as *–ed,* to a verb indicates something happened in the past (such as *mov__ed__*) and adding *–ing* to the verb indicates something is happening in the present (such as *mov__ing__*).

In Chinese, however, there is no system of grammatical morphology for tense. Instead, temporal adverbs such as 昨天 (yesterday), 今天 (today) and 明天 (tomorrow) are used to indicate the time in the past, present and future.[33] It is possible that a Chinese-dominated, English heritage-language speaker would have difficulty learning the English morphological rules related to temporal reference. An American couple living in Beijing, the People's Republic of China, told me that their daughter, who was born and grew up in Beijing, sometimes had problems using English tenses.[34] Below I will address some language-specific morphosyntactic phenomena observed in the development of Léandre and Dominique.

French articles and possessive pronouns

Léandre and Dominique's French **articles** (words that are used with nouns to indicate the types of references being made by the nouns) and **possessive pronouns** (nouns that demonstrate ownership) have generally developed on a par with native French speakers during adolescence. However, in everyday conversation, there are a few gender-related articles that Léandre tended to use incorrectly. For example, Léandre (15; 1; 24) used *la gym* instead of the correct form *le gymnase*.

Also, Léandre and Dominique occasionally made mistakes with French possessive pronouns. For example, during a FaceTime conversation with Philippe from his college dorm, Léandre (18; 7; 22) said *la réputation* instead of using the correct possessive pronoun *sa réputation*.

Despite making mistakes in spontaneous conversations, both Léandre and Dominique did have knowledge about the usage of these articles and possessive pronouns. In other words, when asked, they did know the correct usage, and as time went on, the boys often self-corrected their errors.

Chinese articles

Chinese articles (冠词) are different from the French or English articles in that Chinese articles do not follow a logical pattern. For example, in English, the pattern is *a book*, *the book* or *the books*, whereas in Chinese, the pattern is 一本书 (one book), 这本书 (this book) and 这些书 (these books). Despite this difference, Dominique and Léandre rarely made mistakes using Chinese articles, although they tended to make lots of measurement word mistakes, which will be addressed next.

Chinese measurement words

Chinese measurement words or **classifiers** (量词) are used to count nouns. Because of the variety of classifiers, this is a difficult concept to master, even for native Chinese speakers. Box 5.5 shows some examples. Often a person's education level can be determined by looking at his or her use of the measurement words. Young children and less educated people often use the general measurement word 个 for most things and objects, and well-educated people tend to use more variety of measurement words.

> **Box 5.5 Examples of Chinese Measurement Words**
>
> 台 (e.g. computer, television and radio)
> 群 (e.g. group of people, flocks of sheep and herd)
> 坐 (e.g. mountain, building and bridge)
> 辆 (e.g. car, truck and bicycle)
> 户 (e.g. used with home and household)
> 匹 (e.g. horse and bolt of cloth)
> 把 (e.g. used with toothbrush, chair, knife and umbrella)

As Box 5.5 shows, a single measurement word can be used to count different nouns, and it is not an easy task for heritage-language Chinese learners to attain them. Indeed, it has been a great challenge for both Léandre and Dominique to master Chinese measurement words during adolescence. They tended to use 一个 as a generic measurement word in most situations.

French tenses

During early and mid-adolescence, Léandre and Dominique continued to use some incorrect tenses in French. Box 5.6 shows an example.

Moreover, some French tense forms such as *passé simple* (simple past, one type of past tense) are not usually used in spoken communication (e.g. *'je naquis'*/I was born). In spoken communication, the idea 'I was born' is expressed in *passé composé* (another type of past tense) as *'Je suis né.'* Léandre and Dominique did not know the passé simple tense until they began to learn how to write French in their high school French AP class.

Most interestingly, the boys also produced some grammatical tense forms that do not exist in French. For example, Dominique (15; 7; 9) said, *'Avant que j'oublisse'* (before I forget) instead of *'Avant que j'oublie.'* Although this tense Dominique created is incorrect, it is interesting that it resembles an **imperfect subjunctive** (the French imperfect subjunctive is a literary verb form used in formal writing. One typically does not use the verb form colloquially).

> **Box 5.6 Example of French Tense Mistakes**
>
> [Dominique (16; 6; 22) commented about our neighbour Johannes's cousin's resemblance to Johannes after we were invited to have dinner at Johannes's house].
>
> **Dominique**: Il lui ressemblait (He used to look alike). [Dominique used an imperfect tense here. He meant, 'He looks like Johannes.']
>
> **Philippe**: Il lui ressemblait? (repeated his mistake.)
>
> **Dominique**: Il lui ressemble...

Chinese passive voice use

Léandre and Dominique did not use much passive voice in Chinese until late adolescence. Proportionally speaking, they used less than 2% of passive voice in their daily communications.[35] They tended to use active voice to replace the idea of passive voice. Starting from age 17, the boys began to use the basic passive voice forms, such as '被骂了, 挨骂了, 给骂了 (be scolded).' This phenomenon was perhaps related to my input. In my daily communication with them, I rarely used passive forms. Only when I realised their lack of passive voice use did I begin to add more passive voice forms in my own speech.

The two boys did not have an issue with the passive voice form use in French.

English morphosyntactic influence on French

Because Léandre and Dominique live in an English dominant environment, their French and Chinese morphosyntax sometimes reflected English influence. For example, Dominique (16; 9; 11) told Philippe, *'Je me sens accompli.'* (I feel accomplished) after he completed all his homework. Even though this sentence in itself is not wrong, in the context, what he really intended to say is *'Je suis satisfait de ma journée'* (I am satisfied with what I did). It is clear that Dominique is applying English morphosyntax to French. This instance is comparable to 'The weather is agreeable' by a French speaker, which is a direct translation from the French phrase *'Le temps est agréable.'* The sentence is not wrong, but one can tell the direct influence from French. A more authentic English phrasing would be *'The weather is nice.'* Another example is that Léandre (14; 10; 15) directly translated the English phrase 'make a face' into French phrase *'faire une visage'* instead of *'faire une grimace.'* However, with Philippe's intentional help and more exposure to French during vacations, both teens produced fewer English-influenced phrases and sentences in French by the end of their adolescence.

It is interesting to note that the mistakes Léandre and Dominique made are quite typical for multilingual children as well as adolescents. According to the **multilingual bootstrapping hypothesis**, each of a multilingual's languages develops at a different pace. Consequently, the more advanced language system will boost the development of the less advanced one. Thus, although the grammars of the multilinguals' different languages develop independently, they occasionally produce sentences consisting of grammatical constructions imported into the use of the language that lags behind in development as a 'temporary pooling of resources.'[36] So, in other words, what this means is that while Léandre and Dominique were developing their French morphology and syntax, they temporarily used their stronger language, English, to fill in the gap of their less developed language, French.

Avoidance strategy

As a compensatory measure, Léandre and Dominique sometimes also used avoidance as a strategy when they were not able to express themselves in Chinese; that is, they would use an alternative syntactic structure to express themselves. For instance, if they didn't know how to use the **subjunctive mood** in Chinese (Subjunctive moods are used to express various states of unreality such as wish, emotion, possibility, judgement, opinion, necessity or action that has not yet occurred), they would use an alternative way to express the same concept, such as replacing 假如我住在讲法文的地方，我就不会犯这样的错误 (If I lived in French-speaking places, I would not have made such mistakes) with 我住在讲法文的地方，我就不会犯这样的错误 (I could not make such mistakes; I lived in French-speaking places). In the context, one certainly understood what they meant.

Discrepancy in grammatical knowledge between speaking and writing

Léandre and Dominique acquired French grammatical rules by simply immersing themselves in the French environment with their father. Before they were formally taught how to read and write in French, they were ignorant about some grammatical rules. For instance, even though Léandre (16; 2; 12) knew how to produce them in oral French, he did not know some basic French grammatical rules in writing, such as the rule for *–er* verbs in imperative second person singular. The imperative is easy to construct. With a few exceptions, one takes the indicative present second person singular, first person plural and second person plural without the subject pronouns. For instance, *tu prends* (you take, are taking, do take) becomes *prends* (take), *nous prenons* becomes *prenons* (let's take) and *vous prenez* becomes *prenez* (take). The difficulty is that the most common verbs, verbs whose infinitive ends in *–er*, drop the *s* of the second person singular without any changes in pronunciation; for example, *tu manges* makes *mange* in the imperative. *Aller* (go), though irregular, follows this rule, too. *Tu vas* makes *va* (go) in the imperative. The dropped *s* comes back in front of pronouns *y* and *en*, such as in *manges-en* (eat some) or *vas-y* (literally go there). This is less difficult because the *s* is pronounced. Verbs ending in *–er* including *aller* drop the final *s* in the imperative 2nd singular (for instance, *mange* or *va*). Léandre and Dominique did have issues with this rule before they were taught it formally in their AP French class.

Crosslinguistic morphological awareness and transfer

Research suggests that morphological awareness can be transferred from one language to another. For instance, studies have shown that Chinese children who received Chinese morphological training outperformed the control group on an English morphological awareness task (i.e. there was a transfer of morphological awareness from Chinese to English). Among children who received the English morphological training, only those with high English proficiency outperformed the children in the control group on a Chinese morphological awareness task. Thus, there seems to be a causal link between Chinese and English morphological awareness. Nevertheless, the transfer of morphological awareness is conditioned by the morphological features of the languages involved, and not all morphological features can be transferred. For example, children can transfer English compound awareness to Chinese but not English derivational awareness to Chinese. In addition, there is a reciprocal relationship between English compound awareness and Chinese vocabulary.

Moreover, the aspect of morphological awareness (compound vs. derivational) that transfers and the **direction of transfer** (i.e. from a stronger language to a less strong language vs. from the less strong language to a stronger language) are both influenced by the morphological structures of the languages involved. Transfer tends to occur when the morphological structures of the languages involved are similar. The direction of transfer seems to be determined particularly by the morphological structure of the language; for instance, because reading Chinese requires more compound awareness, cross-language transfer of compound awareness is more likely to be observed from English to Chinese.

Moreover, it seems that the nature of morphological awareness is different from that of phonological awareness. Phonological awareness transfers across languages, regardless of the nature of the script used to represent them.[37] This is considered to be a common underlying competence.[38] In contrast, different aspects of morphological awareness exhibit different transfer patterns. Derivational awareness and inflectional awareness have been observed to transfer between two alphabetic languages that are rich in derivation and inflection.[39] Compound transfers between Chinese and English occur due to shared compounding structures.[40] Furthermore, since Chinese and English do not share any cognates, what transfers is not concrete vocabulary knowledge, but abstract metalinguistic understanding; that is, it could be the understanding of compounding rules or the ability to derive compound meaning from constituent morphemes or both.

This is certainly true with Léandre and Dominique's crosslinguistic morphological transfer patterns during adolescence. As a general pattern, they tended to transfer derivational awareness and inflectional awareness between their two alphabetic languages, English and French; and to make compound transfers between Chinese and English.

Sensitivity to morphological rules

Perhaps as a result of being reminded and corrected all their lives about their heritage-language use, Léandre and Dominique were sensitive to morphological rules when analysing languages and learning a new language. For example, in a restaurant at a rest stop in the south of Germany, we saw an advertisement about homemade strawberry cake. Without being asked, Léandre (18; 11; 13) spontaneously explained the meaning of the word *hausgenachter* (homemade). He explained to me that when looking at this word, one has to consider three aspects: the number, the case and the gender, which all determine the singular nominative masculine adjective ending *–er*. In addition, he recognised that the *ge-* prefix indicates a past participle verb form used as an adjective. This phenomenon has also been touched upon in Chapter 4.

Maze production in Chinese

A **maze** is a false start, hesitation, repetition or a reformulation of a sentence. The following is an example of a maze.[41]

But one time, when I had a b-, when uh, when last Christmas, I, uh uh, my aunt Mary Ann, my aunt, she gave me a bird, and her, and I called him Tweetie Bird.[42]

When people try to organise what they want to say, they sometimes search for words and sentence structure to express themselves, thus producing mazes. Mazes are common for both monolinguals and multilinguals when they are attempting to formulate long, complex utterances. Except for people who have more excessive and consistent maze production, such as those who have language impairment, occasional production of a maze is typical.

As for Léandre and Dominique, they sometimes produced mazes in Chinese, particularly when expressing long and complex ideas. As they became more proficient in Chinese, their maze production gradually faded. Both teens rarely produced mazes in French.

Strategies for Supporting Adolescent Morphosyntactic Development

Given the characteristics and morphosyntactic heritage-language development discussed above, it is important to carefully consider how we interact with our adolescents regarding their heritage-language morphosyntactic development. Based on our experience in working with our own children, it seems that explicitly teaching some targeted morphological skills is especially helpful, considering the teens' limited heritage-language morphosyntactic exposure. Below are some ideas for explicit teaching.

Building morphological knowledge to develop heritage-language reading skills

In Chapter 3, I mentioned that phonemic awareness is important for reading development.[43] This is because readers must have a degree of phonemic awareness to learn that letters usually map onto phonemes (partially in alphabetic languages). In addition to phonological awareness, research shows that morphological awareness is also critical in reading development. **Morphological awareness** refers to the ability to reflect upon and manipulate morphemes (the smallest phonological unit that carries meaning) and to use word formation rules to construct and understand morphologically complex words. In fact, recent research has identified morphological awareness as an important predictor of literacy constructs including vocabulary, word reading and reading comprehension in alphabetic languages among monolingual and bilingual children.⁴⁴ In logographic languages such as Chinese, characters map directly onto individual morphemes. Thus, morphological awareness is even more vital for reading Chinese.⁴⁵

Thus, as discussed in Chapter 4, in your everyday interactions with your teens (whether your teens' heritage language is alphabetic or logographic), you will want to help them build their morphological knowledge in their heritage language by analysing the morphological components of words. I discovered that dinnertime is often a good occasion to do this. You can either prepare a list of complex words and ask your teens to tell you the components, or you can select a page of heritage-language reading material and ask your teens to identify the morphemes. Alternatively, you can also use situational instances (or opportunity teaching) to help them develop morphological knowledge. Box 5.7 shows two examples.

Box 5.7 Example of Morphological Analysis Activity in the Daily Context

Example 1:

[While finishing dinner, I picked five words from a small basket and laid them out on the table.]

Mother: [Putting the cutouts of the Chinese characters on the table: 语, 说, 谚, 谢, 谎] Tell me how these words are related? (告诉我这些字有什么相同的地方？)

Dominique (12; 3; 2): They all have a radical of 讠. (他们都有讠字旁。)

Mother: Can you guess what they might mean? (你能猜猜这些字的意思吗？)

Dominique: I don't know. (我不知道。)

Mother: What does 说 mean? (说是什么意思？)

Dominique: Speaking. (讲话。)

Mother: You are right. 说 has a radical 讠. All these words have something to do with speaking: 语-language, 谚-proverb, 谢-thank, 谎-lie. (对。说有讠字旁。这些字都和说有关系。语言，谚语，感谢，说谎。)

Example 2:

In an ancient town near Shanghai, Léandre (18; 11; 13) noticed that words such as 泗, 渔 were connected with the radical 氵 (water). I seized the opportunity to show him that there were more words that could be related to the radical and they all had something to do with 氵 (water), such as 湖 (lake), 江 (long and river) and 河 (small river).

Building morphological knowledge to develop heritage-language writing skills

Morphological awareness not only benefits reading development but also helps with spelling and writing development. Research in English and other alphabetic languages has shown that children learning to spell and write are sensitive to morphological information, which serves as a resource for them to acquire writing skills.[46] The reason that knowledge about morphemic structure can aid in spelling and writing is because the properties of writing systems are often closely related to morphological relationships within the languages they represent. For example, the knowledge that the spoken forms *horse* and *horses* are morphologically related (i.e. they represent the morphological alternation between singular and plural marking) is relevant to the fact that the correct spelling of the base form is *horse* with a silent *e* rather than *hors*.[47]

Morphological knowledge may be even more critical to the acquisition of writing in Chinese than in alphabetic languages because of the closer relationship between morphemes and basic orthography units (i.e. characters). For example, the morpheme 火 (fire) appears both in the word 火材 (match) and in the word 火巨 (torch). 火材 (match) and 火巨 (torch) are semantically related in a way that is reflected in their shared morpheme 火 (fire).

In addition to the type of word morphemic knowledge structure referred to above, there is an additional kind of systematic structural knowledge in Chinese that is relevant for learning to read and write; that is, knowledge of the structure of Chinese character orthography. Despite its well-known complexity, the Chinese written language is, in fact, highly systematic in its structure. The majority of Chinese characters (around 82%) do represent sound and meaning in a highly systematic fashion. For example, in phonetic compounds, pronunciation information occurs in the phonetic radical, which is usually located on the right side of a character; and meaning information is present in the semantic radical, which is usually located on the left. Take a look at the phonetic compound characters 清 and 晴. The pronunciation information is represented by the phonetic radical on the right, and meaning information is represented by the semantic radical on the left. The first character 清 has the three-stroke (water) semantic radical on the left-hand side and the phonetic radical 青 on the right (which serves as the simple character for *blue*), and so the entire character is pronounced /qing/ (following the phonetic radical) and means 清 (*clear*), as implied by the water semantic radical. The second phonetic compound character 晴 also gets its pronunciation /qing/ from the phonetic radical on the right, and has the semantic radical for 日 (sun) on the left, giving a clue to the entire character's meaning of 'cloudless sky.'

It is important to note here that orthographic structure is different from word morphology. **Orthographic structure knowledge** refers to knowledge that semantic and phonetic radicals are located in specific places in Chinese characters. **Word morphology** refers to knowledge of how a single morpheme with a given meaning may appear in different complex words that have related meanings, as in the example given above, 火材 (match) and 火巨 (torch). These two types of knowledge are conceptually related because both directly pertain to the reader's acquisition and manipulation of semantic information. In addition, these two concepts are even more closely related because the meaning contained in the semantic radicals of phonetic compound characters is, in general, the meaning common to most of the morphemes those characters represent. The semantic radicals in Chinese characters share many of the characteristics of the 'morpheme' construct, because most are associated with a particular meaning.[48]

Chinese writing is a very demanding task for Chinese-language learners; needless to say, it is even more challenging for heritage-Chinese-language-learning children and adolescents. In the first grade alone, Chinese children generally learn to write 436 visually complex characters, with 7.37 strokes each on average. The traditional way to learn a new character is to write it repeatedly. Given the large size of the corpus of characters that Chinese learners must master to be competent readers, learning efficiency is critical. Thus, helping Chinese-language-learning children and adolescents develop insights into orthographic structure can enable them to write characters much more efficiently. For example, in the case of the phonetic compound character 植 (plant), a child or adolescent can be oriented to dissect the character into the semantic radical 木 (wood) and the phonetic radical 直/zhi/. Children can be explicitly taught that the semantic radical represents the semantic category of the character 木 (wood), and that the phonetic radical 直/zhi/ represents the pronunciation of the characters. Understanding the orthographic structure of characters can help learners to choose among characters in their lexicon that have similar pronunciations and/or graphic forms. They can tell, for example, that among the four homophonic characters 植, 值, 埴 and 殖, only 植 is related to wood because of the radical 木. The advantage of drawing teens' attention to multiple features of the orthography is that it can provide them with different sources of information they may need to produce written forms, thereby expanding their ways of decoding a character or a word. When semantic, phonetic, morphological and graphic features of print become transparent, they provide varied information sources for retrieving characters and words that go beyond rote memorisation.

Another advantage of teaching morphological structure is related to motivation. It has been reported that morphological insight makes writing a more engaging task than mechanical repetition. Research shows that those children who were taught the morphological structures were more likely to write because they were able to use creativity and approach writing as a problem-solving task.[49]

Promoting lexical development through morphological awareness

As shown in the previous chapter, morphological development is closely related to vocabulary development because knowledge of root words is necessary to understand and construct compound words.[50] In fact, morphological awareness is often considered to represent vocabulary depth.[51] It offers an effective way to organise morphologically related words in the mental lexicon.[52] Therefore, you may want to focus your teens' attention on root words (in alphabetic languages such as in English and German) and radicals (such as in Chinese) to facilitate their compound word development.

Teaching intra- and intersentential connectives

In Chapter 4, we discussed how teaching certain literate words such as polysemous and double-functional terms, adverbs of likelihood and magnitude, abstract nouns, metalinguistic verbs and factive and nonfactive verbs are important for reading and writing development in a heritage language. Other words such as **intrasentential** (within sentence) words (such as *although, but, since, unless, whenever*), **intersentential** (between sentence) connective words (such as *furthermore, consequently, however, moreover* and *rather*) are also very important because these words are related to syntactic development.[53] Knowing these words will help teens construct more complex sentences.

Reading helps morphology development

Earlier in the chapter, it was mentioned that the largest increase in deviational morphological skills occurs between ages 9 and 14. Some[54] believe that this increase is also correlated to adolescents' increased exposure to written language that contains a great number of morphologically complex words. Thus, engaging your teens in heritage-language reading that contains more morphologically complex words is one advantageous way to help them build their deviational morphological skills. Additionally, reading is the best way to learn complex words. However, in a typical heritage-learning environment, children and adolescents do not usually have opportunities or the ability to read the high-level texts that they read in their dominant language in school. One strategy I found effective in increasing adolescents' opportunities for reading higher-level texts is to select texts that contain more complex words, ask them to identify the complex words in the texts, let them tell you how these words are formed and explain any parts of the words they can recognise. If they cannot read themselves, you read to them. The goal is to consciously draw the teens' attention to these words.

Scaffolding complex sentence use

The appropriate use of subordinate sentences can enhance the efficiency with which ideas are expressed. For example, instead of producing a monotonous string of independent clauses (e.g. 'I went to California. I saw a movie. It was a new movie. Jeremy had recommended it'), a competent speaker can combine them into one complex sentence that is rich in information yet clear in meaning (e.g. 'When I went to California, I saw the new movie that Jeremy had recommended').[55] I found the easiest way to do this is to start such an exercise orally. For instance, during mealtimes or when driving your children somewhere, you can start with a few simple sentences and then ask your children to tell you whether there are ways that they can combine these sentences or phrases into more complex sentences. If you make such oral exercises a routine, your teens can form the habit of producing complex sentences consciously, which will help them in their heritage-language writing.

Modelling complex sentence use in the context

Another important aspect of helping your teens develop heritage-language syntax is modelling. In your everyday conversations with your child, you may want to purposely use more complex sentences. The chances are that the more you expose your children to complex sentences, the more likely it is that they will be able to use complex sentences on their own. If you feel uncomfortable using more complex sentences (after all, it is a little unnatural to speak this way in a typical colloquial context), you can let your teens listen to recorded lectures or debates, which may provide complex sentence exposure in your heritage language in a more contextualised manner.

Increasing input in passive forms

Research suggests that the input in children's environment has an impact on how they acquire passive voice. In a study, young children were asked to listen to stories containing either a high proportion of passive voice sentences or a high proportion of active voice sentences. Children who heard stories with passive sentences produced more passive constructions (with fewer mistakes) and showed higher comprehension scores than children who heard stories with active sentences.[56] Thus, in your interactions with your teens, you may also want to increase passive-voice modelling for them. I found that readings that contain passive forms are the best input for teens. You can read these materials to them or try to incorporate the passive sentences from these readings into your everyday conversations.

Useful Measures to Monitor Adolescent Morphosyntactic Development

To help you monitor your teens' morphosyntactic progress, you may want to try the following measures.

Measures for knowledge of morphological rules

In language studies, researchers often use **nonwords** (or nonsense words) to test children and adolescents' understanding of morphological rules. For instance, psychologists (discussed in Chapter 4) used the nonword *wug* to test young children's understanding of the English morphological rules (e.g. two *wugs*). Using nonwords is a very good way to measure your teens' morphological knowledge in their heritage language because the task requires them to use the correct morphological rules in a language without having previous information about the word. You can make up a list of nonwords and ask your teens whether they know how to apply the heritage-language specific morphological rules to these words. For instance, researcher Bruce Derwing[57] asked his adolescent and adult participants to complete the correct English forms by showing them a picture and reading aloud a sentence such as 'This is a man who knows how to *yurse* (nonword).' He would then pose the question: 'A man who *yurses* is a what?' Participants needed to use their knowledge of English to come up with the correct answer, which was *yurser*. Measures like this may be performed before you teach particular morphological rules to your teens to get a sense of their current morphological levels. This information will help you plan what areas to focus on with regard to their morphological development. You can also use the nonword measure to help you understand how your teens are doing after you teach them the morphological rules.

Although this nonword measure has been used to help understand language learners' knowledge of morphological rules in alphabetic languages, you can certainly use nonwords to help you understand your teens' morphological rules understanding in logographic languages such as Chinese. For instance, I mentioned earlier that the Chinese radical 讠 has something to do with speaking; thus, you can come up with some nonword with the radical 讠 to see whether your children have mastered the general principles.

Measures for syntactic development

As discussed before, two key markers of later syntactic development are sentence length and clausal density.[58] Clausal density measures sentence complexity; it has been recognised as a key marker of syntactic development in conversation and is sensitive to growth.[59] In Chapter 4, I suggested recording teens' narratives to measure their vocabulary development. You can use the same method to measure their syntactic development. You can analyse a sample of your child's conversation or writing with the T-unit and the C-unit.

T-unit

As shown before, a T-unit contains one **independent (main) clause** and any **dependent (subordinate) clauses** or nonclausal structures that are attached to it or embedded within it.[60] For example, the utterance 'Bill bought a new bicycle before he went to Europe' is one T-unit that contains an independent clause ('Bill bought a new bicycle') and a dependent clause ('before he went to Europe'). In contrast, the utterance 'Bill went to France and then he went to Italy' consists of two T-units because it contains two independent clauses joined by the coordinating conjunction 'and'. Whenever a coordinating conjunction (e.g. 'and', 'but', 'so') initiates an independent

> **Box 5.8 An Example of T-Unit Calculation**[61]
>
> As a self-proclaimed web newbie, she learnt that starting an online business was tough. Initially, she was only getting about 25 visitors a month, which in the gardening world is about as beautiful as a pot full of snails.
>
> In this example, there are two T-units and 39 words. The mean words per T-unit are 19.5.

clause, that clause is considered to be a new T-unit. Box 5.8 is an example of how T-units are calculated.

C-unit

A C-unit is identical to a T-unit but includes responses that lack an independent clause when answering a question. For example, the response 'yes' to the question 'Did Jack drive?' is one C-unit.

Once you have a baseline measurement of your adolescent's T-unit and C-unit, you can compare over a period of time to see whether or not your child is making progress. It is also important to note that T-unit length is greater in the expository discourse genre (to explain things) than in the narrative discourse genre.

Summary of Key Points in Chapter 5

- Adolescents make several remarkable advances in their morphosyntactic development.
- As a result of the development in the areas of spoken language abilities, metalinguistic skills and exposure to the morphologically complex words in written language via reading and writing (especially spelling), adolescents show improvement in their deviational morphology development.
- There is a language-specific developmental trend in derivational and compound morphology. For instance, speakers of a logographic language (such as Chinese) may have more advanced compound awareness than speakers of an alphabetic language (such as English), whereas speakers of an alphabetic language (such as English) may have more advanced derivational awareness than speakers of a logographic language (such as Chinese).
- As a general trend, transparent compound words tend to be mastered faster than opaque compound words.
- Adolescents also increase their complex sentence use. Across the board, adolescents' sentence complexity increases considerably over the years, which is demonstrated by the fact that the sentences they produce become increasingly longer with more words, embedded phrases and clauses as evidenced in their:

- increase in sentence length and clause density;
- increase in complex sentences in the expository genre;
- increase in flexibility in adjustment in communication setting, purpose and listener needs;
- increase in the use of sophisticated syntactic structure;
- improvement in conjunction sentence structure;
- improvement in adverbial conjuncts and adverbial disjuncts.
• Adolescents make gradual progress in their passive sentence production.
• There are some language-specific development characteristics in Léandre and Dominique's heritage-language morphosyntax:
  - Errors in French articles and possessive pronouns, but rarely in Chinese articles (冠词).
  - Difficulties in mastering the Chinese measurement words or classifiers (量词).
  - Mistakes in French tenses or inventing French tenses.
  - Less passive voice form use in Chinese in early and mid-adolescence.
  - English syntactic influence on French.
  - Syntactic avoidance strategy in production.
  - Discrepancy in grammatical knowledge in speaking and writing.
  - Crosslinguistic morphological awareness and transfer.
  - Sensitivity to morphological rules.
  - Occasional maze production in Chinese syntax.
• To help teens further develop their heritage-language morphology and syntax, several strategies may be considered:
  - Building morphological knowledge to develop heritage-language reading skills.
  - Promoting lexical development through morphological awareness.
  - Teaching intra-and intersentential connectives to help develop complex sentences.
  - Reading, which helps morphological development.
  - Scaffolding complex sentence use.
  - Modelling complex sentence use in context.
  - Increasing passive form input in everyday conversations.
• Finally, to help you understand your teens' current morphosyntactic levels in their heritage language, you can use the following measures:
  - Use nonwords to measure your children's knowledge of the morphological rules in their heritage language.
  - Use T-units and C-units to measure your children's syntactic complexity.

Recommended Readings

Kuo, L. and Anderson, R.C. (2006) Morphological awareness and learning to read: A cross-linguistic perspective. *Educational Psychologist* 41, 161–80.

Nippold, M.A. (2007) *Later Language Development: School-Age Children, Adolescents, and Young Adults*. Austin, TX: Pro-ed.

Notes and References

1. Kuo, L. and Anderson, R.C. (2006) Morphological awareness and learning to read: A cross-linguistic perspective. *Educational Psychologist* 41, 161–80.
2. Nippold, M.A. (2007) *Later Language Development: School-Age Children, Adolescents, and Young Adults* (p. 53). Austin, TX: Pro-ed.
3. Nippold, M.A. (2007) *Later Language Development: School-Age Children, Adolescents, and Young Adults*. Austin, TX: Pro-ed
4. Green, L., McCutchen, D., Schwiebert, C., Quinlan, T., Evaod, A. and Juelis, J. (2003) Morphological development in children's writing. *Journal of Educational Psychology* 95, 752–61.
   Derwing, B. and Baker, W. (1979) Recent research on the acquisition of English morphology. In P. Fletcher and M. Garman (eds) *Language Acquisition: Studies in First language Development*. Cambridge: Cambridge University Press.
   Levin, I., Ravid, D. and Rapaport, S. (2001) Morphology and spelling among Hebrew-speaking children: From kindergarten to first grade. *Journal of Child Language* 28, 741–72.
5. Carlisle, J. (2000) Awareness of the structure and meaning of morphologically complex words. Impact on reading. *Reading and Writing* 12, 169–90.
   Mahony, D.L. (1994) Using sensitivity to word structure to explain variance in high school and college level reading ability. *Reading and Writing* 6, 19–44.
6. Nippold, M.A. (2007) *Later Language Development: School-Age Children, Adolescents, and Young Adults* (p. 65). Austin, TX: Pro-ed.
7. Nippold, M.A. (2007) *Later Language Development: School-Age Children, Adolescents, and Young Adults* (pp. 58-65). Austin, TX: Pro-ed.
8. Nippold, M.A. (2007) *Later Language Development: School-Age Children, Adolescents, and Young Adults* (p. 58). Austin, TX: Pro-ed.
9. Moats, L. and Smith, C. (1992) Deviational morphology: Why it should be included in language assessment and instructions. *Language, Speech, and Hearing Services in Schools* 23, 312–19.
10. Nippold, M.A. (2007) *Later Language Development: School-Age Children, Adolescents, and Young Adults* (p. 55). Austin, TX: Pro-ed.
11. Carlisle, J. (1988) Knowledge of deviational morphology and spelling ability in fourth, sixth, and eighth graders. *Applied Psycholinguistics* 9, 247–66.
12. Kuo, L. and Anderson, R.C. (2006) Morphological awareness and learning to read: A cross-linguistic perspective. *Educational Psychologist* 41, 161–80.
13. Ku, Y. and Anderson, R.C. (2003) Development of morphological awareness in Chinese and English. *Reading and Writing: An Interdisciplinary Journal* 16, 399–422.
14. Pasquarella, A., Chen, X., Lam, K. and Luo, Y.C. (2011) Cross-language transfer of morphological awareness in Chinese–English bilinguals. *Journal of Research in Reading* 34 (1), 23–42.
15. Miller, J.F. (1981) *Assessing Language Production in Children: Experimental Procedures*. Baltimore: University Park Press.
16. Nippold, M.A., Hesketh, L.J., Duthie, J.K. and Mansfield, T.C. (2005) Conversational versus expository discourse: A study of syntactic development in children, adolescents, and adults. *Journal of Speech, Language, and Hearing Research* 48, 1048–64.
17. Nippold, M.A. (2007) *Later Language Development: School-Age Children, Adolescents, and Young Adults*. Austin, TX: Pro-ed.
18. Pence, K.L. and Justice, L.M. (2008) *Language Development from Theory to Practice*. Upper Saddle River, NJ: Pearson.
19. Wang, X.-L. (2015) *Understanding Language and Literacy Development: Diverse Leaners in the Classroom* (p. 190). Malden, MA: John Wiley & Sons, Inc.
20. Nippold, M.A. (2007) *Later Language Development: School-Age Children, Adolescents, and Young Adults* (p. 259). Austin, TX: Pro-ed.

21 Clause density was calculated by dividing the total number of clauses (main and subordinate) in the sample by the total number of T-units across the sample. See Scott, C. and Windsor, J. (2000) General language performance measures in spoken and written narrative and expository discourse of school-age children with language learning disabilities. *Journal of Speech, Language, and Hearing Research* 43, 324–39.

22 Scott, C.M. and Stokes, S. (1995) Measures of syntax in school-age children and adolescents. *Language, Speech, and Hearing Services in Schools* 26, 301–19.

23 Nippold, M.A. (2007) *Later Language Development: School-Age Children, Adolescents, and Young Adults*. Austin, TX: Pro-ed.

24 Berman, R.A. and Verhoeven, L. (2002) Cross-linguistic perspectives on the development of text-production abilities: Speech and writing. *Written Language and Literacy* 5, 1–43.

25 Berman, R.A. and Verhoeven, L. (2002) Cross-linguistic perspectives on the development of text-production abilities: Speech and writing. *Written Language and Literacy* 5, 1–43.

26 An appositive is originally a Latin word meaning to put near. An appositive is a noun, a noun phrase or a noun clause which sits next to another noun to remake it or to describe it in another way.

27 Nippold, M.A. (2007) *Later Language Development: School-Age Children, Adolescents, and Young Adults*. Austin, TX: Pro-ed.

28 Nippold, M.A. (2007) *Later Language Development: School-Age Children, Adolescents, and Young Adults*. Austin, TX: Pro-ed.

29 Nippold, M.A. (2007) *Later Language Development: School-Age Children, Adolescents, and Young Adults*. Austin, TX: Pro-ed.

30 Owens, R.E. (2012) *Language Development: An Introduction*. Boston: Pearson.

31 Francis, N. (2006) The development of secondary discourse ability and metalinguistic awareness in second language learners. *International Journal of Applied Linguistics* 16, 37–60.

32 http://cowgill.ling.yale.edu/sra/morphology_ecs.htm Retrieved on 10 September 2014.

33 Li, P. (2013) Successive language acquisition. In F. Grosjean and P. Li (eds) *The Psycholinguistics of Bilingualism* (p. 162). Oxford: Wiley- Blackwell.

34 Personal communication, 12 June 2012.

35 Data were calculated based on 8 hours video recordings in 4 years (ages 12 to 16; 2 hours each year).

36 Meisel, J.M. (2006) The bilingual child. In T.K. Bhatia and W.C. Ritchie (eds) *The Handbook of Bilingualism* (pp. 91–144). Oxford: Blackwell.

37 For example, Durgunoglu, A.Y., Nagy, W.E. and Hancin-Bhatt, B.J. (1993) Cross-language transfer of phonological awareness. *Journal of Educational Psychology* 85, 453–65.

38 Genesee, F., Geva, E., Dressler, C. and Kamil, M. (2006) Synthesis: Cross-linguistic relationships, Chapter 6. In D. August and T. Shanahan (eds) *Developing Literacy in Second Language Learners. Report of the National Literacy Panel on Minority-Language Children and Youth* (pp.153–74). Mahwah, NJ: Lawrence Erlbaum.

Genesee, F., Geva, E., Dressler, C. and Kamil, M.L. (2008). Cross-linguistic relationships in second language learners. In D. August and T. Shanahan (eds) *Developing Reading and Writing in Second Language Learners: Lessons from the Report of the National Literacy Panel on Language-Minority Children and Youth* (pp. 153–83). New York, NY: Routledge.

Koda, K. (2007) Reading and language learning: Crosslinguistic constraints on second language reading development. *Language Learning* 57 (1), 1–44.

39 For example, Saiegh-Haddad, E. and Geva, E. (2008) Morphological awareness, phonological awareness, and reading in English – Arabic bilingual children. *Reading and Writing* 21 (5), 481–504.

40 Wang, M., Yang, C. and Cheng, C. (2009) The Contributions of phonology, orthography, and morphology in Chinese-English biliteracy acquisition. *Applied Psycholinguistics* 30, 291–314.

41 Gillam, R.B., Marquardt, T.P. and Martin, F.N. (2011) *Communication Sciences and Disorders: From Science to Clinical Practice* (p. 256). Burlington, MA: Jones & Bartlett.

42 Gillam, R.B., Marquardt, T.P. and Martin, F.N. (2011) *Communication Sciences and Disorders: From Science to Clinical Practice* (p. 256). Burlington, MA: Jones & Bartlett.
43 Foorman, B., Francis, D., Novy, D. and Liberman, D. (1991) How letter-sound instruction mediates progress in first-grade reading and spelling. *Journal of Educational Psychology* 83, 456–69.
44 For example, Nagy, W., Berninger, V., Abbott, R., Vaughan, K. and Vermeulen, K. (2003) Relationship of morphology and other language skills in at-risk second grade readers and at-risk fourth grade writers. *Journal of Educational Psychology* 95, 730–42.
45 Packard, J.L., Chen, X., Li, W.-L., Wu, X.-C., Gaffney, J.S., Li, H. and Anderson, R.C. (2006) Explicit instruction in orthographic structure and word morphology helps Chinese children learn to write characters. *Reading and Writing* 19, 457–87.
Li, W., Anderson, R., Nagy, W. and Zhang, H. (2002) Facets of metalinguistic awareness that contribute to Chinese literacy. In W. Li, J.S. Gaffney and J.L. Packard (eds) *Chinese Language Acquisition: Theoretical and Pedagogical Issues* (pp. 87–106). The Netherlands: Kluwer.
46 Waters, G., Bruck, M. and Malus-Abramowitz, M. (1988) The role of linguistic and visual processes in spelling: A developmental study. *Journal of Experimental Child Psychology* 45, 400–21.
Leybaert, J. and Content, A. (1995) Reading and spelling acquisition in two different teaching methods: A test of the independence hypothesis. *Reading and Writing: An Interdisciplinary Journal* 7, 65–88.
Leybaert, J. and Alegria, J. (1995) Spelling development in deaf and hearing children: Evidence for use of morpho-phonological regularities in French. *Reading and Writing: An Interdisciplinary Journal* 7, 89–109.
Senechal, M. (2000) Morphological effects in children's spelling of French words. *Canadian Journal of Experimental Psychology* 54, 76–85.
47 Examples from Packard, J.L., Chen, X., LI, W.-L., Wu, X.-C., Gaffney, J.S., Li, H. and Anderson, R.C. (2006) Explicit instruction in orthographic structure and word morphology helps Chinese children learn to write characters. *Reading and Writing* 19, 457–87.
48 Zhou, X.-L, Marslen-Wilson, W., Taft M. and Shu, H. (1999) Morphology, orthography, and phonology reading Chinese compound words. *Language and Cognitive Processes* 14 (5/6), 525–65.
49 Zhou, X.-L, Marslen-Wilson, W., Taft M. and Shu, H. (1999) Morphology, orthography, and phonology reading Chinese compound words. *Language and Cognitive Processes* 14 (5/6), 525–65.
50 For example, Chung, W.-L. and Hu, C.-F. (2007) Morphological awareness and learning to read Chinese. *Reading and Writing* 20, 441–61.
51 Kieffer, M.J. and Lesaux, N. (2008) The role of derivational morphology in the reading comprehension of Spanish-speaking English language learners. *Reading and Writing: An Interdisciplinary Journal* 21 (8), 783–804.
52 Ideas from Pasquarella, A., Chen, X., and Lam, K. and Luo, Y.C. (2011) Cross-language transfer of morphological awareness in Chinese–English bilinguals. *Journal of Research in Reading* 34 (1), 23–42.
53 Nippold, M.A. (2007) *Later Language Development: School-Age Children, Adolescents, and Young Adults.* Austin, TX: Pro-ed.
54 White, T.G., Power, M.A. and White, S. (1989) Morphological analysis: Implications for teaching and understanding vocabulary growth. *Reading Research Quarterly* 24, 283–304.
55 Nippold, M.A., Hesketh, L.J., Duthie, J.K. and Mansfield, T.C. (2005) Conversational versus expository discourse: A study of syntactic development in children, adolescents, and adults. *Journal of Speech, Language, and Hearing Research* 48, 1048–64.
56 Vasilyeva, M., Huttenlocher, J. and Waterfall, H. (2006) Effects of language intervention on syntactic skill levels in preschoolers. *Developmental Psychology* 42 (1), 164–74.
57 Derwing, B. (1976) Morpheme recognition and the learning of rules for derivational morphology. *Canadian Journal of Linguistics* 21 (1), 38–66.

[58] Scott, C.M. and Stokes, S.L. (1995) Measures of syntax in school-age children and adolescents. *Language, Speech, and Hearing Services in Schools* 26, 309–19.
[59] Scott, C.M. and Stokes, S.L. (1995) Measures of syntax in school-age children and adolescents. *Language, Speech, and Hearing Services in Schools* 26, 309–19.
[60] Hunt, K.W. (1970) Recent measures in syntactic development. In M. Lester (ed.) *Reading in Applied Transformational Grammar* (pp. 179–92). London RW Holt.
[61] Example from http://users.clas.ufl.edu/rthompso/interactioncombining.html

6 The Development of Multilingual Knowledge and Usage During Adolescence

One day, Philippe was playing *jass*, a Swiss card game, with Léandre and Dominique. When deciding who would begin first, Philippe took out a coin and said, 'Pile ou face' (tails or heads). Léandre (16; 4; 30) joked that he wanted the *battery*, which he intentionally said in English. Léandre was impishly playing with the dual meanings of the word *pile*, which also means *battery* in French. On another occasion, I asked Dominique what kind of tea he wanted after lunch; he (12; 0; 0) kidded that he wanted the *sixteen* tea (十六茶). In Chinese, *pomegranate* (石榴) sounds like *sixteen* (十六). Dominique was toying with the Chinese homophones of 石榴 (pomegranate) and 十六 (sixteen); that is, he was making jokes about the two words that sound alike but have different meanings. I then turned to Léandre and asked what kind of tea he preferred; he (13; 11; 4) put on a poker face and said that he would like the *seventeen* tea (十七茶). Léandre obviously took the hint from Dominique and played along. In these seemingly mindless jokes, Léandre and Dominique demonstrated their sophisticated crosslinguistic knowledge. No wonder a wise acquaintance once commented, 'Anybody can make a joke. But a good joke requires not only one's cleverness but also one's superb knowledge about a language.'

This chapter is about multilingual adolescents' knowledge and use of their ambient languages. It begins with an overview of adolescents' major **pragmatic** (language use) and **metalinguistic** (language knowledge) achievements. It then discusses Léandre and Dominique's specific heritage-language pragmatic and metalinguistic developmental characteristics during adolescence. Next, effective strategies are proposed to help you support your teens' pragmatic and metalinguistic development. Finally, practical measures are introduced to help you monitor your teens' continued pragmatic and metalinguistic progress in their respective languages.

Major Pragmatic and Metalinguistic Achievements During Adolescence

Mastering a linguistic system requires not only grammatical competence but also pragmatic competence and knowledge about the linguistic system. Compared with earlier developmental stages (early childhood and middle childhood), teens have made notable progress in their conversational, narrative and **figurative language** (nonliteral language) abilities. Moreover, adolescent girls and boys have also developed gender-specific speech styles that are termed by some researchers as *genderlect*.[1]

Conversational competence

Conversational competence improves with age and over time as adolescents continue to refine their conversational skills. As shown in Box 6.1, teens demonstrate increasingly polished conversational abilities in peer exchanges. Most notably, adolescents (e.g. 17-year-olds) are more likely to respond to feelings and attitudes expressed by the previous speaker, whereas younger children (e.g. 10-year-olds) are more likely to respond to facts expressed by the previous speaker.[2]

Narrative competence

Narratives are a more complex and more sophisticated discourse genre than conversation. Narratives require speakers to draw on a range of linguistic, cognitive and social abilities. From the linguistic perspective, speakers must use more complex words and sentences to encode information about the characters and events in a story by using the appropriate grammatical devices to articulate the sequence of events and their temporal relations. Narratives also require a complex story grammar. **Story grammar** refers to the elements of a story. A well-formed story grammar (structure) includes an abstract (a summary of the narrative or a title), an introduction (a description of the characters, setting, time and activity to set the stage for the narrative), events (actions that advance the storyline, including the problem), a resolution (a termination of complicating events) and a coda (an ending to the narrative). From the cognitive perspective, speakers in a narrative must infer the motivation for protagonists' actions, the logical relationships between events and the theme of the story. They also need to demonstrate their assessment of the

---

Box 6.1 Areas of Improvement in Conversation

- Staying on a topic longer
- Having extended dialogues with others
- Spending more time conversing with peers
- Making a greater number of relevant and factually based comments
- Shifting gradually from one topic to another
- Being more sensitive to listeners by adjusting to their feelings and reactions
- Offering more support to the conversational partner

Modified from Nippold, M.A. (2007) *Later Language Development: School-Age Children, Adolescents, and Young Adults* (p. 286). Austin, TX: Pro-ed.

meaning or significance of the events in the story. From the social perspective, when telling a story, speakers must engage and maintain the listener's attention.[3]

Adolescents' narratives show several areas of improvement. First, teens progressively increase their narrative length and number of episodes. Second, they begin to use more adverbial conjunctive links (such as *meanwhile, anyway* and *incidentally*) to enhance their narrative cohesiveness. Third, they become more aware of the interlocutor's (conversational partner's) mind in their narratives by including comments on the thoughts, feelings and emotions of the characters.[4]

Figurative language competence

One significant area of metalinguistic achievement during adolescence is their increasing ability to use figurative language. **Figurative language** is language that is used in nonliteral and abstract ways. People often use figurative language to evoke mental images and make impressions in other people. Figurative language competence is an indicator of an individual's cognitive level, creativity and abstract reasoning ability.[5]

There is a clear developmental trajectory in figurative language development. At as young as two years old, children begin to use spontaneous metaphors. However, it is not until age ten that children appear to have the true ability to interpret metaphors.[6] In fact, it is really during adolescence that the understanding of figurative language becomes reliable. Interestingly, there is a U-shaped curve in the production of figurative language. During early childhood, preschoolers are commonly observed using imaginative expressions such as 'The faucet is crying' and 'Pretend the headlights are eyes.' During middle childhood, the use of imaginative expressions decreases, but the expressions increase during adolescence.[7]

Adolescents show a gradual refinement in figurative language comprehension (understanding) and production (usage), as evidenced in their use of metaphor, simile, hyperboles, idioms, irony and proverbs.

Metaphors and similes

A metaphor is a type of figurative speech in which a word or a phrase that is ordinarily used to describe one thing is used to describe another to make a comparison, as in the example *'She is the apple of my eye'*. A simile is similar to a metaphor. A simile, however, uses the words *like* or *as* when comparing, as in *'like water off a duck's back.'* Although teens have already begun to understand some metaphors and similes, they continue to improve their comprehension and usage throughout adolescence and beyond.

Hyperbole

Hyperbole is another form of figurative language that uses exaggeration for emphasis or effect. For example, in the sentence *'I am so hungry, I could eat a horse,'* the speaker exaggerates his/her hunger to emphasise that he/she is very hungry.

Children between ages 8 and 10 may use two kinds of cues to understand hyperbole: paralinguistic cues (the speaker's intonation patterns) or pragmatic cues (the speaker's intent). Adolescents, on the other hand, begin to improve their ability to understand hyperbole both in comprehension and production, therefore limiting their need to use other cues.[8]

Idioms

Idioms are expressions that contain both a literal and a figurative meaning. Examples include *'We are in the same boat,' 'It's raining cats and dogs,'* and *'I've put that issue on the back burner.'* Teens continue to improve their understanding and production of idioms throughout adolescence and beyond.

Irony

Irony means speaking or writing about one thing, but actually meaning another. For example, a person says, *'What a nice day!'* when the day is in fact cold and windy. Although younger children can begin to figure out the meaning by using acoustic cues or contextual information, adolescents are much better at understanding the underlying meaning of an ironic remark. They also begin to use irony in their communication.

Proverbs

A proverb is a conventional saying that usually gives advice. Examples include *'A stitch in time saves nine'* and *'An apple a day keeps the doctor away.'* Proverbs are one of the most difficult types of figurative language to master.[9] During middle childhood, children tend not to use proverbs spontaneously but begin to understand them. Adolescents begin to improve their ability to understand proverbs, and some adolescents can use them in their communication. Proverb attainment during adolescence is associated with adolescents' development in abstract thinking because proverb understanding requires adolescents to know the abstract and metalinguistic aspects of language. Proverb attainment relies on a supportive linguistic environment. If teens are frequently exposed to proverbs in their daily environment, they also tend to use them more frequently in their own communication.

Genderlect

Genderlect is a particular speech or conversation style used by a particular gender. Typically, girls and boys already exhibit differences in their language use from a young age. However, it is during the adolescent period that gender differences in language become more noticeable. The language use and styles of adult women and men begin to be observed in adolescent communication. The gender differences in speech, or genderlect, among adolescents are shown in the areas of phonology (such as pronunciation and intonation), lexicon (word choice) and conversational style.

In phonology, adolescent girls tend to use a higher pitch when speaking than adolescent boys. They also tend to use different intonation patterns in communication from adolescent boys.

There is also a quantitative difference between females and males in lexical use. Males tend to use more swear words and coarse language in conversation, while females use more polite words (e.g. *please*). Females use more descriptive words (e.g. *adorable, sweet, lovely*) and more colour terms than males. In addition, females use emphatic expressions more frequently than males (e.g. *oh dear* and *goodness*), and men use more expletives (e.g. *damn it*).[10] Adolescents begin to adopt these male and female lexicon choices.

Style differences in male and female teens are observed as well. First, using English as an example, adolescent girls typically speak 'standard' English more often than boys. Interestingly, this pattern continues through adulthood. Second, adolescent boys and men tend to be more verbose than adolescent girls and women, contrary to common belief. Third, adolescent girls and women tend to use language that expresses more uncertainty (e.g. they ask more questions) than men. Fourth, adolescent boys and men interrupt to suggest alternative views, to argue, to introduce new topics or to complete the speaker's sentence. In contrast, adolescent girls and women interrupt to clarify and support the speaker.[11] Moreover, women tend to sustain conversation topics longer than men. For example, research shows that 96% of male-introduced topics are sustained by females, but only 36% of female-introduced topics are sustained by males.[12] Finally, males place more value on status and report talk, competing for the floor in conversational interaction, while females value connections and rapport, fulfilling their role as more cooperative and facilitative conversationalists who are concerned for their partner's positive face needs.[13]

Some researchers attribute the gender differences in communication styles to the language socialisation process. Studies show that parents speak to their daughters and sons differently. As early as two years of age, mothers imitate their daughters more and talk to their daughters longer than they do to their sons. Fathers use more imperatives and insulting terms (e.g. *butthead*) with their sons and address their daughters as *honey* and *sweetie*. Fathers also use the diminutive form (adding a smallness suffix to denote affection) more frequently with daughters and interrupt them more often than sons.[14] There are also sociocultural factors that contribute to gender differences. In some cultures, such as in Africa and the Caribbean, women interrupt men far more frequently than in the United States.

Heritage-Language Pragmatic and Metalinguistic Developmental Characteristics During Adolescence

Pragmatic and metalinguistic development in more than one language is an intricate process. There are many complicated factors affecting attainment. Because there are more than one language and culture involved in multilingual development, adolescents who are exposed to more than one language not only have to master how their different languages are used properly within their specific linguistic constraints, but they also have to develop competence in how these languages are used in culturally appropriated contexts. In the process of mastering their respective languages, multilingual children and adolescents may bring their own contributions to the multilingual development process and thus form their own characteristics in multilingual communication.

Multilingual syncretic language use

There are obvious similarities between monolinguals and multilinguals in their use of language. However, there are also noteworthy differences between them. All things considered, multilinguals' language use is syncretic in nature. By syncretic, I mean that they draw multiple resources from their respective languages and cultures to form their nuanced and creative way of communication. In fact, communication in multiple languages is never a pure linguistic event. Instead, it is always organised based on the integration of a speaker's cultural and linguistic experiences. Multilingual speakers tend to incorporate more than one cultural value, belief, emotion, practice, identity and linguistic resource into the organisation of their communication. In other words, when different cultural and linguistic systems interact, multilingual speakers rarely simply replace one linguistic system with another; rather, their communication reflects the integration of more than one system. This unique **syncretic communication** may be the hallmark of multilingual communicative pragmatics.

Several studies have indicated the syncretic nature of multilingual children's innovative ways of using their ambient languages, which are different from their monolingual counterparts. For example, researchers examined the language use of bilingual Spanish-and English-speaking children, and they found that compared to monolingual Spanish speakers, the bilinguals used the progress relative more frequently and used the simple present less frequently than their monolingual counterparts in reference to time, which included the specific moment of speech.[15] Similarly, another study shows that bilingual Norwegian-and English-speaking children used durative expressions in Norwegian, a language that does not mark a progressive aspect like English. They also used the perfect tense in their English narratives more than is reported for monolingual children.[16]

Thus, heritage-language children and adolescents may incorporate their knowledge in different languages in their daily communication. Box 6.2 shows examples of Léandre and Dominique's syncretic expressions in their spoken and written communication.

Example 1 in Box 6.2 suggests that even though Léandre did not know the authentic Chinese expression 蟑螂的卵, he was able to gather his linguistic resources from two of his languages and come up with the expression of *cafards*的鸡蛋

Box 6.2 Examples of Syncretic Communication in Heritage Language

Example 1:

Mother: There is a cockroach outbreak in the neighbourhood.

Léandre (14; 3; 5): If you get rid of the <u>cockroaches' *chicken eggs*</u>, you will solve the problem. (如过把 <u>cafards 的鸡蛋弄掉</u>, 问题就解决了。)

Mother: You mean the cockroach eggs? (你指的是蟑螂的卵？)

...

Example 2:

[Dominique incorporated his cultural experiences into his college application essay. Below is an excerpt].

'I have seen the Great Wall of China, Versailles, Stonehenge, and other historical landmarks where the presence of the past is palpable; I have marveled at panoramas in the Vosges, the Alps, and other boundless vistas where the future lies before me...' [More will be discussed in Chapter 8.]

(cockroaches' *chicken eggs*). Similarly, in Example 2 (Box 6.2), Dominique was able to gather his multicultural travel experiences in his writing. These examples show that Léandre and Dominique were able to creatively transform their communication by using the knowledge in their existing pool of languages and experiences. Their expressions were nuanced and contextually appropriate.

However, when looking at the *cafards*的鸡蛋 example, one may relate it to a phenomenon called **interlanguage**, which has often been used to refer to the language production of nonnative speakers or new-language learners.[17] Because these language learners have not yet become fully proficient in a new language, they have their own unique way of using language by temporarily incorporating elements of other languages into their new-language. I, however, see a fundamental difference between syncretic language use and interlanguage. In interlanguage, nonnative speakers lack the intuition that heritage-language speakers have. Heritage-language speakers like Léandre and Dominique can draw from a wider source of information and transform their expressions in a creative way based on their linguistic intuition. Therefore, language creation is based on the structure of their respective languages, whereas nonnative speakers and new-language learners often lack that ability. Thus, I would like to argue that syncretic language deserves to be recognised as a unique communication system, and it is heritage-language speakers' own version of language use.

Multilingual narrative characteristics

Research on multilingual children and adolescents' narrative development is scarce. However, we are beginning to understand several aspects of their narrative characteristics. First, multilingual children and adolescents' narrative styles may be associated with their language socialisation experiences.[18] The input in the early years of their lives is important in shaping their narrative style. For instance, in some Latino families, parents tell traditional stories which differ from the narrative styles in mainstream North American families.[19] Moreover, multilingual children and adolescents' narrative styles are also influenced by their socioeconomic status[20] such as parental education levels, class and profession.

Second, although narrative styles may be influenced by cultures and socialisation experiences, multilingual children and adolescents' narrative structures tend to exhibit universal characteristics and properties, which are language and culture independent.[21]

Third, multilingual children and adolescents' ability to produce a narrative is more dependent on cognitive processes than on the specific language.[22] In other words, multilinguals' narrative structure in one language may benefit the development of narrative structures in their other language(s). Therefore, narrative scaffolding (support) in one language may boost development in the other language(s). However, narrative transfer does not necessarily happen automatically, and parental modelling is key. For example, one study noticed that Spanish–English bilingual children's English narrative performance did not impact their Spanish narratives.[23] Similarly, another study found that bilingual Russian–Hebrew children who attended the monolingual Hebrew preschool did not show narrative transfer from their Hebrew to their Russian. The reason is likely that these children's parents did not often use Russian to narrate certain events such as birthday parties, and instead, they used Hebrew to converse about such events.[24] In other words, these parents did not provide enough Russian narrative modelling at home. This same study also found that children who attended bilingual Hebrew and Russian preschool programmes developed narrative skills in both of these languages.[25] It seems that linguistic transfer in narratives may occur only when children receive narrative modelling, and only in such an environment can they activate and consolidate their various linguistic knowledge in narratives.

Moreover, multilingual children and adolescents may use different transfer strategies in their narratives. For example, they may use **forward transfer** (i.e. using mainstream-language narrative strategies to process the heritage-language narrative), **backward transfer** (use heritage-language narrative strategy to process mainstream language) and **amalgamation** (a combination of forward and backward transfer).[26]

In general, Léandre and Dominique's narrative style was influenced by English, their dominant language, during adolescence. They used forward transfer strategy in their Chinese and French narratives more frequently; that is, they used their mainstream-language English narrative strategies to process their French and Chinese narratives.

For instance, the data across their adolescent years[27] suggests that the overall story grammar (or narrative structure) in their Chinese and French is similar to their English.

Multilingual metacognitive development

Multilingualism enhances many metalinguistic abilities, such as sensitivity to the details and structure of a language, recognition of ambiguities and correction of ungrammatical sentences. Individuals who are exposed to more than one language are likely to develop metalinguistic awareness earlier than those who are exposed to only one linguistic system. Research shows that multilinguals tend to exhibit more advanced metalinguistic abilities as compared to their monolingual peers.[28] Below are some metalinguistic examples Léandre and Dominique demonstrated during their adolescent years.

Commenting on language-related phenomena and issues

Meta- is a Greek prefix, which means *after* and *beyond*. Metalinguistic ability means the ability to think about the language. Both Léandre and Dominique tended to think and talk about language-related issues and phenomena frequently. Video-recorded naturalistic conversations across seven years[29] have shown that on average, Léandre had 38% and Dominique had 27% comments on language-related issues in naturalistic conversations, which is salient compared with other conversation topics. Box 6.3 lists some examples.

Linguistic sensitivity and knowledge

Growing up multilingual, Léandre and Dominique consistently demonstrated their superb linguistic knowledge and sensitivity about their respective languages as well as the new languages that they encountered. Box 6.4 shows some examples.

Linguistic intuition

I asked Dominique (16; 1; 15) how to say abacus (算盘) in Chinese; he said that he had forgotten. Léandre reminded him. Dominique then commented, '对, 计算的板' (Right, computing panel or computing board). His comments demonstrated that he has a good intuition of the Chinese word 算盘, which literally means computation panel or computation board.

Metalinguistic reflection

Léandre and Dominique often reflected and commented on language-related issues (metalinguistic reflection). For instance, Léandre (15; 3; 26) commented that it was logical to use the measurement words or classifiers for 一杯茶 (one cup of tea), 一壶茶 (one pot of tea), and 一碗饭 (one bowl of rice), because the contents were inside a container. However, he commented that it was illogical to call 一辆车 (one 辆 car) and 一匹马 (one 匹 horse). Even though he was playing devil's advocate, I have to give him credit for constantly thinking about language and not just using a language 'blindly.'

Box 6.3 Examples of Thinking about Language-Related Issues

Example 1:
   We were watching the news while having breakfast in a hotel in Paris. Léandre (17; 0; 9) kept commenting on the anchor's pronunciation and word choices. In the same conversation, Léandre commented that in French, there was always an article in front of the name of a country, except Israel.

Example 2:
   I made shitake noodles for Dominique's lunch. Dominique (14; 8; 22) commented, 'This should not be called *flour thread*. It should be called *bean thread* because it is made with beans.' (这不应该叫面条, 应该叫豆条, 因为这是豆子做的.)

Example 3:
   I asked Léandre (16; 9; 30) to bring extra batteries with him for his SAT Math II subject test.

Léandre: It would not happen that the batteries would run out. (不可能没有电池。)

Mother: One never knows. What would happen if your batteries run out? (不怕一万, 就怕万一。万一没有电池怎么办？)

Léandre: 万一没有电池怎么办 sounds like a subjunctive mood. ('万一没有电池怎么办' 听上去好象 subjunctive mood).

Mother: Yes, it sounds like a subjunctive mood. (对, 听上去好象虚拟语气。)

Example 4:
   When Léandre and Dominique's Swiss friend David visited Basel, he used the word *tiptop* (in French) to compliment Léandre and Dominique's grandmother on her apple pie. Léandre (17; 11; 20) commented that *tiptop* was an English expression and this was the first time he had heard a French-speaking person using it.

Example 5:
   Léandre (18; 4; 20) told me that his French professor in one of his college French classes spoke like a native speaker. However, he betrayed himself by saying *un gifle* (a slap) instead of *une gifle*. He commented that no French native speaker would make such a mistake.

Example 6:
   In Nîmes (France), Léandre (17; 10; 27) commented on whether the î in Nîmes was originally double *ss*.

Box 6.4 Examples of Linguistic Selectivity and Knowledge

Example 1:

While waiting for the ferry from Dover to Calais, a message was announced in English, French and Dutch via the loudspeaker about a delay. Then, the same message was announced in a language that I was not able to identify with certainty. Dominique (17; 0; 17) told me it was Polish. I asked him how he knew. He said that he knew it because he recognised some words and phrases such as *dziękuję* (thank you), *proszę* (please) and *my* (we), and he remembered them from when he visited Poland five years ago.

Example 2:

When we saw a road sign that read *Cherbourg* on our way to Cherbourg (France), Léandre (12; 11; 19) wondered whether the name of the town had something to do with German because of the *-bourg* part of the word.

Example 3:

I could not find the ð symbol in my word file on my computer. Léandre (17; 6; 2) suggested that I Google the Icelandic alphabet.

Example 4:

On a tour bus in Barcelona, Léandre (17; 11; 30) turned the language channel to Catalan. He said that he understood 50% of the explanation because of his Spanish knowledge.

Example 5:

I was reading a story to Léandre and Dominique written by their Chinese grandfather. In the story, it mentioned that different words are used to represent *alley* in different regions in China. In Beijing (北京), alley is called 胡同; in Shanghai (上海), alley is called 弄堂; in Fuzhou (福州), it is called 街坊; and in Jiangsu (江苏) and Anhuai (安徽), it is called 巷子. Léandre (15; 6; 15) commented that the variations are due to dialect differences, just like the differences between English (*alley*) and French (*ruelle*).

Example 6:

On the ferry from France to the United Kingdom, Dominique (13; 0; 4) spoke with a British accent (the BBC accent), joking that 'We are from Westchester*shire*[30] and New York*shire*.'

Linguistic precision and reciprocal correction

In their everyday interactions with Philippe and I, as well as with other people around them, both Léandre and Dominique showed a tendency of correctness and sometimes overcorrectness in terms of language use. Further, correcting others almost became their second nature. Being frequently corrected by us in their heritage languages while growing up, they, in return, correct us as well. I call this **reciprocal correction**. Even when I poked fun by sometimes speaking French to them, they would answer in English (instead of Chinese) to respond to my inappropriateness in using a 'wrong' language. Box 6.5 lists some examples.

Box 6.5 Examples of Linguistic Precision and Reciprocal Correction

Example 1:

When we passed the French side of the Jura mountain range back to Neuchâtel (Switzerland), Philippe pressed the horn. I asked him why he did that. He said, 'I wanted to *see* what it *sounded* like.' Dominique (11; 1; 29) joked, 'Oh, we would like to *taste* what it *sounds* like.' He was indirectly reminding Philippe to use the right verb *hear* for *sound*.

Example 2:

When reading a Chinese text, Léandre (13; 6; 1) commented, 'It sounds better in Chinese and more logical to add an 又 (again) in the sentence "今年我升了一级' (This year, I am promoted to another grade): '今年我又升了一级.' He was absolutely right.

Example 3:

Léandre (14; 11; 9) corrected his Swiss grandmother by telling her that the correct phrasing would be *look for* a hotel, not *look after* a hotel.

Example 4:

Léandre's A.P. French teacher said, 'Il y avait une panne de power' (We lost electric power). Léandre (17; 3; 28) corrected him and said, 'You mean courant?'

Example 5:

Léandre (17; 22; 15) told me that his A.P. French teacher said 'appliquer collège.' Léandre commented that it was not an authentic French expression both from the linguistic perspective and from the cultural perspective. He argued that in French-speaking countries in Europe, the process of going to college is different from the United States. He said that the right term should be something like concours.

(Continued)

Example 6:
When conversing with a French-language professor in French during his visit to his prospective university campus, the French professor used English 'in French' while speaking French. Léandre (17; 8; 4) discreetly rephrased what he said, but deliberately said 'en français.'

Example 7:
In the Bundesbriefmuseum (Federal Museum) in Schwyz (Switzerland), I was asking a staff member at the front desk for a French-language brochure for Léandre and Dominique. I mispronounced *en français* as *en françaises*. Dominique (14; 1; 8) immediately corrected me, '妈妈是 français' (Mother, it's français).

Example 8:
Dominique (14; 2; 25) corrected his Spanish teacher by telling her it is <u>*la pared*</u> (wall) and not *el pared*.

Example 9:
Dominique (15; 9; 28) corrected me when I asked Léandre to fetch Dominique a 勺子 (spoon). Dominique corrected me, '妈妈是叉子不是勺子' (Mother, it is not fork, it is spoon).

Example 10:
Léandre (16; 7; 10) was proofreading one of my book drafts. He asked me whether knowing more than one language would make a person learn another language more easily. I was very excited to talk about it. Apparently, I mixed English with Chinese in the conversation. Léandre interrupted me and said that I was speaking Chinglish. Another time, I asked Léandre, 'Akira 给你写 email, 你有没有回?' (Akira wrote an email to you. Did you return his email?) Léandre (17; 6; 26) deliberately added English to his Chinese to remind me not to mix English: 'Yes, 我给他 reply' (Yes, I replied to his email).

Example 11:
Once an English-language learning friend of Léandre's used the present tense to describe something in the past, saying 'I *stick* something on the wall.' Léandre corrected him immediately, responding 'Yeah, you *stuck* something on the wall.'

Word creation based on multilingual knowledge

In Chapter 4, I discussed how Léandre and Dominique sometimes invented words for communication when they did not have enough words. They also invented words for fun. As young children, Léandre and Dominique already demonstrated talent in inventing interesting words for fun in their heritage languages. For example, they invented *fromage criminel* (criminal cheese) for *cream cheese* to indicate the 'criminal amount of fat in cream cheese' and *violonisateur* to indicate that Dominique played the violin so badly that he violated other people's ears.[31] As time went on, they continued to do so. For example, Léandre (15; 3; 8) invented *pédophage* and *puérivore* (child eater) to make jokes about their school bus. He said, 'The school bus is like a child eater. It eats students in the morning (when students enter the bus) and it spits them out in the afternoon (when students get off the bus).' What is amazing is the way that Léandre invented words. Even though his invention was probably only based on his knowledge in French, he indirectly used Greek and Latin roots via French; *pedo* (child) and *phage* (eater) are Greek roots, and *puéri* (child) and *vore* (eater) are Latin roots. Léandre and Dominique's ability to invent words demonstrated their metalinguistic knowledge about languages.

Linguistic humour

Jokes add fun to life and release tension. Being multilingual, Léandre and Dominique were able to profit from their multilingual knowledge in making jokes and bringing laughter and joy to their and our lives. Some examples are shown in Box 6.6.

Box 6.6 Examples of Linguistic Humour

Example 1:
Philippe said in the car that he was eager to change the *plage* (*track* also means *beach*); that is, he was looking forward to playing the classic music in the car using the iPad (old version) without looking at it. Léandre (15; 7; 25) said, 'Oh you didn't like Jones Beach!'

Example 2:
When hearing on the radio that doctors in New York were soon going to be banned from wearing ties, Léandre (15; 9; 1) commented, 'It is too *female* (formal) for doctors to wear ties anyway.' He purposely pronounced *female* with a French accent (it sounded like *formal*, but means *female*).

Example 3:
Each time we passed Besançon (France), Léandre called it Besan*con* (con is a vulgar word in French).

Example 4:
During dinner, Dominique (16; 0; 2) tested Léandre's knowledge about John the Baptist. Léandre did not know much. However, he (17; 11; 29) joked that 'John Batiste is the person who hit (*batten*) Jesus.'

(*Continued*)

Example 5:
Léandre and Dominique were discussing politics. Dominique said, 'The *left* always has good ideas.' Léandre (17; 11; 21) joked, 'Why then it is the *right way*.'

Example 6:
Dominique (16; 5; 10) put on a red scarf and pretended to be someone from the east side of Manhattan. He said in English, 'I went to see Monet's piece.' He then changed it to *'pièce de monnaie'* (coin) in French.

Example 7:
Dominique (12; 5; 5) joked by saying *Santa claws* instead of *Santa Claus*.

Example 8:
Léandre (15; 7; 18) poked fun at me by saying, '请给我一把碗' (Please give me one 把 bowl; the correct classifier is 只 or 个).

Example 9:
A French-speaking friend, David, called. Before he finished the call, he said, '*Nickel* (ok)' Léandre (17; 11; 20) said, '*Quarter*' (pronounced with French accent).

Example 10:
On the way to St. Malo (near Swiss New Normandie in France), we saw smoke coming from the distant fields where farmers were clearing their fields. Léandre joked, 'Oh it's Bushfire,' speaking with the accent of George W. Bush.

Example 11:

Dominique **(17; 4; 13)**:	今晚吃什么？ (What's for dinner tonight?)
Mother:	虾子, 磨菇, 疏菜炒粉丝 (Stir-fried shrimp, mushrooms, vegetable bean thread.)
Dominique:	噢, 我们吃草。 (Oh, we eat grass.) [Dominique was playing with the homophone of 炒 (stir fry) and 草 (grass).]

As seen in these examples, Léandre and Dominique used their multilingual resources to play with language in humorous ways, which either helped them occupy time on a long-distance trip or release tension in any given situation.

Flexibility in language response
During early childhood, Léandre and Dominique tended not to respond to nonnative speakers in French and Chinese. I remember that each year, when they had their annual

medical checkups, their paediatrician Dr Meyer would speak French to them. Detecting his accent, Léandre and Dominique would always answer him in English. Things had changed as they grew. For instance, Dr Meyer (who is multilingual) spoke Spanish to Léandre. Without any hesitation, Léandre (17; 10; 16) immediately responded to him in Spanish. Similarly, when Dr Meyer spoke German to Léandre, he (18; 10; 12) immediately conversed with him in German.

In Chapter 3, I mentioned that Léandre and Dominique had a neutral Chinese accent. They usually conversed with me in this accent in daily context. However, during adolescence, they tended to adjust their accent when speaking to other native Chinese speakers. For example, when Léandre (15; 5; 24) had a Skype conversation with his Chinese grandparents, they praised him, saying that he had made progress with his Chinese accent. Later, Léandre told me that he purposely pronounced certain words in a super correct way to impress his grandparents.

Self-correction or self-repair

Self-correcting or self-repairing one's mistakes in language use is regarded as a form of metalinguistic awareness.[32] Multilingual children begin to use self-correction or self-repair early in life and they learn early on to correct themselves when they use the 'wrong' language to communicate to an interlocutor or to correct others. For example, at age two years and five months, a German–English bilingual child, Laura, could self-correct, *'Adam gibt-geht auf den tree'* (Adam gives-goes on the tree).[33] Elsewhere,[34] I mentioned that by third grade, Léandre and Dominique began to correct their own mistakes as soon as they detected them in their own speech. When they realised that they made mistakes in their heritage languages, they would say, 'Excuse me, I think I should have said..., I meant to say, or I think I just used the wrong word.' They even joked that 'We need a vacation,' indicating that they needed to be in a French-speaking country or a Chinese-speaking country to refresh their French and Chinese.

During adolescence, self-repair in communication remained part of Léandre and Dominique's self-monitoring in their heritage languages. For instance, while Léandre was writing his college application, I asked him about his strengths. He (17; 3; 23) said, '我的語言能力和我的 travel 经历' (my language abilities and my travel experiences). He realised that he had used an English word, *travel*, and quickly corrected himself with '我的旅游经历.' Proportionally, I have seen an increase in the percentages of self-repair in Léandre and Dominique's self-repairs (Léandre: 10% and Dominique: 13% in adolescence and Léandre: 4% and Dominique: 3% in early and middle childhood).[35]

Regional differences in expressions

Because Léandre and Dominique's French input is mostly from their father and their Chinese is mostly from me, they occasional run into trouble with regional expressions. For example, in the Roman Amhethere in Nîmes (France), people under age 17 had free admission. When the clerk in the ticket booth asked Léandre about his birth year, Léandre said *'Nonante-cinq'* (95 in Swiss French) and the clerk did not understand him because in France, 1995 is *quatre-vingt-quinze*.

Similarly, there are also regional differences in Chinese. As a result, Léandre and Dominique sometimes had trouble understanding some regional expressions or pronunciations. For example, the word garbage (垃圾) is pronounced differently in mainland China, *laji*; and in Taiwan, *lese*. The word *potato* is called differently in different regions: 土豆, 洋山芋, and 马铃薯.

Eagerness to try out other languages

During adolescence, Léandre and Dominique were both eager to try out other languages. For instance, in Barcelona, Léandre (17; 11; 30) helped Philippe and I to communicate in Spanish with the hotel parking attendant, who did not speak English. The next day, he was also eager to help Philippe order his sandwich in Spanish in a restaurant. Sometimes, Léandre went out of his way to find opportunities to try out other languages. For example, a couple of summers ago, Léandre ran to pick up a ping-pong ball for someone in Basel, just to find an opportunity to try out his newly learnt Swiss German phrases.

Using linguistic resource as a 'weapon'

Léandre and Dominique sometimes used their linguistic resource as a 'weapon' to achieve the purpose of gaining the upper hand or for retaliation. For instance, in his senior year of high school, Léandre did not want to work hard on his bass practice – a daily 45-minute torture for him. He hated the written assignments given by his music teacher even more. To show that he was really fed up with the music assignments, Léandre (17; 9; 29) decided to write the assignments in French. His music teacher told Léandre that he had little power over him since he could not read French.

Similarly, using their accents for revenge is quite common for the two teens. For example, during a discussion at dinner about the topic of the news of Dominique Strauss-Kahn's scandal in New York, Léandre mixed lots of English phrases in his conversation. Philippe was irritated and commented that maybe they should all speak English. Léandre (15; 9; 11) began to speak English with a French accent just to mock Philippe and to get back at him for his previous comments.

Pragmalinguistic and sociopragmatic failure

In different cultures, there are different ways that men and woman use language to communicate. For instance, among the Carib Indians in the Lesser Antilles, males and females must use entirely different syntactic and phonological variations. In Japan, women and men's languages are differentiated by formal (syntactic) variations, intonation patterns and nonverbal expression.[36] It is not an easy task for teens to master the pragmatic aspect of their heritage language because they may not know the idiomatic expressions or cultural norms in male and female styles in the heritage language, or they may transfer their mainstream-language rules and conventions into their heritage language.

There are two commonly occurring pragmatic failures among heritage-language learners: pragmalinguistic failure and sociopragmatic failure. **Pragmalinguistic failure** occurs when the pragmatics used by a speaker are systematically different from those of native speakers of the heritage language or when speech-act strategies are inappropriately transferred from mainstream language to heritage language. **Speech acts** are a type of communication function in which speakers apologise, greet, request, promise, congratulate, complain, invite, compliment or refuse. Using speech acts in real-life communication requires not only knowledge of the language but also appropriate use of that language in a given culture. An example of pragmalinguistic failure can be illustrated by the transfer of the Russian word *koneso* (of course) when it is used in place of *da* (yes) in English. For example, one might respond to the question 'Are you coming to the party?' by saying 'Of course.' When *koneso* is transferred into English in the above, it may be interpreted as a peremptory response or even as an insult, as if the first speaker is asking a question that is stupid to ask or for which the answer is self-evident. **Sociopragmatic failure** refers to the social conditions placed on a language caused by different beliefs in social interaction. An example of sociopragmatic failure would be a Russian speaker asking an American for a cigarette based on the assumption that cigarettes are virtually free in the United States, as they are in Russia.[37]

Further, a speaker's emotive communication under any given circumstance is in accordance with cultural expectation. However, many heritage-language speakers tend to transfer their mainstream cultural norms to the heritage language. For example, research about Japanese new-language learners suggests that the Japanese English-language learners tend to have difficulties encoding affect appropriately in English. They frequently employ the following four strategies:

- They accommodate the English patterns.
- They avoid language specific features unique to English. They avoid using hyperbole and curse words in English. When it comes to the situation that requires the use of hyperbole in English, they tend to either simply avoid using it or find that they are not competent enough to express it.
- They overgeneralise English linguistic rules. They hypercorrect the tense match in English, which prevents them from effectively using the historical present as a linguistic expression of affect in English. This is perhaps because tense matching is not part of the Japanese grammar, whereas aspect is more predominant in Japanese.
- They demonstrate negative transfer from Japanese to English. They clearly indicate the negative transfer in the area of correlation between the intensity of aggression and the use of weakeners. **Weakeners** are discourse markers. They are also called 'intensifiers' or 'hedges.' Examples of weakeners are *sort of* and *I think*.[38]
- They use more weakeners when the intensity level of aggression increases.[39]

> **Box 6.7 Cultural Misunderstanding**
>
> **Example 1:**
>
> **American**: What an unusual necklace. It's beautiful!
>
> **Samoan**: Please take it.
>
> **Example 2:**
>
> **American teacher**: Would you like to read?
>
> **Russian student**: No, I would not.
>
> Brown, H.D. (2000) *Principles of Language Learning and Teaching* (p. 258). White Plains, NY: Pearson Education.

Thus, the process of mastering a heritage language is not only a linguistic issue but also a cultural issue. Box 6.7 lists two examples that illustrate cultural misunderstanding beyond the linguistic form.

The development of pragmatics in the heritage language can be difficult in the areas of apologising, thanking, face-saving, conventions and **conversational cooperative strategies** (people cooperate to achieve mutual conversation ends).[40] The conversational cooperative strategy is the most difficult for new-language and heritage-language learners to master. For instance, Japanese learners of English may express gratitude by saying, 'I am sorry,' a direct transfer from *Sumimasen*, because it conveys a sense of gratitude, especially to persons with higher status.[41]

Léandre and Dominique sometimes exhibit pragmalinguistic and sociopragmatic failure in their heritage languages, particularly in their Chinese (perhaps due to vast cultural differences). For example, Léandre (15; 3; 17) saw a Chinese student on his school bus who had just come to the United States. They conversed for a while in Chinese. In a disagreement, Léandre said, '操你妈妈的' (a very vulgar expression in Chinese that is equivalent to the English 'Mother Fxxxx'). In the context, Léandre had an obvious pragmalinguistic failure. He should have said something that was more appropriate, such as 去你的吧 (come on, get out of here).

Moreover, Léandre and Dominique sometimes had difficulty understanding cultural expressions despite the fact that they understood the literal meanings of the heritage language. Box 6.8 presents an example.

This example suggests that Léandre failed in the cultural aspect of communication. In Chinese culture, people often say or state the obvious in order to greet or to establish a relationship. You will often hear people greet each other by asking 'Have you eaten?' (吃过啦？) or 'Going to market?' (买菜去？). People from non-Chinese backgrounds can sometimes be puzzled by such cultural and linguistic behaviour. For example, in a flea market in Shanghai, Philippe wanted to look at some jade carvings.

> **Box 6.8 Example of Sociopragmatic Failure**
>
> When Léandre (18; 9;18) came back from his friend's house, I asked,
>
> **Mother**: You came back. (你回来啦。)
>
> **Léandre**: I did not come back [He said it sarcastically] and is it so obvious? (我没有回来。为什么你要问 这么明显的事?)

When presented with the object (which showed obvious carvings of snake or bat), the seller said, 'This is a snake and this is a bat.' Philippe said, 'I can see' indicating that he knew and there was no need to label them. However, Philippe did not know that this was a way for the seller to establish a relationship with him so that the vendor could do business with him.

Genderlect in French but not in Chinese

Earlier in the chapter, I discussed the genderlect phenomenon during the adolescent period. In French, Léandre and Dominique also followed the typical genderlect development trajectory by speaking like males. They used more swear words in French, such as *merde* (shit). However, in Chinese, their choice of words and overall conversation style tended to be feminine because their major input was from their mother (me). They rarely used curse words, except when joking or trying out some curse words they just learnt.

Linguistic interests and curiosity

Both Léandre and Dominique were fascinated with linguistic issues. However, Léandre was exceptional. He was always fascinated with phenomena that were related to languages. I often found him reading language-related issues online. Box 6.9 shows some examples.

Figurative language comprehension and use

Unlike younger children, multilingual teens may already possess good idiomatic knowledge in their mainstream language with the help of their cognitive advancement. However, they may not be able to understand and interpret the figurative meanings in their heritage language right away. They may first try the literal interpretation, and after that fails, they may begin to try other strategies. Heritage learners' ability to make sense of the figurative language use in their heritage language largely depends on their mastery of the heritage language. They may use cues to understand and interpret figurative language, such as vivid phrasal idioms, in addition to the pragmatic system that they employ in order to construct the appropriate cultural meaning of a given idiom in the heritage language.

Idiomatic understanding in a heritage language is a continuous and interactive as well integrative process. Heritage-language learners extract and produce meaning

Box 6.9 Examples of Interests and Curiosity in Different Languages

Example 1:
  Léandre (17; 3; 16) was fascinated with a *New York Times* article on the French signs in Quebec. He learnt that in 1977, Quebec passed a language law that requires that all large retailers which serve customers to signify their business in French. As a result, in Quebec, one sees the typical American retailers' signs translated into French; for example, *Staples* is *Bureau En Gros*, *Best Buy* is *Meilleur Achat* and KFC is *Poulet Frit Kentucky* (PFK). Léandre spent hours researching this.

Example 2:
  Léandre (17; 3; 15) became interested in Russian. He went online to learn the Russian alphabet. Every morning during breakfast, he used the Russian alphabet to spell people's names.

Example 3:
  During breakfast, Léandre (17; 3; 17) told me that he was interested in the tones in languages and he searched online about the tones in Chinese 吳語 (Wu dialect) and 奧語 (Cantonese). He was also interested in voices, and he found out that the Mongolian language has five voices.

Example 4:
  Léandre (17; 9; 4) told me that for two years, his friend Felipe taught him Portuguese every morning on the school bus, and that he taught Felipe French in return.

Example 5:
  Léandre (17; 10; 29) was fascinated with Chinese characters and tried to figure out how they were related to the meanings. For example, he was particularly interested in the symbols for 入口 (entrance) and 出口 (exit) when getting in and out of subway station in Shanghai.
  Léandre (17; 11; 2) sat in a tea house in 七寶 (an ancient town near Shanghai). He asked his Chinese grandfather many interesting questions about Chinese characters such as 泗, 魚, and 亞 that he could see from the window of the tea house.

Example 6:
  Léandre (17; 10; 22) asked me how to pronounce my brother's name, 砢.
  I told him that some people pronounce it as /ke/ and some as /ge/. He said this is an example of linguistic sound change. He said that he had researched this phenomenon online.

from a text and from what they bring to the dynamic act of reading by way of their prior personal and cultural background knowledge, experience, interests, values, and societal paradigms.[42]

Overall, as time went on, Léandre and Dominique developed a good understanding of figurative languages in French. Their figurative comprehension was on a par with their French counterparts who live in French-speaking environments. However, they rarely used French proverbs in their daily communication (in fact, not many teens who live in the French-speaking environment do this either). Moreover, although Léandre and Dominique understood the French colloquial expressions or idioms, they rarely used these lingos, such as 'C'est pire chiant, mec!' (That sucks, man!). When their Swiss friend David began to use this phrase, they imitated him. They also knew that these are expressions one should know but not use with everyone.

Their Chinese figurative language also made significant improvement. They generally had little issue with Chinese metaphor and simile (比喻词) and irony (讽刺用法). However, they did have issues with Chinese hyperbole (夸张词), such as *I am angry to death* meaning *I am very angry* (气死我了) and *I am hungry to death* meaning *I am very hungry* (饿死我了). They tended to interpret idioms (成語) literally. For example, Léandre (16; 8; 29) interpreted the idiom 拍马屁 literally as *patting on horse behind* (the intended meaning is to please someone). Also, I told Léandre that I was making my '拿手的麦片' (my <u>signature</u> granola). Léandre (17; 8; 3) asked why I wanted to take my hands. The literal meaning of 拿手 is *take hand*. Similarly, when I used the phrase 不对头 (something is not right), he (16; 2; 10) literally interpreted it as *not the right head*. Finally, Léandre and Dominique both had trouble with understanding and using Chinese proverbs (谚語), such as 杞人忧天 (unnecessary worries).

Misuse of culturally related polite forms and honorifics

Every culture has its norms in honorifics and polite forms. For example, in the Korean culture, there is a hierarchical relationship between parents and children, young and old, and husband and wife. There is an expectation about how people should speak to each other in terms of their status to maintain harmony. Social acts, such as the order of eating, greetings and farewell rituals, indicate hierarchical relationships. Korean speakers consciously mark these asymmetric relationships with appropriate linguist features, such as **honorifics** (linguistic features that mark relative social status and index social difference). Korean honorifics are a set of obligatory linguistic markings indicating relational sociocultural status (e.g. generation, age, sex and social status) across a range of speaker relations, including speaker-addressee, speaker-referent (person talked about) and addressee-referent. Koreans are socialised from childhood to display respect and deference to others by using appropriate honorifics. Thus, it is crucial for Korean speakers to use the proper kinship terms.[43] Mrs Kim's Korean relatives criticised her, saying that she had not taught her daughter properly because her 12-year-old daughter addressed her great-aunt as if she was her peer when they visited Korea.[44]

Similarly, not living in the heritage-language speaking environment and lacking models in everyday communication, both Léandre and Dominique had issues with the polite forms of *you* in French (*vous* [polite] and *tu* [casual]) and Chinese (您 [polite] and 你 [casual]).

Awareness of language-teaching strategies

Beginning in middle childhood, Léandre and Dominique became more conscious of our heritage-language teaching strategies. For example, when they came back from school, I made a snack for them. I asked, 'Do you want <u>one chunk</u> of bread or do you want <u>one piece</u> of bread?' (你要一块面包还是一片面包？) and 'Do you want <u>one box</u> of soymilk or do you want <u>one can</u> of soymilk?' (这是一合豆浆还是一罐豆浆？). Léandre (14; 4; 20) realised that I was actually teaching him how to use the correct Chinese classifiers (measurements words). He commented that our 'normal' conversation in Chinese is often Chinese lessons. He agreed that this was a better way to teach Chinese measurement words or classifiers.

Strategies for Supporting Multilingual Pragmatic and Metalinguistic Development During Adolescence

Because a heritage language is usually acquired in a non-heritage-language speaking environment, teens may speak the heritage language but act 'foreign'. Children and adolescents who acquire their language in the typical native environment acquire the style of the language use in the language-learning process. However, children and adolescents who acquire the heritage language in the home environment need to be explicitly taught about the pragmatic rules. Again, overt teaching is essential in helping heritage-language speakers learn heritage-language pragmatics. In the remaining part of this chapter, some explicit teaching strategies are introduced for you to consider.

Teaching cultural knowledge and cultural pragmatics through travel or involvement in local heritage-cultural communities

One effective way to teach cultural knowledge is to expose heritage-language adolescents to authentic interaction with native speakers and become familiar with cultural differences in order to avoid possible mistakes and inappropriateness in language use. Special attention should be paid to those pragmatic areas that are different from the teens' mainstream culture and language. For example, in Paris, Léandre ordered a *café au lait* (larger size). In fact, he wanted to order a *café crème* (smaller size). He was surprised when the coffee came and it was not he wanted. This example speaks to the importance of language and culture.

Therefore, it is important to expose teens to the native-speaking environment. Every summer, we make travel to native-speaking environments a priority and always make sure that Léandre and Dominique have opportunities to be in French- or Chinese-speaking environments. Over the years, we have found that these two- to three-month stays in the French- or Chinese-speaking environments make a tremendous difference in Léandre and Dominique's heritage-language use.

If travelling to a heritage-language-speaking environment is not possible, exposing teens to the local heritage-language community is also useful. For instance, Mrs. Cho took her daughter to her local Korean church weekly and arranged a weekly sleepover night for her daughter with other Korean–speaking families. The key is that teens need cultural contexts to learn cultural pragmatics.[45]

Teaching figurative language use in daily contexts

As discussed in Chapter 2, adolescents have many other things happening in their lives, and as a result, they may not have time for their heritage-language learning, such as figurative usages. One natural way is to support their heritage-language pragmatic development through everyday conversation. You can make a list of the figurative languages that you want to teach your teens and intentionally use them in your conversations with them. Box 6.10 shows two examples of how Chinese idioms can be taught in daily conversations.

Box 6.10 Examples of Teaching Idioms in Daily Conversations and Contexts

Example 1:

Mother: Dominique, did you brush your teeth last night? (昵可,你昨晚有没有刷牙？)

Dominique (13; 2; 20): I always do. (我总是刷牙。)

Mother: You must tell me *from five to ten* [idiom: *the truth*] (你要一五一十地告诉我)

Dominique: Of course. (当然。)

Mother: Did you *add oil and vinegar* [idiom: exaggerate]? (你有没有添油加醋。)

Example 2:

Our neighbourhood was having its water pipes changed. When we turned on the water faucet, the water came out in a thin stream. I commented to Léandre (18; 9; 7) that this reminded me of the Chinese idiom 细水长流 (The literal meaning is 'thin stream is slow but will last for a long time' and the intended meaning is 'If one saves, one will have money for a long time.')

Similarly, Philippe also taught Léandre and Dominique French proverbs when the context was appropriate. For example, he used sayings and proverbs such as *'A bon entendeur, salut!'* (a word to the wise), *'Un tiens vaut mieux que deux tu l'auras'* (half a loaf is better than none), *'Mieux vaut tard que jamais'* (better late than never) and *'Il ne faut pas vendre la peau de l'ours avant de l'avoir tué'* (don't count your chickens before they've hatched). We noticed that both Léandre and Dominique used these proverbs and sayings in their communication also.

Learning via media technology

Teens can learn many colloquial expressions, including foul language, in their heritage language(s) through media technology, such as the internet, movies and television shows. Dominique learnt a lot of French slang and foul expressions (e.g. *enculé, tête de noeud, connard* and *trouduc*) from watching French movies. Thus, you need to expose your teens to these colloquial expressions and even foul language via media technology and help them understand their usage in a proper context.

Engaging in metalinguistic reflection

Adolescents who are developing their heritage language have typically developed metalinguistic knowledge in their mainstream language (through schooling). Thus, you can encourage them to take advantage of this ability to analyse their errors in their heritage language(s). For example, you can ask your teens to identify their errors or you can hint at their errors. Encourage them to reflect on the reasons for these errors.

Moreover, encourage your teens to notice the differences between their mainstream language and their heritage language(s). You can ask them to use their smart phone, for example, to record their own conversation about a topic with you (the native heritage-language speaker), then analyse and compare the differences in language use. You can, for example, draw their attention to how many idioms you and your teen have used and how the use of idioms makes a conversation more vivid. I find family mealtimes are the best occasion for these types of activities and teens usually enjoy them.

Encouraging the use of translanguaging

Translanguaging refers to multilingual speakers' shuttling between their different languages for different communication purposes. The term translanguaging was originally used as a pedagogical practice in Welsh schools, where the language mode of input and output in Welsh bilingual classrooms was deliberately switched.[46] Traditionally, translanguaging is frowned upon in educational settings. However, it has been gradually recognised that translanguaging is a creative, pragmatic and safe practice.[47] Box 6.11 shows some benefits of translanguaging use in classrooms.

As shown in Box 6.11, the use of translanguaging in classrooms can help multilingual speakers make meaning, shape experiences and gain deeper understanding and

> **Box 6.11 Benefits of Translanguage Use in the Classroom Setting**
>
> - Students exhibited the ability to engage audiences through translanguaging and **heteroglossia** (the presence of two or more voices within a text).
> - Students used translanguaging to establish identity positions both oppositional and encompassing of institutional values.
> - Students recognised that languages do not fit into clear bounded entities and that all languages are 'needed' for meanings to be conveyed and negotiated.
> - Students used their languages for different functional goals, such as narration and explanation.
> - Students used translanguaging for annotating texts and had greater access to the curriculum and lesson accomplishment.
> - Using the translanguaging approach can promote both native language and second language development simultaneously.
> - In addition, the practice will make students feel that their native language is valued, and thus they are more likely to continue the development of their native language.
>
> Modified from Creese, A. and Blackledge, A. (2010) Translanguaging in the bilingual classroom: A pedagogy for learning and teaching. *Modern Language Journal* 94, 103–15.

knowledge of the languages in use as well as the content that is being taught.[48] Thus, the well-known bilingual expert Ofelia García[49] extended the scope of translanguaging to refer to processes that involve multiple discursive practices, where learners incorporate the language practices of school into their own linguistic repertoire freely and flexibly. It is clear that the act of translanguaging can create a social space for multilingual speakers by bringing together different dimensions of their personal history, experience and environment, attitudes, beliefs and performance.[50]

In the home context, it may also be necessary to encourage translanguaging; that is, to encourage your teens to use their mainstream language together with their heritage language to achieve different communicative efficiency. For example, teens can use their heritage language in daily conversations with you and use their mainstream language to e-mail or text you or vice versa. My personal experience with my two children suggests that allowing translanguaging in discussing complex topics and in writing has given Léandre and Dominique confidence to express their ideas freely. More will be discussed in the next chapter.

Using humorous materials to teach pragmatics

Teaching pragmatics and the figurative use of language can be daunting and boring. Therefore, choosing funny materials can achieve better results. For instance, Philippe used the jokes from *Le Chat* to teach Léandre and Dominique French figurative use of language.

A caveat to this approach is that jokes sometimes may not be politically correct or appropriate. You need to discuss with your teens the reality that improper jokes may cause offence. In fact, this practice in itself is a form of teaching pragmatics (using language in a proper communication context).

Using story or event recounting to promote multilingual narrative development

Narrative ability is an important linguistic skill for communicative effectiveness and social interaction. In other words, the ability to tell a coherent story and speak to the point affects how a message is conveyed and how the speaker establishes his/her relationship with others. Additionally, narrative ability is also connected to children and adolescents' school success,[51] such as literacy achievements.[52]

Compared to their counterparts who live in the heritage countries, heritage-language-learning teens are likely to be behind in their spontaneous narrative productions due to their limited heritage-language exposure. Hence, additional help is essential. Research has indicated that narrative styles are influenced by input styles and adolescents' familiarity with the story influences their narrative quality.

One effective strategy is to use story recounting to help heritage-language-learning adolescents' narrative development. **Story recounting** is a scaffolding process in which parents and adolescents coconstruct stories/narratives. For example, immediately after an event, such as after watching a television series, you can scaffold (assist) your teen to tell the experience/story to another person (e.g. to a sibling). Story recounting is particularly useful for heritage-language-developing adolescents who otherwise would not be able to narrate their experience on their own in their heritage language(s).

Using nonverbal communication to promote communicative competence

Heritage-language competency is not only restricted to the linguistic aspect but also the nonlinguistic aspect. Every culture has its distinct **emblems** (conventional gestures) that set it apart from others. The same hand gesture, for example, may have different meanings in different cultures. The famous American 'OK' gesture is an obscene gesture in Latin American cultures. Box 6.12 lists some areas of nonverbal communication.

To use a language authentically, a language user must also understand and master these nonverbal behaviours. It usually takes deliberate effort for heritage-language users to achieve nonverbal communication proficiency in their heritage language(s).

In this chapter, I have discussed the pragmatic and metalinguistic characteristics in typical language and heritage-language development as well as the supporting strategies. Although it is important to help your teens to develop pragmatic and

> **Box 6.12 Nonverbal Communication**
>
> **Hand gestures and body movements** Every culture has its distinct emblems (conventional gestures) and body movements. For example, rubbing one index finger on the other index finger means 'shameful' in the United States, whereas in Chinese culture, one scratches an index finger on one's cheek or nose. Nodding one's head means 'yes' among most Europeans and Americans, but among the Ainu of Japan, 'yes' is expressed by bringing the arms to the chest and waving them.[53]
> **Eye behaviour** In American culture, avoiding eye contact is impolite, while in Japan, intense gazing may indicate rudeness.
> **Proximity** The comfortable physical distance between speakers differs from culture to culture. In the American culture, the safe physical distance between people is about 20 to 24 inches. If it is violated, people feel threatened. However, in Latin American and southern European cultures, this distance is too great.
> **Touching behaviour** In some cultures touching signals a personal and intimate interpersonal communication.
> **Olfactory dimensions** In some cultures, odour such as perspiration is considered unacceptable, whereas in others it is acceptable and even attractive.[54]
> **Time orientation** Punctuality is understood differently in different cultures. 'We start the meeting at 8:00 am may mean different timeframes for people from different cultures. For North Americans, it means 8:00 am sharp, but for some Arabs and Latinos, this may mean roughly at 8:00 am.
> **Artefacts** Clothing and jewellery signify a person's sense of self, socioeconomic class and identity. North Americans tend to avoid being seen wearing the same clothes for two consecutive days and tend also to wear different clothing for different occasions. However, this may not be true in many other cultures.

metalinguistic competence, it is also important to stress that these abilities are not all or none. Rather, pragmatic and metalinguistic skills evolve throughout the adolescent period and beyond.

Useful Measures for Monitoring Narrative Development

In this section, I will introduce three useful measures to help you determine your teens' heritage-language overall narrative level: Narrative Assessment Protocol (NAP), High Point Analysis (HPA), and Narrative Scoring Scheme (NSS). Unlike the standardised tests and inventories, these three measures are more user-friendly and cost effective in measuring heritage-language narrative abilities. More importantly, learning how to use them will help you monitor changes in your children's heritage-language narrative skills and know in which specific areas your children will need support.

Narrative Assessment Protocol (NAP) measures the narrative microstructure; that is, how your teens use words, sentences and grammar in their heritage language(s). You can try the following steps listed in Box 6.13.

High Point Analysis (HPA) measures the narrative macrostructure. In other words, HPA measures the story grammar. In general, adolescents should have developed this ability in their mainstream language. Although their story grammar as developed in their mainstream language may be helpful in their heritage-language narratives, some language-stearic and cultural-specific narratives may need attention. For instance, the aforementioned narrative macrostructure is based on the English language. In other languages and cultures, narrative macrostructures may differ. Based on your heritage-language and culture narrative convention, you may want to focus on the quality of the story by analysing your teens' narrative structure completeness and complexity both in personal and fictional narratives. You can first ask your teens to make a personal or fictional narrative. Video- or audio-record the narrative and then transcribe it verbatim. You then analyse their story elements based on a 0–7 point scale (see Box 6.14). The more points your teens get, the better narrative structure development they have.

Box 6.13 Narrative Assessment Protocol (NAP)

Step 1:
Ask your teens to tell (narrate) a story based on the wordless picture book such as *Frog, Where Are You?* by Mercer Mayer. You can also choose your own wordless book or pictures if you think that your teens would resent the fact that the content is intended for younger children.

Step 2:
You either video- or audio-record your teens' narratives (using cell-phone video or audio function is convenient) and transcribe the narrative verbatim. You then examine the microstructure of their narratives by identifying various semantic and syntactic forms such as sentence structure (e.g. complex and negative sentences), phrase structure (e.g. prepositional and elaborated noun phrases), advanced verbs, modifiers and nouns (e.g. copula, auxiliary verbs and pluralised nouns). You then calculate how frequently your teens use each of the linguistic forms. You also calculate the total number of words used in the narrative, the total number of different words, the total number of utterances, and mean length of utterance. You can use this measure throughout the year to see whether your teens make any progress. Generally, you can identify areas of concern in your teens' heritage language and use the NAP to elevate and monitor the changes in their micro narrative structure.

> **Box 6.14 Narrative Scoring Scheme Scales**
>
> (Each of the story grammar elements, such as literal language; lexical, conjunctive, and referential cohesive devices; metacognitive verbs; and metalinguistic verbs, is scored on a five-point scale. Five points indicates proficient narrative skills, three points indicates emergent narrative skills, and one point means inconsistent or immature narrative skills.)
>
> **Introduction:** inclusion and description of character and setting (zero to five points)
> **Character development:** recognition of character's significance in the story (zero to five points)
> **Mental states:** frequent and diverse use of vocabulary to convey characters' thoughts and emotions (zero to five points)
> **Referencing:** correct use of pronouns, antecedents, and clarifiers throughout the story (zero to five points)
> **Conflict/resolution:** inclusion and development of conflicts and resolutions (zero to five points)
> **Cohesion:** sequencing and transitioning between events (zero to five points)
> **Conclusion:** closing the final event and entire story (zero to five points)
>
> Modified from Terry, N.P. et al. (2013) Oral narrative performance of African American pre-kindergarteners who speak nonmainstream American English. *Language, Speech, and Hearing Sciences in Schools* 44, 291–306.

Narrative Scoring Scheme (NSS) also measures narrative macrostructure. However, it evaluates more advanced elements of the narrative quality beyond story grammar such as literal language; lexical, conjunctive and referential cohesive devices; as well as metacognitive and metalinguistic verbs.[55] This measure is designed to be sensitive to changes in the development of narrative skills over time. A modified way of using this measure can look like this: You ask your teens to tell (narrate) a story based on a wordless picture book such as *Frog, Where Are You?* by Mercer Mayer. You can also choose your own wordless book or pictures. You either video- or audio-record the children's narratives and transcribe them verbatim. Then you analyse and score the children's narratives using the scale in Box 6.14.

Although the narrative measures introduced above can be used as a comprehensive way to monitor and assess the overall language and narrative development of heritage-language-developing adolescents, it is important to note that you may also want to become familiar with other standardised tests and inventories and use them to understand your teens' heritage language and literacy development at different levels. Understanding the languages used in these tests and inventories will help you better recognise the nature of your teens' heritage-language development, and the support you provide for them will be more focused and effective. It is beyond the scope of this book to provide a detailed introduction to these standardised language tests and inventories, but the appendix at the end of the book provides some basic information about them.

Summary of Key Points in Chapter 6

- Adolescents demonstrate increasingly polished conversational abilities in peer exchanges. They are more likely to respond to the feelings and attitudes expressed by the previous speaker.
- Adolescents' narratives show several areas of improvement. First, adolescents progressively increase their narrative length and number of episodes. Second, they begin to use more adverbial conjunctive links to enhance their narrative cohesiveness. Third, they become more aware of the interlocutor's mind in their narratives by including comments on the thoughts, feelings and emotions of the characters.
- Adolescents show a gradual refinement in figurative language comprehension and production, as evidenced in the areas of metaphor, simile, hyperboles, idioms, irony and proverbs.
- During the adolescent period, gender differences become more noticeable. The language use and styles of adult women and men begin to be observed in adolescent communication. Gender differences, or genderlect, among adolescents are shown in the areas of phonology (such as pronunciation and intonation), lexicon (word choice) and conversational style.
- When different cultural and linguistic systems interact, multilingual speakers rarely simply replace one linguistic system with another, and their communication reflects the integration of more than one system. This unique syncretic communication may be the hallmark of multilingual communicative pragmatics.
- Multilingual adolescents' narrative styles may be associated with their language socialisation experiences. The input in the early years of their lives is important in shaping their narrative style. Moreover, multilingual children and adolescents' narrative styles are also influenced by their socioeconomic status,[56] such as parental education levels, class and profession. Similarly, although narrative styles may be influenced by cultures, multilingual children and adolescents' narrative structures also exhibit universal characteristics and properties, which are language and culture independent. Furthermore, multilingual adolescents' ability to produce a narrative is more dependent on cognitive processes than on the specific language; that is, multilinguals' narrative structure in one language may benefit the development of narrative structures in the other language(s). Therefore, narrative support in one language may boost development in the other language(s). However, the narrative transfer does not necessarily happen automatically, and parental modelling is key.

- Several metacognitive characteristics have been demonstrated by Léandre and Dominique:
  - Comments on language-related phenomena and issues.
  - Linguistic sensitivity and knowledge.
  - Linguistic intuition.
  - Metalinguistic reflection.
  - Linguistic precision and reciprocal correction.
  - Word creation based on multilingual knowledge.
  - Linguistic humour.
  - Flexibility in language response.
  - Self-correction or self-repair.
  - Regional differences in expressions.
  - Eagerness to try out new languages.
  - Using linguistic resources as a 'weapon'.
  - Pragmalinguistic and sociopragmatic failures.
  - Genderlect in French but not in Chinese.
  - Linguistic interests and curiosity.
  - Figurative language compensation and usage.
  - Awareness of language-teaching strategies.
- Explicit teaching strategies that will help adolescents in their heritage-language pragmatic and metalinguistic skill development include:
  - Teaching cultural knowledge and cultural pragmatics through travel or involvement in local heritage-cultural communities.
  - Teaching in daily contexts.
  - Learning via medial technology.
  - Engaging in metalinguistic reflection.
  - Encouraging the use of translanguaging.
  - Using humorous materials.
  - Using story or event accounting to promote multilingual narrative development.
  - Using nonverbal communication to promote communicative competence.
- To monitor your teens' narrative development level, the following user-friendly and cost effective measures can be used:
  - Narrative Assessment Protocol (NAP).
  - High Point Analysis (HPA).
  - Narrative Scoring Scheme (NSS).

Recommended Readings

Liontas, J.I. (2002) Reading between the lines: Detecting, decoding, and understanding idioms in second language. In J.H. Sullivan (ed.) *Literacy and the Second Language Learner*. Greenwich, CT: Information Age.

Verhoeven, L. and Strömqvist, S. (eds) (2001) *Narrative Development in a Multilingual Context*. Amsterdam, NL: John Benjamins.

Notes and References

1. Owens, R.E. (2012) *Language Development: An Introduction*. Boston: Pearson.
2. Hoff, E. (2009) *Language Development*. Belmont, CA: Wadsworth.
3. Reilly, J., Losh, M., Bellugi, U. and Wulfeck, B. (2004) 'Frog, where are you?' Narratives in children with specific language impairment, early focal brain injury, and Williams syndrome. *Brain and Language* 88, 229–47.
4. Bamberg, M. and Damrad-Frye, R. (1991) On the ability to provide evaluative comments: Further exploration of children's narrative competence. *Journal Child Language* 18, 689–710.
5. Nippold, M.A. (2007) *Later Language Development: School-Age Children, Adolescents, and Young Adults*. Austin, TX: Pro-ed.
6. Hoff, E. (2009) *Language Development*. Belmont, CA: Wadsworth.
7. Nippold, M.A. (2007) *Later Language Development: School-Age Children, Adolescents, and Young Adults*. Austin, TX: Pro-ed.
8. Pence, K.L. and Justice, L.M. (2008) *Language Development from Theory to Practice*. Upper Saddle River, NJ: Pearson.
9. Nippold, M.A. (2007) *Later Language Development: School-Age Children, Adolescents, and Young Adults*. Austin, TX: Pro-ed.
10. Hoff, E. (2009) *Language Development*. Belmont, CA: Wadsworth.
11. Hoff, E. (2009) *Language Development*. Belmont, CA: Wadsworth.
12. Owens, R.E. (2012) *Language Development: An Introduction* (p. 387). Boston: Pearson.
13. Brown, H.D. (2000) *Principles of Language Learning and Teaching*. White Plains, NY: Pearson Education.
14. Owens, R.E. (2012) *Language Development: An Introduction*. Boston: Pearson.
15. Lanza, E. (2001) Temporality and language contact in narrative by bilingual children in Norwegian and English. In L. Verhoeve and S. Strömqvist (eds) *Narrative Development in a Multilingual Context* (p. 46). Amsterdam: John Benjamins Publishing Company.
16. Lanza, E. (2001) Temporality and language contact in narratives by bilingual children in Norwegian and English. In L. Verhoeve and S. Strömqvist (eds) *Narrative Development in a Multilingual Context* (p. 44). Amsterdam: John Benjamins Publishing Company.
17. Selinker, L. (1972) Interlanguage. *International Review of Applied Linguistics* 10, 209–31.
18. Wang, Q. and Leichtman, M.D. (2000) Same beginnings, different stories: A comparison of American and Chinese children's narratives. *Child Development* 71, 1329–46.
19. González, N. (2005) *I Am My Language: Discourses of Women and Children in Borderlands*. Tucson: University of Arizona Press.
    Schecter, S. and Bayley, R. (2002) *Language and Cultural Practice: Mexicanos en el norte*. Mahwah, NJ: Lawrence Erlbaum.
20. Dickinson, D. and McCabe, A. (2001) Bringing it all together: The multiple origins, skills, and environmental supports of early literacy. *Learning Disabilities Research and Practice* 16, 186–202.
21. Kupersmitt, J. and Berman, R.A. (2001) Linguistic features of Spanish-Hebrew children's narratives. In L. Verhoeven and S. Strömqvist (eds) *Narrative Development in a Multilingual Context* (pp. 277–317). Amsterdam: John Benjamins.
22. Schwartz, M. and Shaul, Y. (2013) Narrative development among language-minority children: The role of bilingual versus monolingual preschool education. *Language, Culture and Curriculum* 26 (1), 36–51.
23. Hammer, C.S., Komaroff, E., Rodriguez, B.L., Lopez, L.M., Scarpino, S.E. and Goldstein, B. (2012) Predicting Spanish–English bilingual children's language abilities. *Journal of Speech, Language, and Hearing Research* 55, 1251–64.
24. Schwartz, M. and Shaul, Y. (2013) Narrative development among language-minority children: The role of bilingual versus monolingual preschool education. *Language, Culture and Curriculum* 26 (1), 36–51.

25. Schwartz, M. and Shaul, Y. (2013) Narrative development among language-minority children: The role of bilingual versus monolingual preschool education. *Language, Culture and Curriculum* 26 (1), 36–51.
26. Ideas from Verhoeven, L. and Strömqvist, S. (2001).
27. Data are based on 28 hours of video recordings over a period of 7 years from ages 12 to 19 (4 hours of recordings each year).
28. Bruck, M. and Genesee, F. (1995) Phonological awareness in young second language learners. *Journal of Child Language* 22, 307–42.
29. Data are based on 28 hours of video recordings over a period of 7 years from ages 12 to 19 (4-hours each year).
30. We live in Westchester County in New York (the northern suburb of Manhattan).
31. Wang, X.-L. (2008) *Growing Up With Three Languages: Birth to Eleven* (p. 127). Bristol: Multilingual Matters.
32. De Houwer, A. (2009) *An Introduction to Bilingual Development*. Bristol: Multilingual Matters.
33. Gut, U. (2000) *Bilingual Acquisition of Intonation: A Study of Children Speaking German and English*. Tübingen: Max Niemeyer.
34. Wang, X.-L. (2008) *Growing Up With Three Languages: Birth to Eleven* (p. 161). Bristol: Multilingual Matters.
35. Data were calculated based on 64 hours of video recordings over a period of 16 years from ages 3 to 19 (4 hours per year).
36. Brown, H.D. (2000) *Principles of Language Learning and Teaching*. White Plains, NY: Pearson Education.
37. Baba, J. (2010) Interlanguage pragmatics study of indirect complaint among Japanese ESL learners. *Sino-US English Teaching* 7 (12), 23–32.
38. Baba, J. (2010) Interlanguage pragmatics study of indirect complaint among Japanese ESL learners. *Sino-US English Teaching* 7 (12), 23–32.
39. Baba, J. (2010) Interlanguage pragmatics study of indirect complaint among Japanese ESL learners. *Sino-US English Teaching* 7 (12), 23–32.
40. Grice, P. (1975) Logic and conversation. In P. Cole and J. Morgan (eds) *Syntax and Semantics* (vol. 3). New York: Academic Press.
41. Brown, H.D. (2000) *Principles of Language Learning and Teaching*. White Plains, NY: Pearson Education.
42. Liontas, J.I. (2002) Reading between the lines: Detecting, decoding, and understanding idioms in second language. In J.H. Sullivan (ed.) *Literacy and the Second Language Learner* (p. 211). Greenwich, CT: Information Age.
43. Park, E. (2006) Grandparents, grandchildren, and heritage language use in Korean. In K. Kondo-Brown (ed.) *Heritage Language Development: Focus East Asian Immigrants*. Amsterdam, NL: John Benjamins Publishing Company.
44. E-mail exchange on 2 February 2013.
45. E-mail received on 12 June 2010.
46. Williams, C. (2002) Extending bilingualism in the education system. Education and lifelong learning committee ELL-06-02. Retrieved from http://www.assemblywales.org/3c91c7af00023d820000595000000000.pdf
47. Crease, A. and Blackledge, A. (2010) Translanguaging in the bilingual classroom: A pedagogy for learning and teaching. *Modern Language Journal* 94, 103–15.
48. Cenoz, J. and Gorter, D. (2011) A holistic approach to multilingual education: Introduction. *Modern Language Journal* 95, 339–43.
    Lewis, G., Jones, B. and Baker, C. (2012) Translanguaging: Developing its conceptualisation and conceptualisation. *Educational Research and Evaluation* 18, 655–70.
    Williams, C. (2002) Extending bilingualism in the education system. Education and lifelong learning committee ELL-06-02. Retrieved from http://www.assemblywales.org/3c91c7af00023d820000595000000000.pdf
49. García, O. (2009) *Bilingual Education in the 21st Century: A Global Perspective*. Malden, MA: Wiley-Blackwell.

[50] Wei, L. (2011) Moment analysis and translanguaging space: Discursive construction of identities by multilingual Chinese youth in Britain. *Journal of Pragmatics* 43, 1222–35.
[51] Nippold, M.A. (2007) *Later Language Development: School-Age Children, Adolescents, and Young Adults* (p. 293). Austin, TX: Pro-ed.
[52] Klecan-Aker, J.S. and Caraway, T.H. (1997) A study of the relationship of storytelling ability and reading comprehension in fourth and sixth grade African American children. *European Journal of Disorders of Communication* 32, 109–25.
[53] Brown, H.D. (2000) *Principles of Language Learning and Teaching* (p. 262). White Plains, NY: Pearson Education.
[54] Brown, H.D. (2000) *Principles of Language Learning and Teaching* (p. 265). White Plains, NY: Pearson Education.
[55] Terry, N.P., Mills, M.T., Bingham, G.E., Mansour, S. and Marencin, N. (2013) Oral narrative performance of African American prekindergarteners who speak nonmainstream American English. *Language, Speech, and Hearing Sciences in Schools* 44, 291–306.
[56] Dickinson, D. and McCabe, A. (2001) Bringing it all together: The multiple origins, skills, and environmental supports of early literacy. *Learning Disabilities Research and Practice* 16, 186–202.

7 Multilingual Literacies Development During Adolescence

On the morning of Philippe's 48th birthday, he received a note (see Box 7.1) from Dominique (15; 0; 22).

> **Box 7.1 A Note Written by Dominique**
>
> Moi j'ai un père, et son nom c'est Philippe,
> Il est très vulgaire, et c'est un drôle de type,
> Ses besoins il aime les faire, mais il est propre son slip,
> Car il passe son temps sur terre, avec la goutte qu'il anticipe,
> Il a un énorme nez, plus grand qu'une montagne,
> Visible comme du blé, en milieu de la campagne,
> Il se fâche plus vite, que la vitesse de la lumière,
> Sa générosité est petite, comme les portions d'un resto cher
> Il n'a jamais vécu, donc ce qu'il fait c'est barbant,
> Mais il faut avoir du cul pour faire deux enfants,
> Son regard il menace, plus qu'un chien enragé,
> Mes couilles il me les casse, car il cesse pas de me corriger,
> Pour liu tout le monde est con, et tout le monde le fait chier,
> Quand il dit ton nom, il faut se méfier,
> Mais j'ai pas oublié maman, parce qu'elle aidé à me faire,
> Elle a sacrifié son temps, pour élever moi et non frère,
> Mais joyuex anniversaire, à l'homme de la maison,
> Je ne changerais pas de père, même si t'es un peu con!!!
> Joyeux anniversaire!
> Dominique

I will not translate Dominique's writing into English. If you know French, you know what it says. If you don't know French, please sound out the last word of each line, and you will find that most of them rhyme. Although Dominique's writing contains a few mistakes and is a bit vulgar, it is an amazing piece of spontaneous, funny, vivid, sharp and sentimental composition by a 15-year-old who, at that time, had not formally learnt to write French, did not live in a French-speaking environment, and whose major French input was from his father. In this piece of writing, Dominique knew how to use language to achieve effects in addition to creativity, such as 'He gets angry as quick as the lightning,' 'His nose is as big as a mountain,' and 'His gaze threatens more than an enraged dog'). As Philippe's French-speaking friend Gerald said, 'Chapeau!'(*I take my hat to him*, meaning he has my admiration). Yes indeed, Dominique absolutely earned my admiration!

This chapter is about the development of multilingual literacies. To be in line with the current trend in the field of literacy research, I use the plural form *literacies* instead of the singular form *literacy* to indicate that there are many forms of literacy representations, such as reading, writing, **hypertext** (multimedia text) and **critical literacy** (the ability to read beyond lines by critiquing texts in different formats, challenging the status quo and questioning authorities).[1] The chapter begins with an outline of the general adolescent achievements in literacies. It then focuses on the development and challenges of heritage-language literacies during adolescence. It concludes with some useful strategies and practical measures to help you support your teens' development in heritage-language literacies.[2]

General Developmental Characteristics of Literacies during Adolescence

In a typical language-development environment, reading and writing skills are developed and enhanced in the school environment. These skills gradually improve as teens advance in the academic subject areas. To a larger extent, adolescent reading and writing development is essentially their academic literacy development.

Academic reading

Reading in middle and high school is situated in the disciplines (e.g. in mathematics, biology, English, history and physics). Disciplinary or subject-area literacy is demanding for teens for several reasons. First, subject-area texts at secondary levels are mostly expository (texts that inform or explain things), and adolescents typically have fewer experiences with expository texts. Second, subject-area texts are often denser than narrative texts (texts that describe things). Third, the vocabulary in subject-area texts is often technical, and the organisation is typically harder to follow. For example, the multipart and unusual words found in history or science texts are difficult for adolescents to tackle. Finally, discipline-based texts often require readers to have some prior knowledge of the topic under study.[3] To be a successful reader in academic subjects, a teen must be able to exhibit the characteristics shown in Box 7.2.

Typically, adolescents become increasingly more mature and critical when reading academic texts. With proper adult support (especially teacher support), they are able to handle difficult concepts described in different text genres. They also begin to consider multiple viewpoints. By the end of high school (around age 18), adolescents can usually construct knowledge and understand what others have written.[4]

Adolescents' gradual improvement in their reading skills is the result of the integration of vocabulary expansion, morphosyntactic sophistication and pragmatic and metalinguistic development. By high school, adolescents usually can use higher-level skills such as **inference** (the ability to fill in information that is not overt) and recognition of viewpoint to aid in their comprehension of science and social studies textbooks. Some teens can also use the **theme comprehension strategy** (the ability to derive a more general message from a passage of text) to help their reading comprehension, although this is a more difficult skill to develop than inferential skills.[5]

Academic writing

In general, adolescents' writing abilities develop and improve as they engage in a variety of writing activities in subject-area learning. Some of these activities include writing reports and essays and editing and revising their own or others' writings. By middle school, the length and diversity of teens' writing productions increase, as advanced narratives and expository texts begin to develop. Some adolescents' narrative essays can contain temporal events unified by a topic sentence, elements of story grammar, character development, plot and dialogue. Their expository essays

---

Box 7.2 Characteristics of Successful Readers

- Know how to monitor their comprehension and use a range of strategies when they realise they do not understand what they are reading.
- Are able to explain concepts in the text and relate different concepts within a text to each other and to relevant prior knowledge.
- Can generate self-explanations during reading, ask questions that probe the connections among parts of the text or see explanations.
- Use cues to deduce the logical organisation of a text to guide their comprehension.
- Rely on multiple types of knowledge as they interpret texts by using information about words, concepts, sentence structures, text structures and genres.

Modified from Goldman, S.R. (2012) Adolescent literacy: Learning and understanding content. *The Future of Children* 22 (2), 89–116.

may include a unifying topic sentence, comments referenced to the topic, and elaborations on the comments. In these writings, adolescents' syntax production becomes increasingly more complex. For example, their clause length increases in writing, as shown by the increase in their average sentence length (7.7 words for a 13-year-old and 8.6 words for a 17-year-old). There is also an increase in embedded subordinate clauses and a decrease in coordination or compound sentences. Moreover, the use of relative clauses doubles between ages 7 and 17, and adverbial clauses, especially those signifying time (when...), increase and diversify.

At the phrase level, there is an increase in adolescents' use of pre- and postnoun modifiers. Adolescents can usually modify nouns with adverbs as well as adjectives and use four or more modifiers with a noun. They expand their verb phrases by the increasing their use of modality, tense and aspect; however, it is not until early adulthood that most people develop the cognitive processes and executive functions needed for mature writing. Adolescents still need teacher guidance in planning and revising their writing. By junior year of high school (the third year in high school), teens are usually capable of revising all aspects of writing.[6]

Moreover, adolescents' background knowledge is important in determining their writing complexity. For example, in a study, a group of boys from 9 to 14 years old were asked to write an essay on the topic of football. Half of the boys knew very little about football and the other half knew a great deal about it. The result showed that, in terms of their writing organisation and content, the boys who knew about the sport wrote better essays than the ones who knew little.[7]

Finally, compared with other writing genres (such as narrative and expository writing), **persuasive writing** (writing used to convince others) is more difficult and takes longer to develop. Even though persuasive writing is usually first introduced in elementary grades (typically during the third grade), it remains challenging well into adulthood for many people. The reason for its difficulty is that persuasive writing requires a writer to integrate advanced syntactic, semantic and pragmatic knowledge as well as flexible thinking, metacognitive skills and background knowledge. The writing needs to show organisation, logic and supporting facts. It must also be convincing and show consideration of opposing views.[8]

Hypertext development

As information technology increasingly advances, books and print media are no longer adolescents' sole source of reading materials. Nowadays, many adolescents are actively engaged in hypertext (also referred to as digital text, multimedia text, electronic text, web text, the internet-based system of communication or new literacies). As a *New York Times* article predicts, in a digital future, traditional textbooks could be history. Some educators have already noticed that students today do not engage with textbooks that are finite, linear and rote.[9]

Although hypertext involves the basic processes of reading and writing, it differs from print-based literacy in significant ways.[10] **Hypertexts** are multimedia and are characterised by multisequential text patterns, which present readers with an array of information options online. They are also highly interactive, allowing readers to make choices based on personal interest or purpose. Moreover, in hypertext reading, the reader's purpose and choices, rather than the author's, determine the reading sequence, whereas in conventional text reading, the author determines the reading sequence.[11] The multidimensional nature of hypertext may frustrate readers who are not instantly gratified in their rapid search for immediate answers, because hypertext and interactive features have too many choices and too many animations that may distract and disorient otherwise strong readers.

Reading hypertext involves high levels of visual literacy skills, as well the ability to comprehend multimedia components. Successful hypertext reading requires evaluation of text and nontext (graphics, multimedia and images), as readers must differentiate between important visual images and other information, such as beautification of sites.[12] Overall, successful hypertext reading requires readers to develop sophisticated comprehension-monitoring abilities that involve reviewing, evaluating and synthesising various **lexias** (specific blocks of text).

There are striking differences between reading online text and printed materials. Typically, the interactivity of hypertexts draws out readers' natural curiosity as they forge their own reading paths on the internet. Although some teens monitor their reading sequence and comprehension successfully, many others become disoriented.[13] Box 7.3 illustrates a common experience that many children and teens may encounter when reading hypertexts without adequate adult guidance and monitoring.

In a recent series of studies, researchers instructed adolescents and adults to visit informational, entertainment and commercial websites to complete a series of tasks, including online reading. Adolescents generally performed less effectively (with a 55% success rate) than did adults (with a 66% success rate). The researchers concluded that the difference between the performances of the adolescents and the adults was due to the fact that the adolescents had insufficient reading and information research skills, as well as less patience. Teenagers in the study also exhibited less tolerance for websites that they considered boring or difficult to deconstruct, and they gave more credence to visually appealing sites than adults did.[14]

Thus, although hypertext affords new opportunities for literacy development, it also presents a range of challenges such as the text formats, the speed of information, the purpose of reading and the ways in which to interact with information. All these aspects require a different thought process and skill for making meaning compared with conventional print.[15] It seems that teens may be proficient at using hypertext for a variety of reasons, but they certainly need adult guidance to use it more effectively, particularly in academic learning.

Critical literacy ability

Adolescents are increasingly exposed to readings that offer contradictory viewpoints. This requires them to critically sort through these different viewpoints

> **Box 7.3 Example of Hypertext Difficulties**
>
> Sara, an average reader, used the internet to research how lifestyle and personal attributes influence a person's health. As a starting point, Sara's health education teacher had pointed her to bicycle racer Lance Armstrong's official website. After staring at the screen for several moments, Sara clicked on the link 'About Lance.' She read about Armstrong's training with the US Olympic cycling development team during high school, and then clicked on 'Key Stats' from another menu of topics and discovered such random facts as Armstrong's resting heart rate.
>
> At this point, Sara was feeling confused. She clicked on 'Links,' faced another directory of topics, and aimed for the 'Shimano Components' link, without knowing why or what she might find there. To her surprise, she found a website offering the link 'Which Bike Is Right For You?' Sara's interest was quickly piqued; she had been begging her parents for a new bike for her birthday. Later, after spending time on the Shimano website, Sara realised in frustration that she had not accomplished anything related to her assigned topic.
>
> Sara, a novice hypertext reader with weak hypertext comprehension monitoring abilities, was confused by the many hyperlink options and made decisions that caused her to waste valuable time reading hypertexts unrelated to the assigned research objective. Her learning problem was compounded by the teacher's poor initial website selection.
>
> Example from McNabb, M.L. (2005–2006) Navigating the maze of hypertext. *Educational Leadership* 63 (4), 76–9.

and make their own judgements and conclusions about the messages, in particular the underlying messages. With increasing metacognitive development, teens are better equipped to ask questions spontaneously about what they are reading. However, adolescents still need adult guidance to rethink their identity as readers, and they still need adult support to develop critical literacy ability.

Developmental Characteristics of Heritage-Language Reading and Writing During Adolescence

Because there is little research information on heritage-language hypertext and critical literacy development, I will focus on heritage-language reading and writing development in this section.

Reading and writing in any language are secondary language skills and are built on the foundation of the primary language skills of speaking and listening.[16] Secondary language skills usually do not come as naturally to most children as primary language skills do. Thus, reading and writing requires considerably more effort than oral language in general. Deliberate instruction is often required, even though some exceptional individuals may learn how to read and write on their own without the benefit of instruction.

Although monolingual and multilingual adolescents all need intentional support in their development of reading and writing, heritage-language-speaking teens must double or even triple their effort to acquire their heritage-language reading and writing skills. These youngsters may acquire the conversational skills in their heritage language(s), but it may take them additional years to achieve the same degree of proficiency as their counterparts who live in the heritage-language-speaking countries. If no special support is provided, they may never be able to achieve reading and writing competence in their heritage language(s). Moreover, even with arduous support, the reality is that their heritage-literacy level may never match their mainstream-language (or school language) reading and writing development.

However, this seemingly 'hopeless' outlook should not stop you from trying to help your teens establish a solid reading and writing foundation, which may eventually develop when future opportunities arise. As a case in point, even though Léandre's French reading and writing level was way behind his English reading and writing level during his early adolescent years, Philippe nevertheless focused on helping him lay a firm French reading and writing foundation by frequently exposing him to basic French reading resources, such as reminder notes, advertisements, videogame instructions, newspapers, interesting French books for children and adolescents and popular comic books. Philippe also engaged Léandre in some basic modes of writing such as notes, birthday cards, e-mails, text messages and letters. Because Léandre had built a solid foundation for his French reading and writing, he took a French AP course during his senior year in high school and a French film course during his freshman year in college. Those courses provided Léandre with opportunities to learn to read and write formally in French. In fact, Léandre (17; 10; 11) did well on his AP French exam, and he got the full score on his college French placement test the first month of his freshman year of college. To this day, Léandre continues to improve his French reading and writing competency. In the coming years, Léandre is determined to bring his French reading and writing up to par with his English.

Heritage-language reading

There are several major challenges in the development of heritage-language reading.

Discrepancy between speaking and reading and writing

By the time children reach adolescence, they can usually carry out heritage-language conversations about everyday topics with their parents if the heritage language has been spoken consistently early on in their lives; however, there is typically a discrepancy between these teens' heritage-language speaking skills and their heritage-language reading skills. For example, we were sort of shocked that Léandre (15; 7; 6) wrote 'il y a' (there is) as 'y a,' even though this is a common phrase he had used since he was 18 months of age. This is perhaps because in speech, it sounded liked 'y a.' It is quite common for many heritage-language-speaking children and adolescents to have limited knowledge in terms of their heritage-language reading and writing or to be simply illiterate in their heritage language(s).

Even though parents try to support their children and adolescents' heritage-language reading development by sending them to heritage-language schools, many children's heritage-language reading abilities remain minimal. For instance, I have made tremendous efforts in helping Léandre and Dominique to learn Chinese reading and have sent them to the local Chinese-language school on weekends; however, the result was not ideal. By the time they reached the adolescent period, their Chinese reading levels had barely reached the early elementary level, while their mainstream-language English-reading level was between the 99th and 100th percentile (based on their SAT reading comprehension scores). The discrepancy between Léandre and Dominique's mainstream language-and Chinese heritage-language reading discrepancy was shared by other children who are learning their heritage languages in a place where another language is dominant. One example is Jessica, who is raising her daughter in New York with her husband. Jessica's daughter could speak and read English at a highly proficient level, whereas she could not read Korean at all despite the fact that she could speak Korean quite fluently.[17]

Differences between home and school contexts

The nature of the home context as compared to the school context is another factor that limits children and adolescents' experience with heritage-language reading development. Because of the context differences (mainly everyday communication at home and academic learning in school), it is difficult to for children to reach the same reading level in their heritage language(s) as their school language. Unless special efforts are made in this regard, it is common that heritage-language-speaking adolescents lag behind in their heritage-language reading development.

Language-specific features

Whether children or adolescents are successful in their heritage-language reading attainment is also determined by the similarities and differences between their heritage language and their mainstream language. In the case of Léandre and Dominique's two heritage languages (French and Chinese), their French reading abilities developed better than their Chinese, despite the fact that they had been attending the Chinese-language school on weekends and they never attended any French language school. The reason could be that French and English are alphabetic languages and share more similarities with each other than with Chinese (the logographic language), and it is easier to transfer reading skills from English to French than from English to Chinese.

Heritage-language writing

Like heritage-language reading development, heritage-language writing development also faces the same challenges. In addition, heritage-language writing development involves other unique and complex aspects.

Language-specific challenges in writing systems

Some languages take longer for children to master than others. For example, the Chinese language employs one of the most complex orthographic systems in the world. The complexity of the Chinese writing system has direct implications for those learning to write. The sheer number of characters to be learnt is truly formidable. It has been estimated that knowledge of 3500 characters is required for basic literacy (e.g. to understand newspapers) and a literate adult needs to be able to write more than 6000 characters in daily use.[18]

The mechanics of Chinese character writing is also daunting. The basic unit of character is the stroke, with each character consisting of as many as 32 or more strokes, with a mean number of about 8 strokes per character. Each of these strokes must be correctly positioned for proper production of the character. Moreover, there is a high degree of visual complexity in writing Chinese characters. One must remember the relative position of these components, and the relative order of the strokes used to form them. In addition, one must fit the strokes into the square shape that defines the character. This visual complexity translates into a significant hand-eye motor coordination challenge because of the need to fit relatively large numbers of strokes into a relatively small space.

Learning to write Chinese is further complicated by the fact that Chinese orthography is one of the most phonologically opaque writing systems in the world. A character often contains a graphic element (the phonetic radical) that contributes information about pronunciation. But since there are over 800 phonetic radicals, and because the radicals represent phonetic information in a sometimes irregular and inconsistent fashion, the information provided by the phonetic radicals is difficult for learners to adduce and is often unreliable.[19]

Thus, just learning the Chinese characters alone is a challenging task for Chinese-language learners, especially for heritage Chinese-language learners. It took a tremendous amount of time for Léandre and Dominique to practice writing Chinese characters. Even if they practised writing and remembering Chinese characters intensively for a period of time, they would forget the characters after a few months. Even though I am a native speaker of Chinese, I sometimes forget some Chinese characters because of my infrequent writing in Chinese.

Syncretic writing composition

Writing is never a purely linguistic event; instead, it is always organised based on the integration of a person's cultural beliefs and values. Multilingual individuals will always incorporate more than one cultural value, belief, emotion, practice, identity and resource into the organisation of writing. In other words, when different cultural and linguistic systems interact, an individual rarely simply replaces one linguistic system with the other, and their literacy activities tend to reflect the integration of more than one system. It is likely that multilinguals will use creative forms of literacy practices and transform their literacy experiences by blending their existing pool of languages and cultures. This phenomenon is called **syncretic literacy**.[20] A growing body of research has suggested that syncretic literacy is a common practice among children and adolescents who are exposed to more than one linguistic system and culture.[21]

Up until now, syncretic writing produced by multilinguals has not been fully acknowledged in the research literature. In writing, lexical-, syntactic-, and discourse-level components are integrated in the text generation process. For a multilingual writer, these multiple components not only interact within each language used (e.g. Spanish or English) but may also interrelate between the different languages.[22] Additionally, the development of the various language systems occurs in 'overlapping, parallel waves rather than in discrete, sequential stages.'[23]

Moreover, a writer with more than one language may write as a **conservator** (i.e. stick to the language convention of a particular language) and an **innovator** (i.e. create new ways of writing that integrate more than one linguistic systems). Below (Box 7.4) is an example from Dominique's college application essay, in which he interweaved language, culture, heritage and identity in a syncretic way.

Box 7.4 An Example of Syncretic Writing

I have seen the Great Wall of China, Versailles, Stonehenge, and other historical landmarks where the presence of the past is palpable; I have marvelled at panoramas in the Vosges, the Alps, and other boundless vistas where the future lies before me. However, there is no place where I feel more connected to the past and the future than in the insignificant apartment of my great-aunt, my dear 'tante Sabine,' in the outskirts of Basel, Switzerland.

Every summer, my family visits tante Sabine for an apéritif. She buzzes us in, and with a burst of youthful exuberance, I race up several flights of stairs, arriving breathless at her door. Tante Sabine and the portraits of my ancestors in the hallway genially welcome me inside. Then the magic happens. The portraits of Daniel Bernoulli, who made important discoveries in fluid mechanics, and of other Bernoulli mathematicians on the wall, focus their eyes on me. Looking back at their paintings, I see myself in them. Strangely, their motionless gazes fill me with a yearning for discovery. Despite the centuries that separate us, their intellectual curiosity remains alive in me. Far from frozen on their canvasses, they usher me into the present – tante Sabine's miniature universe.

(Continued)

> I follow the worn path of carpet to a patch littered with tante Sabine's extensive collection of brainteasers that challenge me to find new solutions. Every year, I sit on the floor assembling and disassembling various puzzles, lending only half an ear to the conversation of the grownups. My favourite puzzle is a round tray filled with different shapes in the colours of the rainbow. What I like about this puzzle is that I am free to find my own patterns of colours and shapes. Year after year, this particular brainteaser has taught me to focus, to be persistent, and above all to think 'outside the box' by finding new ways to put the pieces back into the box. It creates a frame of possibilities that I am free to tackle in my own way. Although this puzzle gives me a limited number of pieces to work with, every year I relish the opportunity to make something new and unique out of it. Most recently, I made an image that resembles the Milky Way galaxy. Just as our universe holds more to be explored, this puzzle is only a small, yet meaningful stepping stone for future endeavours.
>
> It is time to go. As we say goodbye in the hallway, I already look forward to next year's visit. Interestingly, tante Sabine's tiny apartment reminds me of the narrow part of an hourglass. Above me, rest my ancestors and their journeys. Below me, lie countless trajectories, one of which I will follow. The visits to tante Sabine's apartment bring a new and different focal point with new directions each time. The ancestors who greet me every year and the puzzles I avidly solve at tante Sabine's have provided me with an understanding of myself within a variety of contexts that are unique to my situation. I am part of something larger that carries me. My aspiration is to keep my awareness of the past I am part of and that lives in me while doing my utmost to reach my goals with the tools at my disposal. Many years down the road, my portrait will perhaps adorn the wall in the hallway of one of my descendants, inspiring a young, eager, and curious mind to make the most of his or her life.
>
> With even more energy than before, I run down the stairs, out the door, and into the larger universe, where infinite possibilities await.

Crosslinguistic writing transfer

It is a common phenomenon that multilinguals transfer knowledge of text-level conventions, such as genre-related text structure in writing.[24] There is evidence that adolescents can transfer spelling skills, strategies for making meaning and text-composition abilities from their stronger language to their less proficient language.[25] For example, research on bilingual Spanish-English adolescents' writing suggests that various levels of transfers were observed among the lexical, syntactic and discourse features within and among languages and genre topics. These transfers can be summarised by three key patterns that emerged from the participants' crosslinguistic writing:

- The impact of topic on rank differences for the various text measures across languages and genres.
- Evidence of language transfer/common underlying proficiencies, as indicated by similar writing performance in Spanish and English across genres.
- The participants' use of a basic, knowledge-telling strategy in writing across languages and genres.[26]

Moreover, research has confirmed that higher-level skills from a stronger language, including knowledge of genre, text structure and general composition skills, can transfer to the less proficient language.[27] Knowledge and application of general academic writing skills can traverse linguistic boundaries. That is, if children and adolescents are able to use more abstract lexical items, compose more complex sentences, and draft a well-organised, genre-appropriate text in one language, they are able to do so in the other. This phenomenon is called **common underlying proficiencies**.[28]

Partial competency in heritage-language writing

Writing is a complex process, and for heritage-language learners, it is even more challenging. Because writing usually does not happen frequently in everyday family communication, it is common that the heritage-language writings produced by many heritage-language speakers may be relatively unsophisticated in the lexical-, syntactic-, and discourse-level domains. The texts they write in their heritage language(s) may be considered incompetent or marginally competent. Nevertheless, even with minimal writing proficiency, the skills involved in heritage-language writing are valuable for their overall heritage-language attainment.

Topics and prompts influence selection of lexical, syntactic and discourse features in writing

Research[29] shows that topics and prompts may influence an individual's selection of certain lexical, syntactic, and discourse features. Certain topics may be more effective in eliciting more productive or more sophisticated writing than others, because these topics may be more engaging for individuals who are better able to identify with them. Moreover, certain prompts may also influence individuals' selection of vocabulary and syntactic structures.

In Léandre and Dominique's early adolescent years, they often spontaneously wrote about topics that interested them. For instance, Dominique was fascinated with the texts written by the French slam artist Grand Corps Malade. He spontaneously composed many verses in French, imitating the style of Grand Corps Malade. His selection of certain lexical, syntactic and discourse features in his French composition was a lot more sophisticated than his Chinese-school homework, the topics of which he had little interest in.

Writing block in Chinese

Because many heritage-language-speaking children and adolescents have limited ability in their heritage-language written communication and they do not have enough heritage-language vocabulary, sentence structure knowledge and writing skills at their disposal, they sometimes experience what I call the **communication block** (i.e. they stop communicating all together because of lack of heritage-language vocabulary or other skills). For example, I once texted Léandre (17; 5; 9) about a change in appointment time for one of his college interviews. Because I had just got a new phone and had not set up the language functions, I had to text him in English. He did not answer me, and I was worried about whether or not he had gotten the message. In fact, he had. The reason he did not answer me (he later told me) was because he did not want to e-mail me in English (at that time, the rule between us was that we wrote only in Chinese to each other), and he did not know the Chinese vocabulary relating to 更换面试日期 (change interview date). Thus, he decided not to answer my e-mail at all. My conversations with several parents who are raising their teens with heritage language confirmed my experience. One of them, Anna, told me that her 16-year old daughter stopped answering her e-mails written in her heritage language (Polish) because she did not have adequate Polish vocabulary to handle the communication with her mother.[30]

Compensating heritage-language limitation

Even though Léandre and Dominique sometimes had Chinese writing communication blocks due to their lexical and syntactic limitations, they were not passive most of the time. Instead, they tried to find creative ways to communicate in written Chinese. For example, Dominique (16; 4; 10) used Siri on his iPhone to text me in Chinese (he spoke Chinese and Siri helped him to write what he was saying). As discussed previously, Léandre used Google Translate to help him compose Chinese. However, Léandre and Dominique never used this kind of shortcut to compose their French. This is perhaps because of the alphabetic and logographic language differences. To write French based on spoken forms (e.g. *Il est facile d'écrire en français*/It's easy to write in French) is more transparent than to write Chinese based on spoken forms (e.g. 写中文很难 – It's difficult to write Chinese).

Chinese homophone spelling errors

It is a common phenomenon among native Chinese speakers to make homophone spelling errors (错别字); that is, they misspell words that sound the same but have different meanings. Often, children and less educated adults tend to make more of these mistakes. Heritage-Chinese-language learners like Léandre and Dominique tend to make even more mistakes. For example, Léandre and Dominique's common errors were misspelling 理 (reason) for 里 (meter), 真(real) for 针(needle) and 吃 (eat) for 痴 (foolish).

Strategies for Supporting the Development of Heritage-Language Literacies

Literacy abilities in more than one language are critical for the 21st century. Developing multilingual literacy skills will allow teens to become effective communicators, critically conscious citizens and active participants in today's globalised world. Despite many challenges, adolescents will have a great chance to develop their heritage-language literacy proficiency as long as they are provided with adequate support.

General principles in supporting adolescent heritage-language literacy development

There are some general principles that you can consider when helping adolescents continue to develop their heritage-language literacies:

- Refrain from criticising adolescents during their language-learning activities. In particular, do not criticise them in front of their siblings or peers. Try to be as positive and supportive as possible. Using humour to replace criticism tends to achieve better results.
- Value your children's opinions and allow choices and freedom when carrying out literacy learning activities.
- Provide opportunities for your teens to take risks in their heritage-language literacy learning and encourage self-exploration.
- Motivate your teens to be self-regulated learners (**Self-regulation** is a form of self-control or self-monitoring in the learning process, which consists of strategies such as setting standards and goals for oneself and engaging in self-motivated learning).
- Encourage your teens to work with other peers who are also heritage-language speakers.
- Help your teens develop critical thinking and critical literacy abilities while carrying out their heritage-language literacy learning.
- Use innovative methods and communication technology to engage your teens in heritage-language literacy learning.
- Link heritage-language literacy development to the needs of future career and life opportunities.

If we can remind ourselves of these general principles often when working with adolescents, we may be more successful in engaging them in their heritage-language literacy learning.

Setting achievable goals

Unlike heritage-language speaking, heritage-language literacy requires careful planning, intentional teaching and opportunities to practice. Thus, setting clear and achievable goals for your teens' heritage-language literacy learning is key. Achievable goals may be determined with some trial and error. For instance, the original Chinese literacy goal I set for Léandre and Dominique was to make them become fluent Chinese readers and writers; however, during their adolescent period, their schedule would not allow them to devote sufficient time for their Chinese literacy learning activities (as indicated in the sample schedule of Dominique's day presented in Chapter 2). Therefore, I adjusted the goals to help them build Chinese reading and writing foundations by working around their busy schedules.

Moreover, to make heritage-language reading and writing possible, adolescents themselves should be involved in the process of determining their heritage-language literacy development goals. Parents and children need to negotiate heritage-language development goals to make them productive. For example, the first year that Léandre was in middle school, I asked him to read and write Chinese every day after he came back from school. He told me that it was too much for him because he had a lot of homework and he also wanted to play and relax when he came back from school. In the end, we agreed to focus on Chinese reading and writing activities on the weekend.

Supporting heritage-language reading development

Because heritage-language-speaking adolescents do not have the same experience as their counterparts who live in heritage-language-speaking countries and are often not educated with the heritage language while learning their school subjects, it is more challenging for them to master heritage-language literacy skills, such as reading. Therefore, you may want to try the following strategies to support their learning.

Selecting age-appropriate heritage-language reading materials

To motivate teens to read their heritage language(s), it is important to select age-appropriate reading materials to make their reading experience meaningful and transformative.

First, reading materials should be enabling, which means that the text moves beyond a sole cognitive focus (such as skills and strategy development) to include a social, cultural, political, spiritual, economic[31] or historical focus. For example, Léandre read *La Nuit* (The Night) in French and found it a meaningful and transformative experience because of the knowledge he gained about the Holocaust.

Second, adolescents' reading materials should address the issues that pertain to them and that they feel are worth exploring, such as texts that help them make decisions, start them on the new path, shape who they are, change the way the behave towards other people, make them feel connected to something important, cause them to think the way they think or change them.[32]

Third, what they read should help them make a meaningful personal connection to their ethnicity, their gender or their peers. Adolescence is the time that they are striving to find their place in the world. Well-chosen reading materials may help fulfil their emotional needs and enhance their identity development.

Fourth, adolescents should be able to select their own reading materials. By doing so, they will feel empowered in their heritage-language literacy development.[33]

Finally, heritage-language reading materials should include a variety of genres such as adventure, science fiction, biographies, mysteries, fantasy, romance, comedy, tragedy and horror to help adolescents find their place in the world, encourage self-discovery (for example, explore identity issues) and build self-esteem and a healthy sense of self.

Adjusting heritage-language reading materials to fit teens' reading levels

Once appropriate heritage-language reading materials are selected, you may also want to make sure that your teens are actually able to read them. Given the limited heritage-language literacy proficiency of many adolescents, the heritage-language text level (such as vocabulary and grammatical structure) is key in determining whether an adolescent can comprehend the text or not. It has been indicated that if readers recognise less than 90% of the vocabulary in a text, then the text is too difficult for them. It is likely that many heritage-language-speaking adolescents will recognise less than 90% of the heritage-language vocabulary in the type of readings that are age appropriate. If the texts are too difficult for your children, you may consider simplifying the original texts to help them understand the content. However, simplification of a text for the purpose of helping comprehension needs to be approached with caution. When you simplify a text, the purpose is to eliminate the barriers to understanding, but you may want to be careful not to make the text too explicit, which will hinder your children's ability to infer while reading. Thus, it has been suggested that you should not insert explicit connectives such as *because* or *although*, so that your children are still able to deduce the relationships between sentences without assistance. When you simplify a text, maintain as much as possible of the quality and structure of the original text and remove only difficult vocabulary and complex sentences.[34]

It is important to mention that this kind of external manipulation of written input (such as text simplification) may have little effect on an adolescents' intake. Research shows that text length has a significant effect on a reader's intake,[35] in particular, for readers with less proficiency. A shorter text length may result in better comprehension. More importantly, a reader's background knowledge, as well as the use of pictures, graphs, charts, maps, highlighting, margin notes, titles and subtitles, plays a more predominant role in determining text accessibility.[36] You can probably try to do all the above and see which strategy works better for your children.

Teaching reading comprehension strategies

Recent research suggests that an explicit approach to teaching literacy skills, such as reading, is effective.[37] There are quite a number of explicit instructional approaches that have been discussed in research literature, among which two seem to be promising in the home environment: strategy-based instruction and discussion-based instruction.[38] Although these strategies are often used in classrooms, I think we can modify them for the home context.

Strategy-based instruction. The major idea underpinning **strategy-based instruction** (SBI) is to teach reading comprehension by focusing explicitly on teaching strategies to aid comprehension. It has been shown that teaching a single strategy tends to have limited effects. Instead, teaching multiple strategies, especially teaching the coordination of different strategies, tends to have better results. Box 7.5 shows some SBI examples that you can try at home.

When implementing SBI to help your children improve reading comprehension, you may want to be mindful of the following: First, effective SBI involves teaching multiple strategies and ways to coordinate them. Some strategies involve explicit attention to features of texts, such as cues to important content and the text's organisation. Other strategies connect pieces of information within the text, while still other strategies build connections to your children's prior knowledge and expectations regarding additional content. Second, coordinating multiple strategies requires your children to assess their successes and failures using particular strategies, understand if they have achieved sufficient understanding and what to do if they have not. Third, explicit teaching of strategies and their coordinated use is necessary for most children, especially when they are reading to learn. Moreover, your children need opportunities to practice the explicitly taught strategies and get feedback on their performances before they acquire these strategies (skills).

However, the drawback of SBI is that it is hard for your children to be able to coordinate multiple strategies. This is because SBI requires readers to engage with texts for a sustained period of time, which children and adolescents sometimes either do not do at all or do only in cursory ways. Moreover, when SBI is taught as generic strategies, children and adolescents may not be able to apply these generic strategies to different text formats such as newspaper articles, research reports, editorials and web texts.[39] Therefore, when implementing SBI, you will want to make sure that your children engage in doing the necessary work, as well as to expose them to a variety of text formats and scaffold their comprehension by using different strategies. This will allow them to generalise the strategies that you teach them to other contexts.

Discussion-based instruction. **Discussion-based instruction** (DBI) is a reading comprehension strategy that focuses on using dialogues to explore ideas and develop understanding of different types of texts. DBI encourages readers to become more active in articulating meaning in and around text and to enhance basic comprehension of the meaning of the text and make inferences based on the text. Box 7.6 shows a couple of examples in using DBI.

Teaching of vocabulary use to facilitate reading comprehension

Explicitly teaching heritage-language vocabulary can facilitate adolescents' vocabulary development and reading comprehension, especially regarding words that are long and uncommon. However, most of these words may be the combinations of

Box 7.5 Examples of Strategy-Based Instruction

Clarification, Questioning, Summarisation and Prediction (CQSP)

The **CQSP strategy** (**clarification, questioning, summarisation and prediction**) can be used for processing both narrative and expository texts. You can work with your children in a heritage-language text. You can help them monitor their reading to clarify that they understand the meaning of the text, encourage them to ask questions they have about the content, summarise the content and predict what will come next in the text.

Structure Strategy Training (SST)

SST (**Structure strategy training**) teaches how to use paragraphing and signalling cues to figure out the overall organisation of the information in a text. For example, paragraph beginning words and phrases (such as *in summary, first, finally, on the other hand* and *the problem is*) can be used to find out whether the text is presenting a problem and solution or is comparing and contrasting ideas.

Explanation Reading Training (ERT)

ERT (**Explanation reading training**) means that you can use explicit, direct instruction to show the purpose and function of different strategies.

Paraphrasing

You can orient your children to understand what the text says, i.e. what the basic structure and meaning of the words and sentences in the text are.

Putting into one's own words

You can help your children to use their own words to substitute the words used in the text and to make the content more familiar.

Elaborating and predicting

You can help your children make inferences that connect what the text says to what they already know or expect based on common sense and general reasoning heuristics.

Bridging

You can engage your children in understanding how different concepts and ideas in the text fit together. You can help your children achieve more sentence-to-sentence connections as well as a more coherent understanding of the overall text.

Comprehension monitoring

You can help your children think about what they do and do not understand and use other strategies to repair problems they detect.

Modified from the ideas in Goldman, S.R. (2012) Adolescent literacy: Learning and understanding content. *The Future of Children* 22 (2), 89–116.

Box 7.6 Examples of Discussion-Based Instruction

Using Cultural Modelling

The cultural modelling method can be used in literature instruction to help children and adolescents become explicitly aware of how they process a literary text. Culture modelling indicates that many of the literary devices that readers need to know to engage critically with literature are already part of their repertoire developed in the everyday context in their mainstream language community. You can help your children realise how the same language techniques used in their mainstream language are also present in their heritage language and how these devices can be used to interpret literature. For example, symbolism is a language device to which your children have been exposed in their mainstream language. Suppose this literary device is critical for understanding a particular type of literary text in the heritage language. You can begin by presenting a more familiar form such as the lyrics of a song, logos or advertisements, since your children already understand them. Building on their prior knowledge, you can then ask your children to discuss what the symbol means and how they know that it is a symbol. Through discussion (first led by you and then by your children), your children have opportunities to give their views and explain the reasoning behind their interpretations. More importantly, by making their reasoning explicit, they are able to apply the same thinking as they approach the texts under study.

Using Translanguaging

Because heritage-language-learning children and adolescents often have to do double work in learning the heritage-language literacy, it may be necessary to encourage them to use their mainstream language (the stronger language) together with their heritage language to achieve heritage-language literacy success. As discussed in the previous chapter, the use of the stronger language and the less proficient language alongside one another is called translanguaging. For example, children and adolescents use their heritage language in discussion about the reading and use their mainstream language (the stronger language) in writing or vice versa. Translanguaging use can promote heritage-language literacy development. In fact, a study[40] on translanguaging use suggested that the participants showed the following knowledge and skills through translanguaging use:

- Participants exhibited the ability to engage audiences through translanguaging and **heteroglossia** (the presence of two or more voices within a text).
- Participants used translanguaging to establish identity positions both oppositional and encompassing of institutional values.
- Participants recognised that languages do not fit into clearly bounded entities and that all languages are 'needed' for meanings to be conveyed and negotiated.

(Continued)

> - The simultaneous literacies and languages used in more than one language kept the pedagogic task moving.
> - Participants were able to skillfully use their languages for different functional goals such as narration and explanation.
> - Participants used translanguaging for annotating texts and other accomplishments.
>
> Moreover, using the translanguaging approach can promote both mainstream and heritage-language development simultaneously. In addition, the practice will make students feel that their heritage language is valued, and thus they are more likely to continue the development of their heritage language.

word parts, such as prefixes, suffixes and roots in alphabetic languages and radicals in logographic languages, with which your children are already familiar. Therefore, deliberately teaching children new words by accessing these words parts can facilitate their vocabulary development. For example, you can create a list for your teens and help them learn the meanings of prefixes, suffixes and roots. Alternatively, you can discuss the meaning of word parts each time they occur in the texts.

Supporting inferencing to facilitate heritage-language reading comprehension

Inferencing is a process of drawing conclusions by connecting related information that may be implicit. There is a connection between inferencing and reading comprehension.[41] Thus, inferencing abilities are crucial for adolescents to understand texts.

Several factors can affect inferencing: vocabulary breadth, grammatical processing and discourse compression (the most important factor). Heritage-language readers may find it difficult to extract information separated by multiple sentences, and in such situations, their text comprehension may break down. Usually, it is less difficult for them to comprehend when the inference is supported by information contained within the same sentence or in an adjacent sentence. Thus, explicit and direct modelling of how to make inferences is beneficial to heritage-language readers.

There are several ways that you can try to help your children develop the capacity to inference. First, teach your children inferencing strategies (see Box 7.7). Research has shown that these strategies, such as lexical inferencing, can improve readers' narrative comprehension.[42]

Second, **shared book reading** activities (reading together with your children and talking about the text) are also useful in helping your children build the capacity to inference. During shared reading activities, you can increasingly ask questions that elicit inferential responses, such as 'What do you think...' and ask your teens to pay attention to predictive inferences,[43] such as 'What do you think will happen based on what you know?'

> **Box 7.7 Inferencing Strategies**
>
> **Lexical inferencing** This strategy teaches students how to search for key words that allow them to understand the text better and the kinds of inferences that can be made from these words.
>
> **Wh-question generation** This strategy encourages students to generate their own queries about the text by asking questions (*who, where, when,* and *why*).
>
> **Predictive inferences** This strategy helps students to focus on sentence meaning by searching for key words surrounding covered sentences. For example, inferring that Simon had hit the ball (the hidden sentence from the surrounding sentences "It was Simon's turn to bat' and 'It was a good hit').
>
> Modified from McGee, A. and Johnson, H. (2013) The effect of inference training on skilled and less skilled comprehenders. *Educational Psychology* 23 (1), 49–59.

Third, thinking aloud can also help improve your children's inferencing abilities.[44] You can ask your teens to verbally explain what they understand about the story after each oral sentence is read to them. The advantage of this strategy is that you can get direct feedback about how well your children are doing with inferencing and what you can do next to help them.

Finally, you can support your teens' inferencing abilities by modelling how to develop a 'map' of events and place the core elements of an event in the middle and the optional or nonessential details in the periphery. This kind of support can help your children develop **script inferencing**[45] (inferencing from written texts).

Supporting expository reading comprehension

Compared to narrative text comprehension, expository-text comprehension is more difficult for heritage-language readers. The challenge of this genre lies in its use of complex syntactic structure, high-level and abstract vocabulary and assumptions of background knowledge.[46]

The **multipass approach** may be useful to support expository-text comprehension. This approach consists of three passes: survey, size-up and sort-out. In the survey pass, children look for information about main ideas and organisation by reading the text title and introduction, reviewing the relationship to adjunct paragraphs, reading subtitles, looking at illustrations and captions, reading summary paragraphs and paraphrasing the information. In the size-up pass, children skim the text to seek specific information for answering questions at the end of chapter or questions they have formulated in their minds. In the sort-out pass, children test themselves by reading each question at the chapter's end and checking off those they can answer immediately. If they cannot answer the questions easily, they return to the text section where the answers might be found and reread until they can answer the questions.[47] In order to make this approach successful, you may want to model it first by **thinking aloud** (verbalise your thinking) so that your children will know what is involved.

Building background knowledge for heritage-language reading comprehension

Reading comprehension does not only depend on the vocabulary size, sentence structure and organisation of the text, but also on readers' background knowledge. Readers are likely to comprehend a text about the Roman Empire if they have knowledge of Roman history. Heritage-language readers may often encounter difficulty in their heritage-language reading comprehension because they lack heritage-cultural background knowledge.

The **reading apprenticeship model** is a teaching method for adolescent literacy development, which is based on an understanding of literacy as a social, cultural and cognitive activity, mediated by settings, tasks, purposes and other social and linguistic factors. This model suggests that if children and adolescents are to become skilled readers, the invisible processes involved in comprehending a text must be made visible and accessible to them as they engage in meaningful literacy activities.[48] Therefore, helping your children build their heritage-cultural background knowledge is critical. For example, to help Léandre and Dominique understand readings about Chinese New Year, I had to help them understand many symbolic terms associated with the traditional Chinese New Year celebration events, such as how eating fish is associated with the symbolic meaning of surplus (the homophone of the words fish/魚 and surplus/余). This cultural background knowledge helped them comprehend readings related to Chinese New Year.

Moreover, you can also use heritage family resources for cultural background knowledge building. For instance, Léandre and Dominique's Chinese grandparents sent the boys stories about their childhood in China. This was a good way for Léandre and Dominique to learn their heritage language, culture, and family history. Most importantly, this was an effective way to build their heritage-cultural background knowledge.

Finally, you can use a **K-W-L** chart to help your children build background knowledge. You can help them answer questions about what they already know before the reading (K), what they want to know about the reading (W) and what they have learnt after the reading (L). If you do this consistently, your children will learn what information they need in order to comprehend what they read.

Providing both intensive and extensive reading experiences

There are two types of reading: intensive and extensive. Both are important for teens to develop their heritage-language literacy skills. **Intensive reading** is slow and careful reading. In many ways, intensive reading is more of a method of language study than a form of reading. Intensive reading is useful for language study because its slow speed allows readers to stop and look up new words in the dictionary and provides them with the opportunity to pause and carefully study long or difficult sentences to get a better understanding. For a heritage-language learner, this experience is necessary.

However, intensive reading alone will not make children and adolescents good readers. In fact, too much intensive reading may actually cause them to develop bad reading habits. For example, because intensive reading requires readers to pay attention to every detail, it often encourages the habit of paying more attention to the vocabulary and grammar of a text than to its overall meaning. It also encourages the habit of reading very slowly, and children and adolescents who become accustomed to reading in this way often never learn to read any faster. Finally, intensive reading tends to be relatively boring, so readers who fall into the habit of reading everything in this manner may ultimately grow to dislike reading.

The main purpose of most reading is to understand the meaning of a text, usually as quickly as possible. This kind of reading is called **extensive reading** – an approach that requires that a reader read quickly and in large quantities. Extensive reading is more like 'real' reading than intensive reading. To become a good reader, one needs to read a lot (entire books or magazines) instead of just short articles or passages from textbooks. Just as a musician must practice sight reading in order to understand the meaning of the musical notes and demonstrate this understanding while playing a musical instrument, a good reader needs to read a lot to recognise the grammatical structure of a text and understand its meaning at the same time.[49]

Moreover, extensive reading skills are essential to functioning in the real world (to obtaining a general understanding of a subject or for pleasure, for example). In a reading, activity, speed, enjoyment and comprehension are closely linked with one another.[50] To achieve in these three areas, proficient readers will not read word by word; instead, they will read a meaningful unit at a time. If they read too slowly, they will forget what they have read.

Research has indicated several benefits associated with reading extensively, such as building confidence, increasing motivation to read, facilitating prediction skills, developing reading automaticity, enlarging vocabulary and increasing knowledge. Thus, although it is useful for children and adolescents to read intensively when studying a text's grammar and vocabulary to get a better sense of their heritage language, it is more important for them to spend time reading extensively, focusing mainly on the meaning of the text, not stopping to look up every new word. Experts have suggested that more access to books leads to more reading, and more reading results in higher levels of grammatical accuracy, a larger vocabulary and greater reading comprehension.[51] Thus, in your children's heritage-language reading activities, you may want to consider balancing intensive reading and extensive reading activities.

Focusing on interests rather than analysis

Many children start as avid readers because they are able to read interesting books. As time goes on, some teens begin to dislike reading because they are 'forced' to read something in which they have no interest. For instance, Léandre and Dominique used to love to read; however, when they entered middle school, their zest for reading disappeared. Léandre (16; 4; 23) told the host of a dinner party we were invited to that he used to like reading, but school killed his interest because teachers always asked him to analyse and overanalyse texts. He was fed up with the literary critics. Likewise, when I asked Léandre to tell me the moral message of one of books in the *Les Aventures de Tintin* (The Adventures of Tintin),[52] he (14; 7; 27) complained that 'this is just like in school and there is no fun in reading any more!' However, teens do read. They read what they like to read. For example, Léandre would spend a lot of time reading popular music news and lyrics because he enjoyed music.

Thus, we may need to make heritage-language reading activities more enjoyable to motivate teens to read. Philippe was a lot more successful in 'luring' Léandre and Dominique to read French than I was in motivating the kids to read Chinese. He would tell Léandre and Dominique one interesting thing from a text that he wanted them to read and urged Léandre and Dominique to find out about the rest on their own. For example, Philippe read Léandre a few excerpts from the French book *La Nuit*, in which Léandre was interested, and Philippe then left the book for him. Léandre read it himself.

Using the everyday context to teach heritage-language reading

The everyday context is the best opportunity for your children to get used to heritage-language reading because it is natural and relevant. Philippe and I often left notes for Léandre and Dominique in their heritage languages, making it a necessity for them to read. For example, I left notes for Léandre (14; 6; 2) about where to find his lunch when I was in my office, and Philippe left notes for Dominique (12; 8; 11) about his soccer tournament schedule.

Also, we often used everyday opportunities and a variety of everyday materials to encourage reading. For example, Philippe asked Léandre (15; 1; 0) to read the *Leckerli*[53] ingredients in French when we bought them from Migros,[54] and he also asked Léandre (16; 1; 21) to read the ingredients of the Engadine nut[55] cake in French while eating it. Similarly, while driving to Le Mans (France), we received some French advertising materials from the ticket booth. Philippe asked Léandre (14; 11; 18) to read the advertisements to him. Over the years, we realised that this everyday reading has contributed to the boys' heritage-language reading development.

Encouraging the habit of reading

Reading, including heritage-language reading, should not be a chore and it should become a habit. To make reading a habit, the best thing is to make reading materials available. For example, you can put heritage-language newspapers and other reading materials on the dining table and in the bathroom. I noticed both Léandre and Dominique read the materials, such as newspapers, that we intentionally left on the dining table. Dominique usually read the sports section and Léandre liked to read the business section, especially when it included news on technology.

Supporting heritage-language writing development

Writing in one's heritage language is challenging but essential if children and adolescents are to become more advanced in their heritage language. As they enter the adolescent period, children gradually move from learning to write to writing to learn. Heritage-language learners have quite a bit of work to do in order to increase their literate vocabularies, acquire more sophisticated syntactic structures and shift from a knowledge-telling to a knowledge-transforming composition strategy.[56] Thus, you need to support them in the development of these areas by trying the following strategies.

Teaching writing skills

Although grammar is an important component in writing, learning how to write is a very difficult skill to develop. Research in writing instruction has indicated that children and adolescents do benefit from direct teaching in writing strategies and structured writing practice rather than just being given time to write or to engage in free writing activities.[57] Generally speaking, when children and adolescents are engaged with personally meaningful topics and are supported with detailed prompts, they can produce authentic writing.

Thus, supporting teens' heritage-language writing development requires direct teaching and guided practice in all stages of the writing process: planning, composing and revising. In the planning stage, you can teach your children how to organise their main ideas by using graphics, or you can utilise computer software such as Inspiration and Kidspiration to help them organise what they want to write about. Moreover, it is helpful to provide your children with a template so that they can use it as a guide to organise their ideas before writing. Furthermore, they need to consider the text genre, purpose and audience of their writing. At the composition stage, you can provide direct teaching and meaningful heritage-language vocabulary and sentence and text structures, using, for example, sentence or paragraph frames and sentence-combining activities. Finally, in the interactive revision stage, you can use strategies such as parent–child collaborative sentence editing. This will provide opportunities to review and practice key lexical, syntactic and discourse structures as your children revise their writing. The writing skills that you help your children develop in their heritage language will also benefit their writing skills in their mainstream language.

Being cognizant of possible cultural rhetorical style differences

Earlier research[58] in writing styles suggests that writers from different cultural and linguistic backgrounds exhibit different writing styles. For example, Arabic-speaking writers made extensive use of coordination, which was considered excessive by English academic standards. Chinese- and Japanese-speaking writers tended to circle around a topic and argument, rather than approach it head on or introduce an explicit argument, as is the expectation of English academic writing. Speakers of French and Spanish tended to digress in exposing a topic or argument in writing, often introducing extraneous material more frequently than did English-speaking academic writers. Subsequent studies[59] found that Anglo-American essay writers generally prereveal their purposes or arguments quite early in their texts, adhering to a predominantly deductive rhetorical structure. In contrast, Japanese and Korean writers consistently delay revealing their purposes for writing until the end of their texts, preferring an inductive rhetorical pattern.

In recent years, some researchers have challenged the findings of the earlier studies. They argued that the previous studies were culturally deterministic,[60] and the texts produced by writers from different cultures were treated as static.[61] In fact, some studies found that Japanese speakers could successfully transfer deductive features from Japanese into their English writing.[62]

Whether we agree or disagree with these studies, what we can learn from them is that we should not presuppose that children from a given linguistic or cultural background will necessarily experience the same challenges of the rhetorical style in their other language writing. However, knowing how patterns of organisation in written language differ crossculturally and crosslinguistically can help our children and us understand the diverse ways in which writers make meaning in and across languages and literacies. This requires talking about and making our children aware of the possible differences in the rhetorical styles in different languages (the mainstream language and the heritage language) and helping them become authentic and creative writers in their respective languages.

Encouraging crosslinguistic comparison

Shared linguistic and conceptual structures may serve as common underlying proficiencies[63] that can transfer across languages. These common underlying proficiencies may include phonological awareness,[64] vocabulary depth,[65] and knowledge of text-level conventions in writing, such as genre-related text structure,[66] although syntax has been viewed as a language-independent structure.[67] Thus, these common underlying proficiencies may help expedite adolescents' ability to compose texts in their heritage language(s).

Research[68] in bilingual writing suggests that children are able to transfer knowledge and skills from their stronger language (first language) writing to their less proficient language (second or new language) writing in both elementary and secondary grades, and older children can transfer spelling skills, strategies for making meaning and text-composition abilities in their first language to their second (new) language.[69] When older children experienced difficulty with writing, their difficulty was most likely due to faulty composing processes (e.g. difficulty with paragraph and text structure and text organisation in both languages) rather than language-specific factors (e.g. vocabulary or syntax). These findings show that text-related common underlying proficiencies may be present in writing across both languages and also suggest that higher-level cognitive processes (such as phonological processing, spelling and concepts of print) and concepts are likely to transfer across languages.

Thus, to help your teens transfer the various linguistic features (i.e. lexical, syntactic and discourse) in their mainstream-language literacy (in which they are often more proficient) to their heritage language (in which they are often less proficient), it may be helpful to provide them with opportunities to make explicit comparisons and contrasts between lexical and morphosyntactic features across the mainstream-language and heritage-language systems. Research suggests that structured translation activities may support this process. For example, in the area of writing, understanding of communicative functions, genre conventions and text organisation and structure may be emphasised. These aspects of language knowledge might serve as general linguistic resources that your teens can apply to writing in both their mainstream and heritage languages.[70]

Scaffolding and modelling heritage-language writing

Writing is a long, gradual, successive and continuous process. Even though heritage-language-speaking adolescents typically have developed abilities in planning, organising and revising their writing in their mainstream language, which is taught in school, they will still need parental scaffolding and opportunities to write in their heritage language. You can try the following steps when scaffolding your teens' heritage-language writing development:[71]

- Give teens writing tasks that are appropriately challenging for their level. If a writing task is too easy, they will not make the necessary effort, and if a writing task is too difficult, they will give up quickly.
- Encourage adolescents to take ownership of what they are writing and inspire them to write about things that matter to them.
- Help adolescents focus on the most important parts of the writing task by first simplifying the writing task and then letting them practice and perfect the skills that they can manage; this is called **reducing degrees of freedom**. However, it is important to remember that you must help your children move on to new challenges as soon as they master the skills that they initially try to master. The goal of reducing degrees of freedom is to use simple writing tasks as a stepping stone to more challenging tasks.
- Provide direct feedback that prompts your children to pay attention to areas that need improvement so that they can continue to make progress. Your feedback should not only focus on surface level corrections, such as punctuation, grammar, words or phrases; rather, your feedback should aim to help improve the overall quality of their writing. For example, you can help your children understand which parts of their writing need attention and provide guidance and examples of how they can revise.
- Help your children understand important aspects of their writing and assess why they have difficulty. You can guide your children to the parts of the composition that have potential but are not yet quite there yet. Help them figure out which sections or parts need to be expanded and which need to be

shrunk, and then determine various possible arrangements and rearrangements of these sections.[72]
- Provide good samples of writing for your children. There are different ways to do this. You can model how to write. For example, Léandre and Dominique's Swiss friend David once sent Dominique (13; 2; 23) a message from his Facebook in French. Although Dominique could read it, he could not write back to David in French in the way he wanted (or in 'good French,' to use Dominique's words). Philippe helped Dominique return messages to David. This type of scaffolding and modelling not only helps teens to observe and learn the heritage-language writing but also helps them to build confidence. You can also use exemplary writings from a newspaper, commentary and peers. The goal is to show what exemplary writing should look like. For example, each time I found a good sample of writing in Chinese, I drew Léandre and Dominique's attention to it. I pointed out the places where I liked the writing and the way the author used the vocabulary. Some parents choose to do what I did regularly as a way of helping their teens develop heritage-language writing. For instance, Karen,[73] whose family lives in Beijing, developed a routine to analyse one exemplary article in the *New York Times Sunday Review* per week as a way to help her 14-year-old daughter to develop her English writing competency. You can also encourage your children to copy sentences, words and paragraphs from an exemplary piece of writing in a notebook and emulate these aspects of the text in their own writing.
- Help your children to integrate what they know and what they will learn and to avoid concentrating on writing skills that are irrelevant to the current task.

Encouraging writing by focusing on teens' interests

Parents of adolescents (including myself) often complain that our teens do not write or write enough. However, 93% of teens do write, and they write for their own pleasure.[74] For example, Léandre spent many hours during his high-school senior year writing lyrics for his band, and Dominique spent even more hours writing play scripts and rap lyrics. Many adolescents like Léandre and Dominique are already engaged in literacy activities and spend a considerable amount of time composing digital texts. In fact, adolescents nowadays write more than ever in history,[75] despite the fact that their writing may not be valued as formal or academic writing. Thus, if we encourage teens to build on what they are interested in writing about or what they are already doing, they may become more involved in the writing process. It is a general principle that people learn by pulling themselves into new understanding using their existing knowledge as a framework. It is more effective if we acknowledge teens' activities and interests when supporting them in developing their heritage-language writing.

One efficient way to engage adolescents in writing is through popular culture since most of them have special interests in that topic already. For example, fan fiction has recently been introduced and discussed in educational literature.[76]

Fan fiction is a text written by fans of the original work, but these fans add their own versions of creativity and twist to the original piece. Fan fiction can appear as stories, novels, comics, games or other media properties. Fan fiction writers post their work on the internet (www.FanFiction.net). Encouraging and scaffolding adolescents to participate in fan-fiction writing in their heritage language can make adolescents more interested in writing and help them develop skills necessary for their heritage-language writing development.

There are several unique advantages to fan-fiction writing.[77] First, fan-fiction writing motivates adolescents because it offers multiple modes of representation (e.g. stories, cartoons, novels, musicals) and diverse pathways to participation (participatory culture building as a writer, reader or critic). Second, it fosters an excellent learning community in **online affinity spaces** (virtual space where informal learning takes place),[78] in which adolescents can share their work, build peer social networks and develop collaboration abilities. Third, it helps adolescents to see the real purpose of writing. Fourth, it helps adolescents to identify their strengths and the areas of writing in which they need improvement through peer critique and interaction. Finally, it can help teens develop literacy abilities such as creatively using supportive dialogue, strong vocabulary, cohesive storylines and critical literacy.

Support emotional development via writing

As indicated in Chapter 2, the adolescent period is a time when adolescents are learning how to cope with many changes. Writing in their heritage language(s) can be used as a medium for them to express their emotions and vent frustrations and anger in a more constructive manner. More importantly, learning to use precise words to describe specific emotions can help with successful communication. Children and adolescents sometimes do need to be helped to use language to recognise and express their feelings and learn how to identify and label them.[79] Thus, you may want to intentionally help your teens identify their emotions and label them using their heritage language(s). For instance, when your children express frustration, joyfulness or anger, you can help them write down their feelings and think about the accuracy of the words they use to label how they feel. For example, once Léandre (17; 1; 22) wrote to me that he was angry with me because I shouted at him when he did not want to compose his college application essay. He said he was 很气 (very air). I helped him use the right word (生气) to label his emotion and also taught him a different variations of the expression, 'Yes, I know you are very *angry, enraged and furious.*' (对，我知道你很生气，你很气愤，你很愤怒。)

When your children feel the power of words, they will use them to express emotions more accurately (e.g. *moody* is not necessarily *depressed*). Identifying emotions through precise language use can help both you and your children understand each other's emotions, which is important during adolescence.[80]

Talking about writing

Because of the challenge of time limitations during adolescence, sometimes it is very hard for adolescents to spare time to write their heritage language(s). I have found that talking about writing may be especially useful. For instance, I talked with Léandre and Dominique in the car about the structure differences between Chinese and English writing; we talked about how words were sometimes used differently in Chinese and English to achieve different effects, and we discussed the differences in punctuation usage in Chinese and English. Also, when Dominique's Chinese grandparents wrote an e-mail to wish him a happy birthday, I read the e-mail with Dominique (16; 0; 0) and talked about the vocabulary use, idioms and writing style.

Moreover, you can also talk about ideas and discuss how your teens can write about them. For example:

- Talk about what happened that day in school or in their activities. Hint to them that some of these situations could be very good material for writing.
- Find out their interests and discuss what these events might mean to them. Suggest how these can be put into a very nice piece of writing.
- Discuss what they want to write and their plans for writing. Suggest how they can begin the writing process.

Practising metalinguistic feedback

Providing feedback for children, such as comments on their writing, is important in their heritage-language writing development. There are two kinds of feedback: *direct* (explicit) and *indirect* (implicit) feedback. In direct feedback, you point out your children's mistakes directly. In indirect feedback, you only provide hints as to where your children can find their mistakes. Indirect feedback can also be called **metalinguistic feedback**, which refers to a process that results from error/contrastive analysis on the part of the parent, who hints at the type of error the child may have made but does not provide explicit correction. Research on this type of feedback has proven it to be successful with older children who are learning a new language.[81]

In my own practice, I have found that metalinguistic feedback is equally beneficial to heritage-language writing development. For example, instead of correcting Léandre on his mistakes in an e-mail, in which he wrote 'I want electric guitar want other things' (我想要电子吉它其它想要的东西), I told him that I was not clear about what he wanted exactly, the guitar or other things. After our discussion, Léandre went back and fixed his sentence: 'Electric guitar is what I want most' (电子吉它是我最想要的东西).

Choosing writing topics that interest teens

A study[82] found that significant differences in lexical, syntactic and discourse production were generally based on the topic of the writing sample rather than the genre. For example, writings related to the topics such as 'first day of school' and 'a person I admire' were significantly better than the other topics such as 'a letter to a new student.' Perhaps because these topics dealt with a potentially emotional memory, the participants were more apt to include a variety of words related to thoughts and feelings, leading to the selection of more abstract vocabulary and sophisticated syntax.

It seems that the topic choice may play a pivotal role in engaging adolescents in heritage-language writing. When teens are familiar with a topic or when they are interested in the topic, they are likely to be more involved in the writing. Therefore, before you ask your teens to write in their heritage language(s), you may want to discuss what topic they want to write about. Even if you have a definite topic in mind that you want them to write about, you still need to negotiate with them. The key is that they need to feel empowered in their own writing.

Increasing the frequency of complex sentence use in writing

Research suggests that discourse genre and communication context often determine the frequency of complex sentence use.[83] Adolescents tend to produce the most words per T-unit in persuasive and descriptive genres. These two types of genres are more sensitive to developmental growth in T-unit length than the narrative genre.[84] Therefore, you may want to create opportunities to engage your teens in complex sentence use through activities such as asking them to persuade you about something, to report on a book they have read or to research a topic of their interest. It may be more effective for you to model presentation styles, focusing specifically on complex sentence use.

Supporting figurative language use in writing

As discussed Chapter 6, figurative language comprehension and usage demonstrate an individual's high-level metalinguistic ability. Figurative language use can help a writer evoke mental images, create impressions and make writing more interesting and persuasive. Therefore, you may want to provide teens with some words that have different meanings and ask them to play with the words to come up with jokes, sarcasm, advertisements and comic strips. For example, each time Philippe was listening to popular French songs, he would show Léandre and Dominique how to play with the French words figuratively. If you do this often, your children's ability to use figurative language will improve.

Encouraging the use of the informal language register

During the adolescent period, peer influence is very important. Taking advantage of peer influence can help teens develop their writing skills. With the availability of Facebook, Twitter and texting, adolescents have more opportunities to socialise with a wider variety of their peers. You can take advantage of these informal language registers in online social networks and communication platforms and encourage your children to use digital print to discuss ideas and thoughts about what they read. You can also take advantage of their favourite communication forms to encourage them to write. For example, text messaging is a popular communication tool among many teenagers. Despite the debate on whether or not text messaging prevents children from writing formally, many literacy experts now believe that it can promote overall literacy development. Moreover, communicating through text messages can support friendship, intimacy and social networking, which are all vital for adolescent development. Furthermore, text-messaging vocabulary in different languages is linguistically interesting, and it provides an opportunity for children to study the features in the 'texting language.' For instance, discuss the interesting features in abbreviated words (e.g. *lol* – laugh out loud, *brb* – be right back, *gg* – gotta go, *mwah* – kiss, *yt* – are you there, *Gr8* – great and *Db8* – debate) with your children and let them tell you the rules involved in the texting language. Then, compare the abbreviations to the words used for formal writing. By treating text messaging as a legitimate form of communication, you can actually help your children understand that informal registers (such as texting) and formal registers (conventional writing) serve different purposes.

Encouraging unconventional means in aiding writing

Some people despise Google Translate and deem it unfit for language learning. However, whether we like it or not, some teens such as Léandre and Dominique are using it to support their heritage-language writing. Even though Google Translate is not accurate, it can serve as an initial step for heritage-language learning teens to develop their heritage-language writing. For instance, Léandre (15; 3; 27) tried to write a Christmas wish list in Chinese. However, he did not have enough Chinese vocabulary to complete the task. Google Translate provided him with a helping hand. When Léandre emailed me his wish list by copying the Google-translated phrases, it gave me a good opportunity to teach him some Chinese words and phrases. For example, I helped him change the Google-translated sentence '这个礼物不是在号码序' (This gift is not number in order) to a correct sentence 这些礼物不分顺序 (These gifts are not in order). Allowing teens to experiment with different ways to learn their heritage language can only help them move forward with their heritage-language writing.

Using innovative approaches to engage teens in writing

Using family photographs is an innovative approach to engage teens in heritage-language writing in a purposeful and meaningful way. For example, writing about family photographs is a good opportunity for teens to explore their identities, especially their cultural identities. They can use family photos (including photos from older generations) to write in different genres, such as a commentary about a historical event, a memoir, an autobiography, a short story or an essay. It is likely that adolescents will be interested in this kind of writing if you offer them the opportunity. Initially, it may be difficult, but they can begin by labelling the photos and then writing a sentence, then a paragraph and eventually a narrative or an essay.

Keeping a writing journal

Another effective way to help teens improve their writing in their heritage language(s) is to encourage them to keep a journal. For example:

- Keep a journal about their ideas and possible writing topics.
- Think about and write down what words and sentences can express what they really want to communicate.
- Write down what ideas they want to return later.
- Write down their reflections on where in their writing they did well and where they need to change and improve. Reflect on their writing experiences and express their joys and frustrations in writing.

The advantage of keeping a notebook or writing journal is that it can help your teens to reflect on the writing process and make it more conscious and transparent. This will help facilitate their heritage-language writing development.

Teaching self-regulation in heritage-language writing

The importance of teaching your teens self-regulation strategies in heritage-language writing should also be emphasised. Your teens need to develop the ability to self-monitor their heritage-language writing progress for continued growth. For example, you can try the **EmPOWER method** to help your teens develop expository-text production abilities through self-regulation. Your teens need to learn to *evaluate* a writing assignment by first reading the instructions carefully (E), then to *make a plan* that is based on communicative purpose that will help them get started (MP), *organise* their ideas graphically using templates specific to the intended genre (O), *work* from the plan to represent the idea with written language (W) and *evaluate and rework* the draft with the purpose and audience in mind (ER).[85]

Being flexible in communicative language use

Ideally, it is important for heritage-language-speaking teens to write consistently in their heritage language. However, for communication purposes, it is important to be flexible and to allow teens to write in the language in which they are most competent. For instance, when we got our new iPhones, Léandre (16; 2; 5) asked me in which language he should text me. I told him that he should write in Chinese; however, if it was an emergency or he did not know the Chinese words, he could write in English. Since Léandre went to college, I have let him text me in English. I found it is a lot easier for communication, even for myself. In fact, the flexibility I gave Léandre has not affected his desire to write in Chinese; rather, it gave him the power to decide which language to write and for what purposes.

Encouraging writing by hand

In today's society, writing using a computer has become the norm in our everyday lives. However, psychologists and neuroscientists suggest that it is far too soon to declare handwriting a relic of the past. Children not only learn to read more quickly when they first learn to write by hand, but they also generate ideas and retain information more easily.

A study[86] by psychologist Karin James presented children who had not yet learnt to read and write with a letter or a shape on an index card and asked them to reproduce it in one of three ways: trace the image on a page with a dotted outline, draw it on a blank white sheet of paper, or type it on a computer. They were then placed in a brain scanner and shown the image again. When the children had drawn a letter freehand, the brain exhibited increased activity in three areas of the brain that are activated in adults when they read and write: the left fusiform gyrus, the inferior frontal gyrus and the posterior parietal cortex. By contrast, children who typed or traced the letter or shape showed no such effect. In fact, the activation was significantly weaker. In short, when learning to write by hand, children are more able to generate ideas and retain information. It is the actual effort that engages the brain's motor pathways and delivers the learning benefits of handwriting.

Moreover, psychologist Virginia Berninger suggested that printing, cursive writing and typing on a keyboard are associated with distinct brain patterns and each results in a distinct end product. When children in this study composed text by hand, they not only consistently produced more words more quickly than they did on a keyboard, but they also expressed more ideas. Additionally, brain imaging in the oldest participants suggested that the connection between writing and idea generation was even more advanced. When these children were asked to come up with ideas for a composition, the ones with better handwriting exhibited greater neural activation in areas associated with working memory and increased overall activation in the reading and writing networks.

There may even be a difference between print and cursive writing in terms of brain activity. Cursive wiring may train one's self-control ability in a way that other modes of writing do not. The benefits of writing by hand extend beyond childhood. For adults, typing may be a fast and efficient alternative to longhand, but that very efficiency may also diminish our ability to process new information. Not only do we learn letters better when we commit them to memory through writing, memory and learning ability in general may benefit. Psychologists Pam A. Mueller and Daniel M. Oppenheimer found that children learn better when they take notes by hand than when they type on a keyboard. Writing by hand allows students to process a lecture's content and reframe it, which is a process of reflection and manipulation that can lead to better understanding and memory encoding.

Given all of the research evidence, it is important that you provide opportunities for your children, including your teens, to practice writing by hand during the heritage-language writing development process. In languages such as Chinese, handwriting appears to be even more crucial in remembering the characters. I noticed that Léandre and Dominique tended to remember the Chinese characters better when they first learnt them through handwriting than when they were typing them in *pinyin*.[87]

Supporting heritage-language literacies development

So far, I have discussed the strategies for supporting heritage-language reading and writing separately. There are some general points that need to be made about overall heritage-language literacies development.

Supporting syncretic literacy

To be able to participate successfully in literacy activities, heritage-language-speaking teens must learn to utilise resources from their respective cultural and linguistic communities. They must be able to integrate or synchronise their different cultural values, beliefs, emotions, identities and other resources into the organisation of their literacy activities. Even though heritage-language speakers, like Léandre and Dominique, spontaneously practice syncretic literacy (as shown earlier in this chapter), it is still important for you to value the practice and encourage your teens to draw on their different cultural and linguistic resources to make sense of what they are writing. By encouraging your teens to practice syncretic literacy, tap into their rich cultural and linguistic resources and connect their heritage culture to their mainstream culture, you will help them engage in meaning construction at a deeper level. In fact, research shows that when adolescents are encouraged to practice literacies by drawing on all their resources, or, in other words, by drawing on all points on the multilingual continua, they tend to have better chances for successful multilateral development.[88]

It should be noted, however, that practising syncretic literacy does not just involve blending different aspects of different languages and cultures. Rather, the goal is to help your children to transform their literacy practices and make new meaning by drawing on their multilingual and cultural resources. Moreover, it should also be noted that the literacy behaviours of children with more than one linguistic and cultural system are not static; they are always fluid, dynamic, multiplex and changing. Thus, the syncretic literacy process is always evolving, and there are no final products.

Promoting a multimodal approach to heritage-language literacies development

Meaning making should not rely solely on reading print-based texts but rather needs to be expanded to reading multiple text formats as well as composing various text types. This is especially critical for adolescents in the 21st century. **Multimodality** refers to the modes of representation beyond print, including such things as the visual, auditory, gestural and kinesthetic.[89] Adolescents make meaning through multiple expressions. For today's adolescents, multimodality is central to their everyday lives. They have access to information and entertainment at the click of a mouse, the touch of an iPad screen and the sounds from an iPhone.

Therefore, providing adolescents with varied ways to 'read' text, whether it is a book, hypertext, image or song lyrics, is important. This whole range of modes in representation and communication can help adolescents to think about topics from multiple vantage points and eventually help them in meaning making. Different modes have their own potentials for heritage-language literacy development and understanding. Images, movements, gestures, gaze, facial expressions, music, speech and sound effects are all modes that can provide opportunities for adolescents to interpret and construct a richer meaning.[90]

With the advancement of communication technology, multilingual children and adolescents have more opportunities to access heritage-language digital print or hypertexts. When they are exposed to heritage-language hypertexts, children and adolescents develop knowledge and concepts about the language's structure and other elements. Even though language and cultural conventions are different, the digital print that children and adolescents have built in their mainstream language may transfer easily. Thus, they can make an intuitive guess about the meaning. One of the advantages of exploring digital print is that it allows children and adolescents to be exposed to different terminologies in different languages. This is a good opportunity to learn a heritage language. Mrs Zhou from New Jersey shared with me a good practice that she used with her son. She changed the search engine on her son's computer to Chinese so that her son could guess and get used to Chinese web terminologies.[91] Likewise, Philippe set the all the electronic device instructions in our home to French. Interestingly, when updating or installing new programs on their computers, Léandre and Dominique automatically set them to French.

Supporting critical literacy development through pop culture

Multilingual children and adolescents do have advantages in their development of critical literacy. Because they are exposed to more than one language (often also more than one culture) early in life, they are accustomed to looking at things in more than one way. This habit is helpful in the development of critical literacy.

Using popular culture reading materials may motivate teens to read and grow. Popular culture materials (e.g. cartoons, comic strips, lyrics of rap, hip hop, rock or metal music) are often deplored by some parents and educators and denounced as a cause of violence and moral corruption by cultural watchdogs.[92] Nevertheless, pop culture materials have a strong appeal to adolescents from all socioeconomic and cultural/linguistic backgrounds. In fact, pop culture materials are routinely appropriated by youngsters for pleasure, identification and a sense of personal power.

Moreover, pop culture materials can help adolescents circumvent limits on learning and meaning. Despite some negative findings from research on pop culture materials and their association with violence and other behavioural problems, a growing body of literature examining the impact of such media on children's literacy development suggests that bringing pop culture, including pop music, into the classroom can motivate students' learning as well as support critical literacy development. It is now generally recognised among literacy researchers that critical literacy ability should be a part of every student's literacy pathway.[93] Pop music provides an ideal opportunity for adolescents to cultivate critical literacy abilities because the content and language used in the lyrics of pop music are often sophisticated and intellectually demanding. Despite the potential for improper language and messages in their content, popular culture materials may be a way to get heritage-language-learning adolescents interested in reading and writing. Using pop culture reading materials can help you understand how your teens construct meaning based on their personal interests and provide you with a window into how they form their identities.

Retelling procedure as a comprehensive support for literacy development

The retelling procedure is an effective way to engage children in literacy learning by asking them to 'spill over' what they read or what they hear when parents read aloud.[94] The retelling procedure helps teens develop their heritage-language literacy abilities in listening, reading, speaking, thinking and writing simultaneously. The approach is easy to implement and can be used with children of different ages. There are four forms of retelling, and you can use any of them when you engage your children.

- *Oral-to-oral retelling* A child listens to you reading aloud a text and then retells it orally.
- *Oral-to-written retelling* A child listens to you reading a text aloud and then retells it in writing.
- *Written-to-oral retelling* A child reads a text and retells it orally.
- *Written-to-written retelling* A child reads a text and retells it in writing.

You can begin by either reading to your children or asking them to read to you; they then tell you either orally or in writing what they have heard or read. You can remind them to relax and disregard spelling and neatness. The goal is to tell or write whatever they are able to remember or understand. Initially, your children's retelling (orally and in writing) may be very brief. Over time, their writing will become more sophisticated. You can also model the procedure by retelling the text yourself orally or in written form. After your children retell, you may ask them to reread or relisten to the original texts and compare their version with the original texts. It is important to note that the purpose is not to make your children feel bad about their version but to expose them to a more sophisticated version. To avoid boredom, you can vary your request to retell by asking them to retell the texts to their peers.

Children who are immersed in the retelling procedure can gradually spill over the vocabulary, phrases, sentences and other 'accoutrements' of the text structure. This approach to literacy learning is natural in the sense that it is similar to how a child acquires oral language in a natural learning environment.[95]

Supporting the development of theory of mind and emotional intelligence through literature

Every culture has great classic and contemporary literature that can inspire readers to reflect on their lives as well as influence their emotions and behaviours. Literature not only can promote heritage-language learning by enriching teens' vocabulary and modelling new language structures, it can also provide a motivating and low-anxiety context for heritage-language learning. Moreover, research has shown that participants who read literary fiction can better assess others' feelings and reading others' minds than those who read nonfiction or popular fiction.[96] Literature seems to have the potential to foster emotional intelligence as well by providing vicarious emotional experiences that shape the brain circuits for empathy and help the children gain insight into human behaviour.[97]

Adolescence is the time that teens further develop their **theory of mind** (the ability to read others' minds) and **emotional intelligence** (the ability to identify and manage one's own emotions and the emotions of others). Thus, reading good literature will help teens learn how to decode the world around them and interact with people to function well in their future life and career.

Measures for monitoring heritage-language reading and writing progress

It has been shown in the past that linguistic measures were better predictors of holistic writing outcomes than standardised test scores, which did not correlate with the holistic results.[98] Even now, there is still concern regarding the effectiveness of standardised language evaluations.[99] This suggests the need to continue to explore the interaction of linguistic features of heritage-language speaker's writing as potential tools to assess the language proficiency of these children.

The best method to assess and monitor whether your teens have made progress in their heritage-language reading and writing is to use their naturalistic production. In reading, you can choose a heritage-language text with which your children are not familiar (but is at the reading level of your children) and ask them to read it to you. You can record it and compare it with a later recording in an interval you determine (e.g. one month). In writing, you can ask your children to write a paragraph on a topic and calculate the vocabulary diversity, density and complexity (see Chapter 4); the syntactic complexity (see Chapter 5); and the figurative language use (see Chapter 6) as well as the organisation. Compare it with their later writing after an interval you determine to see their progress.

Summary of Key Points in Chapter 7

- As a general developmental trend, adolescents become increasingly more mature and critical in academic reading. With proper adult support (especially teacher support), they are able to handle difficult concepts described in different text genres. They also begin to consider multiple viewpoints. By the end of high school

(around age 18), adolescents usually can construct knowledge from readings that others have written.
- During adolescence, teens' writing ability develops and improves as they engage in a variety of writing activities. By the middle-school years, the length and diversity of teens' writing productions increase. Advanced narratives and expository texts begin to develop. In these writings, the syntax production becomes increasingly more complex. There is also an increase in embedded subordinate clauses and a decrease in coordination or compound sentences. Moreover, the use of relative clauses doubles between ages 7 and 17, and adverbial clause usage increases and diversifies. At the phrase level, there is an increase in pre- and postnoun modifiers. Their verb phrases are expanded by the increasing use of modality, tense and aspect. By junior year of high school (the third year in high school), teens are usually capable of revising all aspects of writing. Compared with other writing genres (such as narrative and expository), persuasive writing (writing used to convince others) is more difficult and takes longer to develop and show consideration of opposing views.
- Although adolescents are actively engaging in hypertext activities, they may still have insufficient reading and information research skills, less patience and less tolerance for websites that they considered boring or difficult to figure out. Additionally, they tend to give more credence to visually appealing sites than adults do.
- With increasing metacognitive development, adolescents are more able to ask questions spontaneously about what they are reading. However, adolescents still need adult (especially teacher) guidance to rethink their identity as readers, and they still need teacher support in developing critical literacy ability.
- There are several major challenges and characteristics in the development of heritage-language reading. These include:
  ○ Discrepancy in speaking and reading and writing competence.
  ○ Differences in school and home contexts.
  ○ Heritage-language-specific features.
- There are also different characteristics in the development of heritage-language writing. These include:
  ○ Language-specific challenges in different writing systems.
  ○ Syncretic writing.
  ○ Crosslinguistic writing transfer.
  ○ Partial competence in heritage-language writing.
  ○ Topic and prompts influence lexical and syntactic differences.
  ○ Writing block in the heritage language.
  ○ Finding ways to compensate heritage-language limitation.
  ○ Chinese homophone spelling errors.
- There are some general principles that you can consider when helping adolescents continue to develop their heritage-language literacies:
  ○ Refrain from criticising adolescents in their language-learning activities. In particular, do not do it in front of their siblings or peers. Try to be as positive

and supportive as possible. Using humour to replace criticism tends to achieve better results.
- Value your children's opinions and allow choices and freedom when carrying out literacy learning activities.
- Provide opportunities for your teens to take risks in their heritage-language literacy learning and encourage self-exploration.
- Motivate your teens to be self-regulated learners. Self-regulation is a form of self-control or self-monitoring in the learning process, which consists of strategies such as setting standards and goals for oneself and engaging in self-motivated learning.
- Encourage your teens to work with other peers who also are heritage-language speakers.
- Help your teens develop critical thinking and critical literacy abilities while carrying out their heritage-language literacy learning.
- Use innovative methods to engage your teens in heritage-language literacy learning.

- Moreover, when supporting your teens in their heritage-language literacies development, it is important to set clear and achievable goals. Be flexible in changing plans if the goals do not work out.
- When supporting heritage-language reading development, you may consider the following strategies:
    - Select age-appropriate reading materials.
    - Adjust heritage-language reading materials to the teens' reading levels.
    - Teach reading comprehension strategies.
    - Teach vocabulary use.
    - Support inferencing in heritage-language comprehension.
    - Support expository reading comprehension.
    - Build background knowledge for reading comprehension.
    - Provide both extensive and intensive reading materials.
    - Focus on reading interests rather than analysis.
    - Use everyday context to teach heritage-language reading.
    - Encourage the habit of reading.
- When supporting your children in their heritage-language writing development, you may consider the following strategies:
    - Teach writing skills.
    - Be cognizant of possible cultural rhetorical style differences.
    - Encourage crosslinguistic comparison.
    - Scaffold and model heritage-language writing.
    - Encourage writing by focusing on adolescents' interests.
    - Support emotional development via writing.
    - Talk about writing.
    - Practice metalinguistic feedback.
    - Choose writing topics that interest teens.
    - Increase the frequency of complex sentence use in writing.

- Support figurative language use in writing.
  - Encourage the use of the informative language register.
  - Encourage unconventional means in aiding writing.
  - Use innovative means for writing.
  - Encourage the use of a writing journal.
  - Teach self-regulation in heritage-language writing.
  - Be flexible in using the communicative language.
  - Encourage writing by hand.
- Overall, when supporting heritage-language literacies development, you may want to do the following:
  - Support syncretic literacy development.
  - Promote multimodal heritage-language literacies.
  - Support critical literacy development.
  - Use retelling activities to help multilingual development.
  - Support teens' emotional development through literature.
- Finally, to monitor your teens' progress, you may want to sample your teens' reading and writing periodically and compare the samples to previous writing.

Recommended Readings

Fitzgerald, J. (2006) Multilingual writing in preschool through 12th grade: The last 15 years. In C.A. MacArthur, S. Graham and J. Fitzgerald (eds) *Handbook of Writing Research* (pp. 337–54). New York, NY: Guilford Press.

Wang, X.-L. (2011) *Learning to Read and Write in the Multilingual Family*. Bristol: Multilingual Matters.

Notes and References

[1] Critical literacy ability has been widely recognised to be as essential as the ability to decode texts.
[2] For complete information on how to help children and adolescents develop multilingual and heritage-language literacies, please consult Wang, X.-L. (2011) *Learning to Read and Write in the Multilingual Family*. Bristol: Multilingual Matters.
[3] Marchand-Martella, N.E., Martella, R.C., Modderman, S.L., Petersen, H.M. and Pan, S. (2013) Key areas of effective adolescent literacy programs. *Education and Treatment of Children* 36 (1), 161–84.
[4] Pence, K.L. and Justice, L.M. (2008) *Language Development from Theory to Practice*. Upper Saddle River, NJ: Pearson.
[5] Nippold, M.A. (2007) *Later Language Development: School-Age Children, Adolescents, and Young Adults*. Austin: Pro-ed.
[6] Owens, R.E. (2012) *Language Development: An Introduction*. Boston: Pearson.
[7] Nippold, M.A. (2007) *Later Language Development: School-Age Children, Adolescents, and Young Adults*. Austin: Pro-ed.
[8] Nippold, M.A. (2007) *Later Language Development: School-Age Children, Adolescents, and Young Adults*. Austin: Pro-ed.
[9] Lewin, T. (2009) In a digital future, textbooks are history. *New York Times*, August 9.
[10] McNabb, M.L. (2005–2006) Navigating the maze of hypertext. *Educational Leadership* 63 (4), 76–9.
[11] McNabb, M.L. (2005–2006) Navigating the maze of hypertext. *Educational Leadership* 63 (4), 76–9.
[12] Kress, G. (1997) *Before Writing: Rethinking the Paths to Literacy*. London: Routledge.

Sutherland-Smith, W. (2002) Weaving the literacy web: changes in reading from page to screen. *Reading Teacher* 55 (7), 662–9.

[13] McNabb, M.L., Thurber, B.B., Dibuz, B., McDermott, P.A. and Lee, C.A. (2006) *Literacy Learning in Networked Classrooms: Using the Internet with Middle-Level Students*. Newark, DE: International Reading Association.

[14] McNabb, M.L. (2005–2006) Navigating the maze of hypertext. *Educational Leadership* 63 (4), 76–9.

[15] Sutherland-Smith, W. (2002) Weaving the literacy web: Changes in reading from page to screen. *Reading Teacher* 55 (7), 662–9.
Coiro, J. (2003) Reading comprehension on the internet: Expanding our understanding of reading comprehension to encompass new literacies. *Reading Teacher* 56, 458–64.

[16] Hoff, E. (2009) *Language Development*. Belmont, CA: Wadsworth.

[17] Personal communication, 3 April 2010.

[18] Packard, J.L., Chen, X., LI, W.-L., Wu, X.-C., Gaffney, J.S., Li, H. and Anderson, R.C. (2006) Explicit instruction in orthographic structure and word morphology helps Chinese children learn to write characters. *Reading and Writing* 19, 457–87.

[19] Packard, J.L., Chen, X., LI, W.-L., Wu, X.-C., Gaffney, J.S., Li, H. and Anderson, R.C. (2006) Explicit instruction in orthographic structure and word morphology helps Chinese children learn to write characters. *Reading and Writing* 19, 457–87.

[20] Curdt-Christiansen, X.L. (2013) Implicit learning and imperceptible influence: Syncretic literacy of multilingual Chinese children. *Journal of Early Childhood Literacy* 13 (3), 348–70.
Gregory, E., Long, S. and Volk, D. (eds) (2004) *Many Pathways to Literacy: Young Children Learning with Siblings, Grandparents, Peers and Communities*. London: Routledge.

[21] Curdt-Christiansen, X.L. (2013) Implicit learning and imperceptible influence: Syncretic literacy of multilingual Chinese children. *Journal of Early Childhood Literacy* 13 (3), 348–70.
Gregory, E., Long, S. and Volk, D. (eds) (2004) *Many Pathways to Literacy: Young Children Learning with Siblings, Grandparents, Peers and Communities*. London: Routledge.

[22] Berninger, V.W. (2000) Development of language by hand and its connections with language by ear, mouth, and eye. *Topics in Language Disorders* 20 (4), 65–84.

[23] Berninger, V.W. (2000) Development of language by hand and its connections with language by ear, mouth, and eye. *Topics in Language Disorders* 20 (4), 65–84.

[24] Durgunoglu, A.Y. (2002) Cross-linguistic transfer in literacy development and implications for language learners. *Annals of Dyslexia* 52, 189–204.

[25] Fitzgerald, J. (2006) Multilingual writing in preschool through 12th grade: The last 15 years. In C.A. MacArthur, S. Graham and J. Fitzgerald (eds) *Handbook of Writing Research* (pp. 337–54). New York, NY: Guilford Press.

[26] Danzak, R.L. (2011) The integration of lexical, syntactic, and discourse features in bilingual adolescents' writing: An exploratory approach. *Language, Speech, and Hearing Services in Schools* 42: 491–505.

[27] Danzak, R.L. (2011) The integration of lexical, syntactic, and discourse features in bilingual adolescents' writing: An exploratory approach. *Language, Speech, and Hearing Services in Schools* 42, 491–505.

[28] Cummins, J. (2000) *Language, Power and Pedagogy: Bilingual Children in the Crossfire*. Bristol: Multilingual Matters.

[29] Berman, R.A. and Nir-Sagiv, B. (2009) Clause-packaging in narratives: A crosslinguistic developmental study. In J. Guo *et al.* (eds) *Approaches to the Psychology of Language Research in the Tradition of Dan I. Slobin* (pp. 149–62). Mahwah, NJ: Lawrence Erlbaum.

[30] Conversation on 16 November 2012.

[31] Tatum, A.W. (2014) Texts and adolescents: Embracing connections and connectedness. In K.A. Hinchman and H.K. Sheridan-Thomas (eds) *Best Practice in Adolescent Literacy Instruction* (pp. 3–19). New York: The Guilford Press.

[32] Ideas inspired by Taturn, A.W. (2014) Texts and adolescents: Embracing connections and connectedness. In K.A. Hinchman and H.K. Sheridan-Thomas (eds) *Best Practices in Adolescent Literacy Instruction* (pp. 3–19). New York: The Guilford Press.
[33] Many ideas from this section are from Boyd, F.B. and Tochelli, A.L. (2014) Multimodality and literacy learning. In K.A. Hinchman and H.K. Sheridan-Thomas (eds) *Best Practices in Adolescent Literacy Instruction* (pp. 291–307). New York: The Guilford Press.
[34] Nuttall, C. (1996) *Teaching Reading Skills in a Foreign Language*. London: Heinemann.
[35] Sullivan, J.H. (2002) The second language educators' challenge: Learning about literacy. In J.H. Sullivan (ed.) *Literacy and the Second Language Learner* (pp. ix–xi). Greenwich, CT: Information Age.
[36] Sullivan, J.H. (2002) The second language educators' challenge: Learning about literacy. In J.H. Sullivan (ed.) *Literacy and the Second Language Learner* (pp. ix–xi). Greenwich, CT: Information Age.
[37] Alfieri, L., Brooks, P.J., Aldrich, N.J. and Tenenbaum, H.R. (2011) Does discovery-based instruction enhance learning? *Journal of Educational Psychology* 103 (1), 1–18.
[38] Note that most of the ideas discussed in this section are based on Goldman, S.R. (2012) Adolescent literacy: Learning and understanding content. *The Future of Children* 22 (2), 89–116.
[39] Goldman, S.R. (2012) Adolescent literacy: Learning and understanding content. *The Future of Children* 22 (2), 89–116.
[40] Creese, A. and Blackledge, A. (2010) Translanguaging in the bilingual classroom: A pedagogy for learning and teaching. *Modern Language Journal* 94, 103–115.
[41] Silliman, E.R. and Scott, C.M. (2009) Research-based oral language intervention routes to the academic language of literacy. In S. Rosenfield and V. Berninger (eds) *Impletions in School Settings* (pp. 107–45). New York: Oxford University Press.
[42] McGee, A. and Johnson, H. (2003) The effect of inference training on skilled and less skilled comprehenders. *Educational Psychology* 23 (1), 49–59.
Silliman, E.R. and Scott, C.M. (2009) Research-based oral language intervention routes to the academic language of literacy. In S. Rosenfield and V. Berninger (eds) *Impletions in School Settings* (pp. 107–145). New York: Oxford University Press.
[43] Silliman, E.R. and Scott, C.M. (2009) Research-based oral language intervention routes to the academic language of literacy. In S. Rosenfield and V. Berninger (eds) *Implementing Evidence-Based Academic Interventions in School Setting* (pp. 107–45). New York: Oxford University Press.
[44] Silliman, E.R. and Scott, C.M. (2009) Research-based oral language intervention routes to the academic language of literacy. In S. Rosenfield and V. Berninger (eds) *Implementing Evidence-Based Academic Interventions in School Setting* (pp. 107–145). New York: Oxford University Press.
[45] Nuske, N.J. and Bavin, E.L. (2011) Narrative comprehension in 4–7-year-old children with autism: Testing the Weak Central Coherence account. *International Journal of Language Communication Disorders* 46 (1), 108–19.
[46] Nelson, N.W. (2010) *Language and Literacy Disorders: Infancy through Adolescence*. Boston: Allyn & Bacon.
[47] Nelson, N.W. (2010) *Language and Literacy Disorders: Infancy through Adolescence*. Boston: Allyn & Bacon.
[48] Litman, C. and Greenleaf, C. (2014) Traveling together over difficult ground: Negotiating success with a profoundly inexperienced reader in an introduction to chemistry class. In K.A. Hinchman and H.K. Sheridan-Thomas (eds) *Best Practices in Adolescent Literacy Instruction* (pp. 308–29). New York: The Guilford Press.
[49] Wang, X.L. (2011) *Learning to Read and Write in the Multilingual Family*. Bristol: Multilingual Matters.
[50] Nuttall, C. (1996) *Teaching Reading Skills in a Foreign Language*. London: Heinemann.
[51] McQuillan, J. (1998) The use of self-selected and free voluntary reading in heritage language programs: A review of research. In S.D. Krashen and J. McQuillan (eds) *Heritage Language Development* (pp. 73–87). Culver City, CA: Language Education Associates.

52 *Les Aventures de Tintin* (The Adventures of Tintin) is a series of comic albums created by Belgian cartoonist Georges Remi, whose pen name is Hergé.
53 Leckerli is a cookie that is a specialty in Basel, Switzerland.
54 Migros is a chain grocery store in Switzerland.
55 Engadine nut cake is a specialty in Engadine, Switzerland.
56 Bereiter, C. and Scardamalia, M. (1987) *The Psychology of Written Composition*. Hillsdale, NJ: Lawrence Erlbaum.
57 Lenski, S. and Verbruggen, F. (2010) *Writing Instruction and Assessment for English Language Learners K-8*. New York, NY: Guilford Press.
58 Kaplan, R.B. (1966) Cultural thought patterns in intercultural education. *Language Learning* 16, 1–20.
59 Hinds, J. (1990) Inductive, deductive, quasi-inductive: Expository writing in Japanese, Korean, Chinese, and Thai. In U. Connor and A.M. Johns (eds) *Coherence in Writing: Research and Pedagogical Perspectives* (pp. 87–109). Alexandria, VA: TESOL.
60 Casanave, C.P. (2003) *Controversies in Second Language Writing: Dilemmas and Decisions in Research and Instruction*. Ann Arbor: University of Michigan Press.
Kubota, R. (2010) Cross-cultural perspectives on writing: Contrastive rhetoric. In N.H. Hornberger and S.L. McKay (eds) *Sociolinguistics and Language Education* (pp. 265–89). Bristol: Multilingual Matters.
61 Kubota, R. (2010) Cross-cultural perspectives on writing: Contrastive rhetoric. In N.H. Hornberger and S.L. McKay (eds) *Sociolinguistics and Language Education* (pp. 265–89). Bristol: Multilingual Matters.
62 Hirsch, E. (2003) Reading comprehension requires knowledge of words and the world: Scientific insights into the fourth-grade slump and the nations' stagnant comprehension score. *American Educator* 27 (1), 10–29.
Kubota, R. (2010) Cross-cultural perspectives on writing: Contrastive rhetoric. In N.H. Hornberger and S.L. McKay (eds) *Sociolinguistics and Language Education* (pp. 265–89). Bristol: Multilingual Matters.
63 Cummins, J. (2000) *Language, Power and Pedagogy: Bilingual Children in the Crossfire*. Clevedon: Multilingual Matters.
64 Bialystok, E. (2007) Acquisition of literacy in bilingual children: A framework for research. *Language Learning* 57 (1), 45–77.
65 Ordóñez, C.L., Carlo, M.S., Snow, C. and McLaughlin, B. (2002) Depth and breadth of vocabulary in two languages: Which vocabulary skills transfer? *Journal of Educational Psychology* 94 (4), 719–28.
66 Durgunoglu, A.Y. (2002) Cross-linguistic transfer in literacy development and implications for language learners. *Annals of Dyslexia* 52, (1), 189–204.
67 Francis, N. (2006) The development of secondary discourseability and metalinguistic awareness in second language learners. *International Journal of Applied Linguistics*, 16, 37–60.
Francis, N. (2005) Cross-linguistic influence, transfer and other kinds of language interaction: Evidence for modularity from the study of bilingualism. In J. Cohen, K.T. McAlister, K. Rolstad, and J. MacSwan (eds) *Proceedings of the 4th International Symposium on Bilingualism* edited Somerville, MA: Cascadilla Press.
68 Fitzgerald, J. (2006) Multilingual writing in preschool through 12th grade: The last 15 years. In C.A. MacArthur, S. Graham and J. Fitzgerald (eds) *Handbook of Writing Research* (pp. 337). New York, NY: Guilford Press.
69 Fitzgerald, J. (2006) Multilingual writing in preschool through 12th grade: The last 15 years. In C.A. MacArthur, S. Graham and J. Fitzgerald (eds) *Handbook of Writing Research* (pp. 337). New York, NY: Guilford Press.
70 Danzak, R.L. (2011) The integration of lexical, syntactic, and discourse features in bilingual adolescents' writing: An exploratory approach. *Language, Speech, and Hearing Services in Schools* 42, 91–505.
71 Ideas based on Benko, S. (2012/2013) with modification to adapt to heritage-language speakers.

72 Ideas are from Boyd, F.B. and Tochelli, A.L. (2014) Multimodality and literacy learning. In K.A. Hinchman and H.K. Sheridan-Thomas (eds) *Best Practices in Adolescent Literacy Instruction* (p. 156). New York: The Guilford Press.
73 Email communication on 4 December 2013.
74 Lenhart, A., Arafeh, S., Smith, A. and Macgill, A. (2008) Writing, technology, and teens. Washington, DC: Pew Internet and American Life Projects. http://files.eric.ed.gov/fulltext/ED524313.pdf
75 Lenhart, A., Arafeh, S., Smith, A. and Macgill, A. (2008) Writing, technology, and teens. Washington, DC: Pew Internet and American Life Projects. http://files.eric.ed.gov/fulltext/ED524313.pdf
76 (e.g. Kell, 2009)
77 Ideas inspired mostly by Kell, T. (2009) Using fan fiction to teach critical reading and writing skills. *Teacher Liberian* 37(1), 32–5 and Curwood, J.S., Magnified, A.M. and Lammers, J.C. (2013) Writing in the wild: Writers' motivation in fan-based affinity spaces. *Journal of Adolescent & Adult Literacy* 56 (8), 677–85.
78 Gee, J.P. (2005) *Why Video Games Are Good For Your Soul: Pleasure and Learning*. Melbourne: Common Ground.
79 Greenspan, S.I. (2007) *Great Kids: Helping Your Babies and Children Develop the Ten Essential Qualities for A Healthy, Happy Life*. Philadelphia: PA: Da Capo Press.
80 Ideas from Wang, X.-L. (2011) *Learning to Read and Write in the Multilingual Family*. Bristol: Multilingual Matters.
81 Mourssi, A. (2012) The impact of reflection and metalinguistic feedback in SLA: A qualitative research in the context of post graduates. *International Journal of Language Learning and Applied Linguistics* 1 (1), 128–46.
82 Berman, R.A. and Nir-Sagiv, B. (2009) Clause-packaging in narratives: A crosslinguistic developmental study. In J. Guo *et al.* (eds) *Approaches to the Psychology of Language Research in the Tradition of Dan I. Slobin* (pp. 149–62). Mahwah, NJ: Lawrence Erlbaum.
83 Nippold, M.A. (2007) *Later Language Development: School-Age Children, Adolescents, and Young Adults*. Austin: Pro-ed.
84 Nippold, M.A. (2007) *Later Language Development: School-Age Children, Adolescents, and Young Adults*. Austin: Pro-ed.
85 Nelson, N.W. (2010) *Language and Literacy Disorders: Infancy through Adolescence*. Boston: Allyn & Bacon.
86 Konnikova, M. (2014) What's lost as handwriting fades. *NY Times Science Section*, June 3.
87 Pinyin is the official phonetic system for transcribing the pronunciation of Chinese characters into the Latin alphabet. Pinyin is used in the People's Republic of China and is now also used in other Chinese-speaking regions.
88 Hornberger, N.H. (ed) (2003) *Continua of Biliteracy: An Ecological Framework for Educational Policy, Research, and Practice in Multilingual Settings*. Clevedon: Multilingual Matters.
89 Boyd, F.B. and Tochelli, A.L. (2014) Multimodality and literacy learning. In K.A. Hinchman and H.K. Sheridan-Thomas (eds) *Best Practices in Adolescent Literacy Instruction* (pp. 291–307). New York: The Guilford Press.
90 Ideas borrowed from Boyd, F.B. and Tochelli, A.L. (2014) Multimodality and literacy learning. In K.A. Hinchman and H.K. Sheridan-Thomas (eds) *Best Practices in Adolescent Literacy Instruction* (pp. 291–307). New York: The Guilford Press.
91 E-mail exchange on 20 September 2013.
92 Wang, X.-L. (2010) A comparative study of how moral values are conveyed in contemporary Chinese, English, and French children's books. Paper presented at the 5th Conference of Asia Pacific Network for Moral Education, Nagasaki, Japan, June 11–13.
93 Martello, J. (2002) Many roads through many modes: Becoming literate in early childhood. In L. Makin and C.J. Diaz (eds) *Literacies in Early Childhood: Changing Views, Changing Practice* (pp. 35–52). Sydney: MacLennan & Petty.
94 Brown, H. and Cambournes, B. (1990) *Read and Retell*. Portsmouth, NH: Heinemann.

[95] Brown, H. and Cambournes, B. (1990) *Read and Retell*. Portsmouth, NH: Heinemann.
[96] Kidd, D.C. and Castano, E. (2013) Reading literary fiction improves theory of mind. *Science* October 2013.
[97] Ghosn, I.K. (1999) Nurturing emotional intelligence through literature. *http://digilander.libero.it/mgtund/nurturing_emotional_intelligence.htm,* retrieved on 16 April 2015.
Ghosn, I.K. (2015) Emotional intelligence through literature. http://files.eric.ed.gov/fulltext/ED432925.pdf, retrieved on 16 April 2015.
[98] Perkins, K. (1980) Using objective methods of attained writing proficiency to discriminate among holistic evaluations. *TESOL Quarterly* 14, 61–9.
[99] Bailey, A.L. (2010) Implications for assessment and instruction. In M. Schatz and L.C. Wilkinson (eds) *The Education of English Language Learners: Research to Practice* (pp. 222–47). New York, NY: Guilford Press.

8 Developing Multiple Identities During Adolescence

For a middle-school class assignment, Dominique's English teacher asked students in her class to identify themselves with an animal and a colour. Dominique (13; 2; 17) responded with the following:

> If I were an animal, I would be a bear, because the bear is the symbol of Bern (the Swiss capital and also the Canton of Bern). I am also Swiss...If I could describe myself as a color, I would be the color yellow. I choose the color yellow because it is my favorite color and I am yellow, as in Asian. Just like yellow, I am very bright. I am proud of my Asian heritage. I am yellow...[1]

On another occasion, Dominique (14; 2; 25) drew a yellow figure wearing a Swiss watch. He named it *'Jaune-Man de Neuchâtel'* (Yellow-Man from Neuchâtel). This spontaneous illustration reflected his identification with his two cultural heritages. The yellow man symbolised that he was 炎黄子孙[2] (the descent of yellow emperors – Chinese), and the yellow colour also symbolised the yellow stone buildings of the Swiss town of Neuchâtel, famously described by the 19th-century French writer Alexandre Dumas as looking 'like a toy town carved out of butter,' where Dominique spent every summer. The watch symbolised the watch industry that Canton Neuchâtel is known for.

It is fascinating to peer into Dominique's identity through these two examples in which he explicitly (in the first example) and implicitly (in the second example) identified himself using his two heritages: Switzerland and China.

This chapter is about the development of multiple identities in multilingual and multicultural adolescents. It begins with a brief discussion about the definition of identity. It then examines several specific features of Léandre and Dominique's identity development to illustrate how the teens navigated, negotiated and explored their multiple identities while switching between different languages and cultural realities. The chapter concludes with some thoughts and suggestions on how to help multilingual teens positively construct their multilayered identities.

Definition of Identity

Identity refers to our sense of who we are and our relationship to others.[3] Contrary to past beliefs, our identity is not fixed; instead, it is constructed and reconstructed over time and in different contexts. In other words, identity is always a process[4] rather than an end result. Many aspects of our 'selves' such as language, culture, race, gender, age and social class contribute to our understanding of our identities (who we are). Which of these aspects become the salient features of our identities depends on contexts and changes over time.[5] For multilingual adolescents such as Léandre and Dominique, what they choose to be the visible part of themselves (identities) is ever evolving.

Negotiation of multilingual identities

Multilingualism provides a much more complicated reality for identity development.[6] Multilingual adolescents are developing many identities, such as an adolescent, a student, a son or daughter and a person who communicates with more than one language and who may be familiar with more than one culture. While adolescents explore their possible selves, the process of being immersed in more than one language will either help or impede their self-development,[7] and thus, they need to constantly negotiate their multiple identities. As such, multilingual adolescents may not associate themselves with a singular identity group, and their sense of identity may be complex, multiple and intersecting,[8] with a unique position between their different languages and cultures.

In general, identity includes two important parts: our own awareness of ourselves and how others perceive us. In other words, the process of our identity positioning reflects the negotiation outcome of who others perceive us to be and who we believe ourselves to be and imagine we can be. In essence, identity reflects the interplay between **interactive positioning** (others' attempts to position us) and **reflective positioning** (our own attempts at self-representation). Thus, identity negotiation happens on two levels: between the individual and others and within the individual, regarding which of a number of possible identity positions they can elect to take up.[9]

An examination of the period from the ages of 12 to 19[10] suggests that the following areas of Léandre and Dominique's identities were noticeable during adolescence: multilingualism (linguistic identity), multiculturalism (cultural identity), binationalism (national identity), biracialism (racial identity), local identity (St. Blaise, Neuchâtel), global identity (international travels) and name representation (effects of their names on their identity). In the following sections, the discussions of Léandre and Dominique's identities are situated in these areas. The purpose is to show how the two teens negotiated and managed[11] their multilayered identities in the process of defining who they were during adolescence.

Linguistic identity

Some researchers consider the process of learning the grammatical rules of a language to be the process of making the language part of oneself.[12] If language acquisition is indeed a process of making language part of oneself, it is an interesting identity formation process for children and adolescents like Léandre and Dominique who grow up with multiple languages. How these children navigate and manage to make the different languages part of themselves is certainly important to understand.

Moreover, language is not only a medium of communication, but it is also a mode by which the identity of a speaker is conveyed. In other words, the language choice by a speaker is an act of identity. Multilinguals may choose a language according to factors such as participants and situations, as well as the theme and purpose of the conversation.[13] As multilingual children enter the adolescent period, the process of how to represent themselves in different languages becomes more intricate and interesting. According to the social constructionist view, the identity options are viewed as constructed, validated and offered through discourses available to language users at a particular point in time and place. The relationship between language and identity is mutually constructive in at least two ways: (1) Language supplies the terms and other linguistic means with which identity is constructed and negotiated. (2) Ideology of language and identity guide ways in which individuals use linguistic resources to index their identities and to evaluate the linguistic resources used by others.[14] Because Léandre and Dominique grew up with three languages simultaneously, it is essential to explore how their identities were conveyed through their different languages and how they chose to enact themselves with their different linguistic repertoires.

English as a neutral language

Since English was not Léandre and Dominique's home language and they did not grow up speaking it with their parents, it functioned as a neutral (impersonal and detached) language for them in the family context. When Léandre and Dominique wanted to distance themselves from something, find excuses, try to get away with something or make a comment that appeared to be from others, they often used English as a medium to convey ideas. In fact, Dominique (14; 0; 9) commented that when he spoke English, he felt neutral (less emotionally involved). We can glimpse the neutrality aspect of their English use from the examples in Box 8.1.

Even though English is their most proficient language, Léandre and Dominique only treated it as their neutral language (in particular, in the family context). In fact, research has indicated that speaking a language does not necessarily mean to identify with the language. For instance, many Iranians in the United States exhibit high competence in the English language, yet they show low identification with the American culture.[15]

Moreover, because we, the parents, had not spoken English to Dominique and Léandre in the family context since their birth, they often felt punished if we spoke English to them during early and middle childhood (see discussion elsewhere[16]). This phenomenon continued into adolescence (though to a lesser degree). For example, Dominique (13; 2; 12) cried when Philippe said, 'Now, let's speak English' after

Box 8.1 Examples of English as a Neutral Language

Example 1:

On the way to Braga (Portugal), we were listening to a French disc we bought at a rest stop regarding the history of the region. Dominique kept on commenting on the disc. Annoyed by Dominique's constant talking, Léandre (15; 11; 19) said to Dominique in English 'Shut up!' instead of saying to Dominique, *'Tais-toi'* (shut up) in French as he usually would. By doing so, Léandre tried to create an impression that it was not just him who resented Dominique's constant rambling but that the others in the car also shared the same resentment.

Example 2:

Dominique and Léandre were hitting each other in the car for fun. I asked them to stop because it was distracting and that could be dangerous. Instead of speaking Chinese to me, Dominique (14; 1; 3) said in English, 'I am sorry.' He, in fact, did not really want to apologise for what he did.

Example 3:

Sometimes Léandre and Dominique would use English with an extremely strong American accent to make a comment on things as if they wanted to use another's voice to comment on things. For example, on the way to St. Malo (France) to take a ferry to Jersey (one of the UK Channel Islands), Philippe lost the way (because Léandre had not put the direction in the GPS as I suggested). Léandre was complaining that we wasted our time finding St. Malo. I said to him, Don't complain. You didn't look at the directions I emailed you. (不要抱怨。因为你没有好好准备我寄给你的路线). Léandre (18; 11; 25) replied in English with a strong American accent, 'Who is doing the complaining?' This was a way for him to blame me without being regarded as the person who was blaming me.

Example 4:

On the way to Aachen (Germany) from Oxford (the United Kingdom), I wanted to make sure that Léandre (18; 11; 18) knew how to convert English miles to kilometers. I asked him to check how many kilometers were in a mile; he said that I could check myself. I handed him my iPhone. He said everything in Chinese, except one word, '你真的不知道怎么用你的电话?' Seriously? (You really don't know how to use your iPhone? Seriously?). Léandre used the English word 'seriously' to show his astonishment; yet, at the same time, he tried to detach himself from the comment.

(Continued)

> **Example 5:**
> In Jersey, we saw a house that resembled the American plantation style we had seen in American movies. Dominique (17; 0; 10) said in English with an accent he just picked up from some locals in restaurants and shops, 'However, we don't import slavery.' He was commenting as if he was a local from Jersey.
>
> **Example 6:**
> We were joking that Dominique's name could be a girl's name. Léandre said in English, 'If I had a little sister, she would have to be a pest. I already have a little brother who is a pest.' Dominique (15; 0; 11) replied in English, 'me or Jean Luc?' (Jean Luc was a nickname for an imaginary figure that Dominique made up). Both of them were speaking to each other in other people's voices.
>
> **Example 7:**
> On the way to his community service in the literacy centre, I tried to prepare Léandre for his college interviews. I had to speak to him in English because interviewers would ask these questions in English. Léandre (17; 3; 10) commented that it was so *unnatural* to speak English with me.

Dominique 'scolded' Philippe in English. It is interesting to notice the teens' double standards; that is, they themselves were entitled to use English to achieve their purposes (such as in the examples in Box 8.1), but when their parents used English to achieve their purposes, the teens' feelings were hurt.

For the same reason (the fact that English was not a family language), both teens felt that English was an unnatural language to use to communicate with their parents. They continued to feel uncomfortable speaking English even with their English-speaking friends when we were around. For example, normally Léandre was talkative either in French, Chinese or English; however, he (16; 8; 18) was quiet when his friend Felipe was in my car. Similarly, Léandre (18; 4; 26) was abnormally silent at the dinner table when his high-school friend Daren was having dinner with us when they both came back from college. Obviously, Léandre felt ill at ease speaking English with his friend in his parents' presence.

French as an emotional core language

As their father tongue and one of their home languages from birth, French functioned as a soul language for the two teens. Box 8.2 shows some examples.

The reason French became Léandre and Dominique's soul and emotional language perhaps can be explained by the following four reasons. First, in their formative years, Philippe spent a lot more time with the boys. For example, Philippe was the only father who walked his children to the school bus stop every day from kindergarten to high school. The daily close interactions through the

> **Box 8.2 Examples of Using French**
>
> **Example 1:**
> In our routine annual good luck game on New Year's Eve (I invented this game for everyone in the family to write down their good wishes for a New Year and put them in a basket for others to pick by tossing a dice), both Léandre and Dominique always chose to write in French, even though they could write a lot better in English.
>
> **Example 2:**
> Sabine (the great aunt of Léandre and Dominique) always spoke to the boys in French. Once she got confused when many languages were used, and she spoke English to Dominique. Dominique (15; 0; 6) almost felt insulted and replied, 'I don't speak English.'
>
> **Example 3:**
> When Léandre registered for the Swiss vote from abroad, he (17; 9; 6) requested that the voting materials be sent to him in French instead of English or German. Dominique followed suit.
>
> **Example 4:**
> Léandre (18; 1; 19) told Philippe that he felt freer to write his ideas and express his emotion and passion in French than in English, even though his English writing was more advanced than his French.

French language exchanges enabled the boys to form a strong emotional bond with Philippe and the French language. Second, being all males, Philippe, Léandre and Dominique shared many common conversation topics, such as musical instruments, games, life and sports as well as rough-and-tumble physical activities. The common interests and activities between Philippe and the boys had also strengthened their bond through the use of the French language. Third, the conversations between the boys were often humorous. Unlike most of my conversations with the boys, which often centred on life's necessities, such as hygiene and work, the conversations between Philippe and the boys were often enjoyable. I was kind of jealous about the laughter that Philippe was able to elicit from the boys. Fourth, research[17] has suggested the crucial role that fathers play in the development of their children. Philippe's role in the boys' growing-up process through the medium of the French language had impacted them in profound ways, a process some may call language socialisation.[18]

Because the emotional bond established through the use of French among Philippe, Léandre and Dominique was deep, any violation of it (meaning not using French to communicate with each other) would generate emotional reactions. For example, when Philippe joked with Léandre in English, Léandre (14; 3; 2) got visibly angry. When Philippe joked in English to Dominique (12; 4; 7), Dominique did not answer. Instead, he said to Léandre in French, *'Tu connais ce con?'* (Do you know this idiot? A vulgar French word).

Additionally, Léandre and Dominique sometimes thought they owned the French language, and other people (particularly non-French native speakers) had 'no right' to use it. For example, Dominique (13; 6; 14) disliked his eighth-grade English teacher. To improve the relationship with Dominique, the teacher wrote to him in not-so-perfect French and asked him where he put the post-its (*'où est post-its?'*). Dominique was offended that the teacher 'dared' to write French. He corrected the teacher's note with the proper French, 'Où sont les post-its?' (Where are the post-its?).

Chinese as a 'moral' language

As their mother tongue and one of their home languages from birth, Chinese often served as a 'moral'[19] language for the two teens. Since language is a cultural way of thinking,[20] the 'moral' aspect of Chinese language use can perhaps be linked to their Chinese language socialisation process. In my general interactions with Léandre and Dominique, I frequently imparted many cultural wisdoms and values to them. Moreover, the interactions with their Chinese grandparents often entailed moral elements (for example, the story in Box 8.7). Furthermore, most of the Chinese stories I read to the kids had something to do with value and moral teaching. Taken together, Léandre and Dominique's Chinese language socialisation had a sort of moral tone, such as 'If one does not work hard when one is young, one will regret it when one grows old' (如果一个人年轻时不努力, 当他老的时侯, 他会后悔) and 'hard work is the mother of success' (勤奋是成功之母). Through such daily interactions, children gradually internalise culture-specific ways of defining themselves and remembering personal experiences.[21]

As a result, the Chinese language became a language of judging a person's moral standing and value. For example, Dominique (14; 3; 7) said to me, 'Mom, it's not right to gossip behind others' backs' (妈妈, 在背后说人坏话不好) when I was complaining to Philippe about an acquaintance. Table 8.1 shows the frequency of Léandre and Dominique's use of their heritage languages to make moral judgements. As shown, Chinese was used more often to make judgements.

Table 8.1 suggests that both Léandre and Dominique tended to use Chinese to evaluate and judge others more than their French.

Table 8.1 Frequency of using language as judgement[22]

	Chinese	French
Léandre	20%	1%
Dominique	26%	1%

Effect of the reaction of others on the development of linguistic identity

Earlier in the chapter, I mentioned that identity includes two important parts: our own awareness of ourselves and how others perceive us. Thus, the process of our identity positioning reflects the negotiation outcome of who others perceive us to be and who we believe ourselves to be and imagine we can be. Box 8.3 presents some examples of how Léandre and Dominique negotiated their Chinese linguistic confidence and identity.

The examples shown in Box 8.3, together with the opening vignette in Chapter 3 about the compliments of the cyclist about Léandre's native French accent (though it caused misunderstanding initially), suggest that a person's self-confidence and self-esteem largely depend on the positive and negative experiences they have in the environment, as well as the ways in which others perceive them and how the individuals see themselves.[23] It is clear that others' reactions to teens' heritage-language abilities boost their confidence and confirm their linguistic identities.

Box 8.3 Examples of Positive Experiences with Chinese

Example 1:

When Léandre (17; 11; 13) was in Shanghai, he heard that there was a famous market called 七浦 where one can bargain for things for a good price. He asked his grandfather to take him there. I showed him a few bargaining tricks. He quickly got the art of bargaining. Initially, he was at a disadvantage; that is, he did not look Chinese. The sellers often gave him a price for an item that was three times more than they would charge a Chinese person. But, as soon as Léandre began to speak Chinese, things took a different direction. At the end of each bargain, the sellers always commented, 'This foreigner speaks very good Chinese.' This kind of experience really boosted Léandre's self-confidence with his Chinese.

Example 2:

Léandre (17; 11; 15) went with his Chinese grandparents to the neighbourhood club house. His grandparents' friends had conversations with him. Léandre conversed with people (who had different backgrounds) in Chinese with ease. People were surprised that this foreign-looking young man could speak such good Chinese. Léandre was very excited to tell me about the praise he got about his Chinese ability. This was indeed quite helpful in his confidence about his Chinese.

Example 3:

Once I received a call from Dominique (14; 2; 13). In the background, I heard some giggles. I asked Dominique what was going on. He told me that he had put me on the speakerphone so that his friends could hear what Chinese sounded like. Apparently, he was very proud to be able to speak Chinese.

Input languages and their impact on linguistic identities

Taking together, if an input language is present early on in a child's life, the child seems to identify with it deeply. Since French and Chinese were the two home languages that Léandre and Dominique grew up with, and since their father and mother had spoken these two languages with them since birth, they identified with French and Chinese in a special and unique way. It has been suggested that the language a person is brought up with is the language one uses to express deep feelings.[24] A recent study also indicates that moral logic (something so fundamental to one's core) is determined by the language that one was brought up with. For example, in an experiment based on a hypothetical moral dilemma (the trolley problem) about sacrificing one person to save five others, the choice was different depending on whether the experiment was made in a native tongue (involving more intuitive emotional concerns) or in a foreign language (involving less intuitive emotional concerns).[25] Similarly, it has also been suggested that people tend to use curse words more casually when using a second language than when using their native language.[26]

Even though English (compared with Chinese and French) is a more proficient language for Léandre and Dominique, they acquired it with input from others in their environment. Thus, their relation to it is different from the two home languages that they acquired from their parents. Overall, both Léandre and Dominique regarded their multilingual abilities as their strengths and something of which they could be proud. For example, when I asked Léandre (17; 1; 8) what his strength was, he did not hesitate to tell me that his strength was his ability to speak more than three languages. In their college application materials, both boys mentioned their multilingual abilities.

Cultural identity

The process of acquiring and developing multiple languages is not only a linguistic process but also a process of acquiring and developing one's cultural identity. Language learning is thus a powerful device for activating and reinforcing associated cultural constructs, and it plays a critical role in the construction, maintenance and expression of a dynamic cultural self.

Special feelings towards Switzerland

Over the years, we have made efforts to bring Léandre and Dominique back to our heritage countries. In particular, frequent visits and long stays in Switzerland created a subjective feeling of belonging for both Léandre and Dominique. Each time when it was time for us to return to New York, Léandre and Dominique would always make a scene. For example, on the eve of leaving Switzerland one year, Dominique (14; 1; 26) told his Swiss friend David to kidnap him and Léandre so that they did not have to go back to New York. Also, when driving back to Neuchâtel, Dominique (14; 1; 23) expressed his sentiment by pretending to be an American country singer, mixing French words with English, 'I don't want to go back to États Unis (United

States).' Similarly, when we returned to New York from Switzerland, I asked Léandre to take a shower. Léandre (16; 0; 24) said that he did not want to take a shower because he did not want to wash away the scent of the Swiss soap. Likewise, Léandre (15; 1; 15) asked me to give him a piece of soap for his shower. I offered him one. He did not want it because he said it did not smell good. I told him that I bought this soap (Les Petit Marseille) in Migros. He immediately changed his mind and took the soap. These kinds of romanticised feelings towards Switzerland permeated their childhood and adolescence. For example, I asked Dominique (14; 3; 16) whether the Tête de Moine cheese I bought in Whole Foods tasted the same as in Switzerland. He answered, 'It does not taste like the one *at home*.' Once when we stepped out of the plane at Geneva airport, Dominique (13; 0; 10) was overjoyed and said, 'We are finally *home!*'

Complex association with the Chinese culture

Both Léandre and Dominique had a firm association with their Chinese heritage culture. Both of them showed pride in being partially Asian. One year, Dominique (13; 11; 14) brought back his middle-school yearbook. I saw that many of his classmates had written about the 'Asian Club for Men.' I was curious and asked what that was. He said that he had formed an 'Asian Club for Men' in school and he 'converted' all his male friends (all of them, except one Asian, were white) into 'Asians.'

Moreover, both Léandre and Dominique were familiar with and observant of traditional Chinese holidays, cultural rituals and customs. For instance, Dominique (16; 9; 23) reminded me that I needed to eat noodles for my birthday because it is a Chinese ritual to eat noodles for one's birthday to symbolise longevity.

Furthermore, the boys were also interested in and curious about Chinese history and cultural events. For example, when I read Léandre a story written by his Chinese grandfather, Léandre (15; 2; 18) wanted to know more about the Chinese cultural revolution, about which he only had a little knowledge from his social studies class.

However, unlike their romanticised, unitary feelings towards Switzerland and the Swiss culture, Léandre and Dominique had an ambivalent and binary feeling towards China and the Chinese culture. On the one hand, as you read above, they do have a firm association with the Chinese culture. On the other hand, they also exhibited some negative feelings about China and its culture. When they observed certain behaviours by some Chinese, they tended to generalise them. For instance, when observing people pushing each other to get seats in the subway in Shanghai, they would make some negative comments about the culture. Even though I have discussed with them the many reasons why some Chinese people behave in certain ways, they continued to hold their beliefs about the culture. I believe that their negative feelings towards Chinese culture were in part also a result of the media in the West in addition to their direct observations.

Multilingual and multicultural identity revealed through autobiographical memories

Autobiographical memory is the ability to recall episodes, experiences and events in an individual's life. It is central to an integrated and functioning self-system.

Given that different cultural beliefs, socialisation practices and meanings are so deeply embedded in the different languages of multilingual adolescents, and given that different languages may entail different cognitive systems and possess separate self-structures associated with their different languages, multilinguals may reveal their different cultural selves through their autobiographic memories. For example, one study suggests that when bilingual young adults from Hong Kong were asked to describe themselves, those who responded in Chinese used more collective and fewer individual terms than those who responded in English.[27] In addition, in a study of autobiographical memory in Russian–English bilingual adults, it was found that memories recalled in English tended to be more self-focused, whereas memories recalled in Russian were more other-oriented.

The phenomenon whereby different languages trigger different autobiographic memories suggests that the use of a language may serve as a cue that makes salient and accessible the cultural belief system chronically associated with that language.[28] The activated cultural belief system may further activate self-concepts congruent with the belief system. In daily life, language, no matter whether it is used privately in thinking or overtly in communication, may serve as a constant reminder of cultural knowledge and beliefs, which can further lead individuals to adopt self-concepts consistent with these knowledge structures. The culturally endorsed self-concepts or cultural self-construals may remain chronically active, salient and accessible given the constant reinforcement of the linguistic-cultural context in which individuals reside. In turn, they may drive cognitive resources into the privileged processing and retrieving of autobiographical information that confirms the goals and motivations associated with the self-concepts,[29] thus giving rise to culture-specific ways of autobiographical remembering.[30]

It is fascinating to learn that the cultural selves revealed in the autobiographic memories of Léandre and Dominique during adolescence positioned them as different cultural selves through using different languages. In their spontaneous recounting of their past experiences in their different languages, Léandre and Dominique revealed their different selves. In French, they tended to position themselves as funny and cheerful. For example, in a 40-sentence spontaneous narrative about his past, Léandre (15; 9; 10) used the word *rigolo* (funny) 19 times. In Chinese, Léandre and Dominique tended to portray themselves as reflective moral beings. For example, in a 32-sentence spontaneous narrative about his past, Dominique (16; 3; 0) used the phrases 我学了 (I learnt) 10 times. In English, both teens tended to reveal themselves as rational beings. For example, in a 23-sentence conversation with his peers, Léandre used the phrase 'my point is' 4 times. Research has indicated that the use of a particular language may activate a specific cultural frame or belief system to which this language is chronically connected in everyday life. The use of a particular language may elicit associated culturally desirable beliefs, self-concepts and memory.[31]

Thus, language is critical to the development and maintenance of a cultural self. For multilingual children, learning to speak different languages equips them with multiple tools with which they can construct their cultural selves in relation to the sociocultural world. Developing different representations of the self in relation to different languages may further provide them with the flexibility to respond effectively to myriads of cultural and linguistic contexts that they transition in and out of in everyday life.[32]

Different representations of selves

Germane to their different cultural selves discussed above, multilinguals' self-representations may be different when different languages are used. Elsewhere[33] (see Box 8.4), I discussed how Léandre and Dominique tended to represent themselves differently in different languages, and these selves were not represented unitarily. Rather, they often enacted different kinds of selves in different linguistic contexts based

---

Box 8.4 Examples of Different Presentations of Different Selves in Different Languages

Dominique (10; 1; 13)

[In English] 'We lived in a hotel called the Splendid Hotel the first night. It was not splendid at all! I don't recommend it. The rooms were too small . . . The breakfast was bad. We then moved to the Hilton Hotel the next night; it was the best in all of Europe...' [the poster on the wall says it's the best in Europe.]

[In French] '... J'ai visité le Louvre et j'ai vu la Joconde. C'était super. Je vais pouvoir dire à mes copains d'école que j'ai vu la vraie! Papa m'a même pris un photo devant elle. Je n'oublierai jamais cette journée . . . J'ai aussi vu la Vénus de Milo. Tu sais pourquoi elle n'a plus ses bras? C'est un 'hobo' qui les lui a mangés'.' ('I visited the Louvre and I saw the real painting of the Mona Lisa. It's fabulous. I can now tell my classmates in school that I finally saw the real thing. Father took some pictures of me in front of her [the painting]. I'll never forget that day . . . I also saw the statue of the Venus de Milo. [Laughing] Do you know why her arms were missing? They were eaten by a hobo ...'). [Dominique wanted to make the similar kind of joke as the Belgian cartoonist Philippe Geluck in one of his comic books.]

[In Chinese] 我们到一个中国人开的泰国饭店吃晚饭。我叫了咖啡冰淇淋，可是那个中国招待员给我巧克力的。她可能想小孩子不能吃咖啡，可是她没有告诉我。她假装要给我，可是她没沒给我...

(We ate dinner in a Thai restaurant opened by two Chinese people. I ordered coffee ice cream, but the Chinese waitress gave me chocolate instead; she probably thought that children should not have coffee [caffeine]. She didn't tell me that I couldn't have coffee ice cream. She pretended to take my order and then gave me a different kind of ice cream...).

From Wang, X.-L. (2008) *Growing Up With Three Languages: Birth to Eleven* (pp.184–85). Bristol: Multilingual Matters.

on their understanding of what kinds of self-representation could best capture their audience in a particular language (and culture). For example, in French, they tended to represent themselves as humorous, passionate and emotional. In English, they tended to represent themselves as linear, rational and neutral. In Chinese, they tended to represent themselves as judgemental and scrupulous. During their adolescent period, they continued to show such tendencies; that is, in French, jokes and humour were more salient; in Chinese, a moral tone was more prominent; and in English, rational and linear description was more evident.

In sum, management of multicultural identity requires overt and conscious flexibility. It requires the presentation in or emphasis on the desirable aspect of the self in context. It seems that both Léandre and Dominique were able to adjust their multilingual and multicultural identities in the changing environment during adolescence.

One word of caution: it would be a mistake to assume that individuals who process the knowledge of a particular cultural tradition will necessarily identify with it. Learning and acquiring knowledge of certain cultural traditions does not necessarily entail identification with them. Nevertheless, even though some multilinguals may not identify with a particular culture, one important advantage is that they can cognitively place the different cultures in juxtaposition and attempt to integrate them to foster a creative synthesis. Thus, exposure to more than one cultural tradition can increase cognitive and behavioural flexibility.[34]

National identity

In my book *Growing Up With Three Languages: Birth to Eleven*, I mentioned that during their early and middle childhood, the boys developed a sense of belonging to the countries of which they were citizens (the United States and Switzerland). They consistently used the collective pronoun 'we' when they referred to Americans and Swiss, but used 'they' when they referred to Chinese. During adolescence, they continued to feel this way. Interestingly, when cheering for national sports teams in competitions, both boys revealed their national identity. For example, during the 2010 World Cup in South Africa, Léandre and Dominique felt bad when the Swiss team lost the game to Chile. They felt the same when the Swiss soccer team lost to the French team in the 2014 World Cup in Brazil. Also, Léandre and Dominique cheered for the US soccer team and accused the Brazilian team of cheating in the 2011 US v Brazil soccer match.

Their Chinese identity is particularly complex. On one hand, they were very proud to be associated with the Chinese culture and be partially Chinese racially. On the other hand, because they did not hold a Chinese passport, they also felt that they did not belong to China. In the case of team sports competitions, they would cheer for the Chinese team only when Swiss and US teams were not involved.

Being a citizen of both Switzerland and the United States, Léandre was eager to register as a voter as soon as he reached the age of 18. On 27 August 2013, 20 days after he turned 18, he voted for the first time as a Swiss abroad. Dominique did the same thing.

Another interesting aspect of Léandre and Dominique's national identity is their knowledge about Switzerland. When I saw a number plate in Switzerland that had an 'M,' I asked Dominique what 'M' means. Dominique (16; 0; 1) joked, 'It's the 27th canton in Switzerland' (there are 26 cantons in Switzerland). He knew that the number plate was for the Swiss military.

Being citizens of more than one country and being able to speak more than one language also can cause some confusion for others. For example, once, in Basel, Léandre brought a sim card for his iPhone. The salesperson was puzzled when Léandre showed him a Swiss ID card, while speaking Chinese to me and French to his father, and then telling the salesperson that he lived in New York. Box 8.5, which tells of an encounter

---

Box 8.5 Example of Puzzlement Concerning Nationalities

Immigration
Officer (IO): Hello, passports please.

Xiao-lei (XL): Hello. (Handed him three Swiss Passports [Philippe, Léandre, and Dominique usually travel with their Swiss passport in Europe] and one American passport.)

IO: You are on vacation?

XL: Yes.

IO: The American in the car needs to fill in the form [handed XL the form].

Léandre and
Dominique: [Made some comments in French in the back of the car].

XL: [Jokingly] So, the American is in trouble? [meaning they had to fill in a form].

IO: [Jokingly] Yes, the American is in trouble. So, where do you live?

XL: In New York.

IO: [looking at Léandre and Dominique]

IO: So, they [Philippe, Léandre and Dominique] live in Switzerland?

XL: No, they live in New York also.

IO: [Puzzled].

XL: [Explained why].

IO: It's too complicated…Have a good vacation.

with an immigration officer in Jersey while we stopped at the booth, demonstrates another example of puzzlement for others.

Local and global identity

Over the years, Léandre and Dominique have formed an emotional attachment with the local community in Neuchâtel, especially St. Blaise. Dominique even composed an excellent music piece named *St. Blaise* to express his sentiment towards the place where in summer he sat for hours on his grandparents' terrace, admiring the panoramic view of the Alps, Lake Neuchâtel, and the steeples and roofs in the distance; and hearing the bells of cows from nearby farms and birdsong from the Jura Mountains. Dominique's sentiment or oversentimental feelings towards Neuchâtel were sometimes exaggerated. For example, we were once driving from France to Neuchâtel. Dominique was playing a video game in the car. While going through a tunnel on the French side, we told Dominique that we were almost in Neuchâtel. Still playing with his video game, he (13; 1; 4) said, 'C'est beau' (It's beautiful), without realising we were still in the tunnel in the French part. Similarly, I asked Dominique (14; 0; 9) whether he wanted to go with us to Geneva to get something to drink. He said, 'No, I want to stay at *home* (St. Blaise).'

Having been travelling with us internationally since they were infants, Léandre and Dominique were (and still are) very interested in global affairs and the world in general. Léandre put a world map on the wall next to his bed when he was in fifth grade. Every morning when he woke up, he would look at the world map, dreaming of the next place he would like to visit. Both Léandre and Dominique were genuinely interested in world history and both got excellent scores on their SAT world history subject test and the AP world history test.

Moreover, both boys were also knowledgeable about the world. They were (and still are) curious about world events and eager to read about world affairs in the *New York Times*. In fact, one of both Léandre and Dominique's college majors is international studies. Moreover, both children are knowledgeable about their surroundings in different counties. For example, I once asked Philippe which route was faster from Lyon (France) to Basel (Switzerland). Philippe said that if we use the *interstate*, it would be faster. Léandre (17; 0; 12) immediately reminded Philippe that we were in France, not in the United States, and that the correct term was *autoroute*. In short, both Léandre and Dominique are globally minded and have accumulated global knowledge as a result of being multilingual and having travelled the world.

Racial identity

Sometimes, there might be a discrepancy between who we are and how others perceive us to be. Here is an episode to illustrate the relationship between identity as seen by oneself and that seen by others. A few years ago, our family drove through Canton Bern (Switzerland) in our French rental car, which had a French number plate. At a pedestrian crossing, Philippe stopped the car to let an older gentleman cross. The man was grateful and said to us loudly, 'Vive la France!' (Long live France). Apparently, the old man thought we were French from our number plate, even though we knew clearly that none of us in the car was French (as I am American, and Philippe, Léandre and Dominique are Swiss-American). This example suggests that others often determine who we are by what we appear to be or not to be. In real life, our racial identity is often judged by others based on what we look like or not like. For instance, Léandre does not look like a Chinese. Therefore, others do not place him as Chinese or Asian. For example, when we visited Léandre in his college, Léandre (18; 3; 22) told me that his friends thought he was either Italian or Portuguese; it was not until they saw me (his mother) in the cafeteria that they realised that he was half Asian. Also, at an international conference in Shanghai in 2013, Léandre co-presented a paper with me. A man from Sweden approached Léandre and told him that he had just been to Spain (he thought Léandre was Spanish). Similarly, on a flight from Shanghai to Zurich, the flight attendants addressed Léandre in Swiss German because they thought he was Swiss German. People were often surprised when Léandre spoke Chinese because he did not look Chinese.

As for Dominique, he looked more Asian when he was younger. As he entered the adolescent period, his look changed, and he looked like a more typical White-Asian mixture. More and more often, he was placed in the racial category of a South American. Being able to speak Chinese was often less shocking than the reactions to Léandre. However, when both Léandre and Dominique were together (for example in China), they were identified as foreigners. For example, once in a store in Shanghai, Léandre and Dominique were in front of me, and I heard the shop assistants telling each other, 'The foreigners are coming...'

People tend to associate a person's look (in a racial sense) with their language ability as well. Box 8.6 is an excerpt from an article that was featured in the *New York Times*. This describes an episode during a visit by New York mayor Bill de Blasio to Italy.

This is a telling example of how people judge a person's linguistic ability often through his/her racial identity. People with mixed racial identities frequently encounter misjudgement. They are easily put into racial categories. From my observations, both Léandre and Dominique are comfortable with their racial identities and they are comfortable in their own skin. However, this is not true for some teens. Karen's daughter Melisa, whose parents are African (Black) and American (White), wished that she was either Black or White and not a mixture of different races (as she termed herself).[35]

Name identity

What's in a name? Obviously, our names are a very important part of our identities. Throughout our lives, our names are associated with us and are part of our being, and thus our names embody who we are.[36] The boys have three sets of

> **Box 8.6 Race and Language**
>
> Maisha Grispino, a college-age daughter of Cécile Kyenge, Italy's first black national official, was sitting on an immaculate terrace of one of this city's most exclusive social clubs on Monday when a white woman approached.
>
> 'Are you Chiara?' the woman asked, mistaking Ms Grispino for the biracial daughter of Bill de Blasio, the mayor of New York City, who was meeting with Ms Kyenge inside.
>
> Ms Grispino shook her head no. The Italian woman, realising her mistake, excused herself, but not before offering a bright smile. 'You speak Italian almost better than I do!' the woman said cheerfully.
>
> Ms Grispino, 21, was born in Italy and is a native speaker, but she has heard remarks like this all her life…
>
> Quotes from Grynbaum, M.M. (2014) In Italy de Blasio meets with 'Mirror Image.' *New York Times*, 21 July.

names corresponding to the languages they speak. Their official names are Léandre and Dominique (spelt in French way), their Chinese names are 理昂 and 昵可 and their English names are Leander and Dominick. In their school and other official documents, the French spellings are used. As a result, Léandre and Dominique were often treated as girls' names in the United States because of the French spelling. For example, once I got an e-mail from a soccer coach politely asking me whether I made a mistake by registering Dominique on a boys' team instead of on a girls' team. Also, Léandre (15; 9; 15) had to change the spelling of his name from Leander to Léandre in order to register for his SAT. Similarly, when colleges and universities began to send information and e-mails to solicit applications from Léandre and Dominique, they were always addressed as Ms rather than Mr. When Dominique received a letter from the White House on 8 August 2014 – a reply from President Obama because Dominique had written to him about a gun control issue for a class assignment (even though this was a kind of standard letter probably sent to everyone who wrote) – Dominique was very excited. However, upon opening the letter, he was disappointed that he was addressed as Ms. The initial thrill diminished a bit because he had been called Ms rather than Mr.

During adolescence, Léandre and Dominique's school friends called them Dre and Dom respectively in English.

In retrospect, we do have some regret about our choice of names for our two children. We realised that we probably should have given them different names that sound less 'feminine' in the United States. If the boys decide to continue living in the United States, they will have to constantly deal with the issue of their names being regarded as female names.

Put it all together

Research suggests that there are three forms of multicultural identity negotiation: integration (blended and merged into one coherent cultural identity), alternation (switching back and forth among cultural identities depending on the context), and synergy (an entirely new, unique identity, not the sum of two cultures).[37] As shown in the discussion so far, Léandre and Dominique's negotiation of their multilingual identities does not work in a single way. Rather, their identity negotiations are complex, elastic and sometimes inconsistent.[38] In other words, their negotiations of their identities may lean towards one or other of the three depending on the context.

Moreover, multilinguals' identity negotiation can be viewed at two levels: one as a group or collective (the numerical level) and the other as an individual (the qualitative level).[39] At the collective level of identity, multilinguals identify with one another on account of shared characteristics or features of other multilinguals. At the qualitative (individual) level, a specific multilingual person, such as a Chinese-French-English speaker who lives in New York, has his or her own characteristics. The person may choose to identify with other multilinguals but also with Swiss and Chinese. The matter of priority or salience, when it does arise, is highly contextual.

Finally, from the above discussions, it seems that the poststructuralists' view on identity can explain some of what Léandre and Dominique went through in their multilingual identity development and negotiation. According to **the poststructuralist view**, identity may include notions of the self as imposed, assumed or negotiated.[40] The imposed self is the label *trilingual* that has been given to them since birth. Along the way, they assumed the trilingual identity. Most of all, they were negotiating their multilingual identity and constructed self as they want themselves to be viewed by others (the negotiated self). Overall, both Léandre and Dominique were successful in negotiating their different identities during adolescence. Their identities will continue to evolve in the years to come. I look forward to documenting the process and sharing it with you in my future books.

Strategies for Supporting Multiple Identity Development During Adolescence

Parenting and adolescent identity development

Psychologist James Marcia categorised identity in four statuses: **identity achievement** (individuals have explored meaningful life directions prior to their commitments, and they show high levels of achievement motivation and self-esteem), **identity foreclosure** (individuals have formed commitments without significant prior explorations), **identity moratorium** (individuals are in the process of searching for meaningful adult roles and values but have not yet formed firm commitments), and **identity diffusion** (individuals are not interested in finding personally expressive adult roles and values).[41] Researchers have linked parenting styles with the different identity formations. For example, identity-achieved and moratorium adolescents have been associated with parenting styles that encourage free and independent behaviour and emphasise both individuality and connectedness in family relationships instead of controlling and regulating. Adolescents who show the characteristics of foreclosure identity tend to be from families that are very close, involved, protective and child-centred. Parents of adolescents with diffusion identity tend to be distanced and rejecting and provide no guidance. Also, the communication patterns are often inconsistent.[42]

Thus, to foster your teens' positive identity formation and development, you may want to encourage them to explore different opportunities to find out who they are, to trust them and to offer support when they need it. Sometimes, you will be surprised how competent your teens can be. I recall here the example I used in Chapter 1 about putting Léandre (14; 11; 0) in charge of planning a family trip to Ireland, Northern Ireland and Scotland. One episode from that trip is intriguing. When we drove from Belfast to Edinburgh, Léandre told us that he had found us a little hotel in Killin. As we drove in the direction of the hotel, it became dark. For a while, we did not see any hotels around. Both Philippe and I became doubtful whether we were right to trust a 14-year-old to arrange a hotel for us. We kept asking Léandre whether he was sure about what he had reserved for us. Léandre assured us, 'Don't worry. We will get there.' Just as we were beginning to think that there was no hope of finding the hotel and were telling ourselves mentally that we would never let Léandre take charge of this sort of thing again, a nice little white house under the hanging dark clouds came into view. This was one of the cosiest and most pleasant little hotels we ever stayed in. Our praise of Léandre boosted his confidence as a competent trip planner. He has since assumed the role of trip planner for our family.

Motivation does not necessarily translate to language learning

The common belief is that if a person is motivated to learn a language, she or he will learn that language well. Although motivation is important in heritage-language learning, Bonny Norton's research and work[43] have shown that while sometimes learners can be highly motivated to learn a language, they will not necessarily invest in a given set of language practices if they feel marginalised by the target language speakers (in our case, the native heritage-language speakers).

Therefore, when interacting with your heritage-language-learning teens, you must create an environment and opportunities where teens feel they are valued as heritage-language speakers. The examples shown previously about Léandre's experiences with the Chinese merchants validated him as a Chinese language speaker, and he was encouraged by his ability to speak Chinese.

Positive experience and positive identity development

Self-efficacy (belief in one's ability to do things) is important for teens in their overall confidence about themselves and their abilities, including their heritage-language abilities. If teens frequently have successful experiences with their heritage language(s), they are likely to keep learning it or them. If they constantly feel incompetent in their heritage-language use, they may have anxiety, which will lead to self-doubt, uneasiness, frustration, apprehension and tension.

Therefore, it is important to provide them with successful experiences in their heritage-language use. For example, the merchants' praise of Léandre's ability in Chinese (Box 8.3) boosted his self-confidence. Sometimes, teens also have self-doubt about their ability in their heritage language(s). For example, Dominique commented that he read and wrote Chinese poorly. In situations like this, showing teens what they have achieved is helpful for them to believe what they can do with their heritage language and that they would do even better if they continue learning it.

However, negative experiences are also necessary for teens to learn and grow. For example, once we visited a town near Braga (Portugal). As usual, Dominique (13; 0; 19) bought himself a local soccer jersey (in this case, the Braga soccer team jersey). Ignorant about the rivalry between Braga and Guimarães, Dominique wore the Braga soccer jersey to Guimarães. When Dominique stopped in a shop to get himself an ice cream, he heard some young men shouting at him with the curse word 'Merda' from several corners. Obviously, these young people thought Dominique was openly challenging them by wearing the Braga soccer jersey to their town. Dominique quickly left town. Although this experience was unpleasant, he learnt a big lesson in life.

Active involvement with heritage cultures

The key to establishing a close tie with teens' heritage culture(s) is to help them engage with those culture(s). For instance, each time Philippe received his Swiss voting booklet from the Swiss government, he would read the information to Léandre and Dominique and discuss his opinions on the issues. Adolescence is an optimum time to discuss ideas.

Moreover, our experiences show that keeping constant contact with the heritage culture(s) is a must if teens are to understand and feel connected to the heritage culture(s). One way of achieving this kind of contact is through frequent visits. Many things cannot be taught until a child experiences them first hand. Hence, creating opportunities for your children to be with their heritage families or visit their heritage countries is essential. Both Philippe and I have witnessed how our two children made tremendous progress in their heritage languages and knowledge about their heritage cultures after their stays in their heritage countries. Therefore, it is important to make travelling to their heritage countries or involvement with their heritage communities a priority in your children's lives.

Heritage-family stories

Knowing their family stories and understanding their roots can help teens' identity development. Through stories told by extended family members in the heritage culture(s), teens not only can learn about the customs in their heritage culture(s) but they can also learn about their cultural roots and family history. Since Léandre and Dominique entered adolescence, I have requested that their Chinese grandparents write about their lives and send these family stories to us. Over the years, I have found these family stories represent valuable Chinese cultural and family history education for Léandre and Dominique and have helped the two teens understand their family's past. Box 8.7 is such an example.

This family story has taught Léandre and Dominique many things. From the cultural perspective, Léandre and Dominique learnt the rituals of birthday celebrations in the Chinese culture as well as the symbolic meanings associated with the practices. From the family history perspective, the teens learnt about their great- great- great-grandfather, their great- great- grandmother, and their grandfather's childhood, as well as their socioeconomic status. From a Chinese moral education perspective, they learnt the Chinese value (or their grandfather's value) of showing respect to mothers and appreciation of mothers. From an identity development perspective, the teens learnt their association with the Chinese family past.

Thus, if you have the opportunity, you may consider requesting that your relatives from the heritage culture(s) write about or tell stories about themselves. I think this is an excellent way to help teens' identity development.

Identity development is an ongoing process

Even though the aspects of identity are more salient during adolescence because this is the period when teens begin to consciously explore their identity issues, identity development is an ongoing process. As discussed earlier, the current understanding is that identity development is a process rather than an end result. Multilingual adolescents (later on youths) will continue to explore their different identities in different contexts. As parents, we need to continue to provide support for our children while they are exploring and negotiating their identities in a new environment. When Léandre recently told us that he had decided to spend his senior year in college in Berlin, both Philippe and I enthusiastically supported his decision. Léandre certainly felt that his choice was respected and his parents were willing to work together with him to enhance his exploration. The advice to parents given by the author of *Uncommon Sense for Parents with Teenagers*, Michael Riera, (mentioned in Chapter 2) is wise: As a consultant (rather than a manager), our job involves more trust and 'back up' and less direct decision making. Adolescents must been seen as individuals who are able to make decisions with the support of parents and other adults.

Box 8.7 A Story Shared by Léandre and Dominique's Chinese Grandfather

English Translation

Remembering Birthday Celebration in the Old Times

Nowadays, when people celebrate their birthdays, they usually have a birthday party, invite some friends to light candles, cut the cake, and sing happy birthday... But when I was a child, birthdays were called 'celebrating longevity'. Many rituals in the birthday celebration were related to 'longevity'; for example, eating was called 'longevity banquet,' gifts were called 'longevity gifts', and the person who was celebrating the birthday was called 'longevity star'. Chinese believe that life is the accumulation of years and respecting longevity is the respect of life. That is why people are so serious about birthday celebrations. In the past, adults always hung the character 'Longevity' in the living room, lit two red longevity candles, and decorated the room with two bowls of longevity noodles and flour-made longevity peaches. During the birthday celebration, the birthday 'longevity star' sat at the head of the table, accepting congratulations and bows from the younger generation. Then the whole family sat around the table and ate longevity noodles.

One year, my grandfather had his 60th birthday; during that era, living to that age was a longevity, so the birthday celebration was especially grand. The birthday celebration was arranged in a restaurant. The hall was covered with silk scrolls made with the silk cover of quilt given by friends and family. Later on I heard from adults that the family had used these quilt covers for many years. After the birthday celebrations began, the MC (master of ceremonies) read aloud the words praising my grandfather's good deeds and ways of managing the family. Then, his children and grandchildren lined up to kowtow (bow at him). After the ceremony, guests and family were treated with banquets and they were also entertained with a special performance – *tanghui* 堂会 (a type of private performance for individual families). We kids were so excited that we could not fall asleep that night.

At that time, children's birthday celebrations were not so grand as adults'. However, children's birthdays were not ignored. I remember my mother taught me since I could remember that one should not only remember one's own birthday but also remember the birthdays of other family members. When we were kids, each year on our birthday, a new set of clothes was made for us. I remember when I was seven, the year when I went to elementary school, my parents bought me a suit, as well as straps and tie on my birthday. They also took me to the studio to take a photo. I felt very proud. Unfortunately, this picture was not preserved.

(Continued)

When we were kids, on the morning of our birthdays, our mother would boil us a special kind of egg with rock sugar, which was her hope for her children to live a sweet life. Cooking noodles was also essential, which was her blessing for her children to live long lives. All these rituals and the symbolic meanings associated with them fully expressed our mother's love for us. Years later, an elder told me, when recounting my mother's life: 'In her 44 short years of life, she gave birth to 13 children, raised 9 children. She sacrificed everything for you, not easy!' I was deeply moved by these words. I realised that our birthday is the day of our mother's day of suffering. Therefore every child should remember the sacrifice of their mother in raising them. Every child should not forget his/her mother's love! Since then, I always remember my mother's birthday every year – September 8 in the lunar calendar.

Original Chinese Text

生日旧事

现代人过生日一般都是开个生日派对，邀请一些好朋友来点蜡烛、切蛋糕、唱生日快乐歌……。但是在我们小时候过生日叫做'祝寿'。生日聚会上的很多内容都要和寿字挂上钩，吃饭叫'寿宴'，送礼物叫'寿礼'，过生日的人大家都尊称为'寿星'。中国人认为寿是生命年代的积累，对寿的重视，就是对生命的尊重。所以家家都非常重视过生日。过去大人们每年过生日都要在家里正厅里贴一个大大的'寿'字，桌上点起两支红红的寿烛，还要摆上两大盘寿面和面制的寿桃。过生日的寿星端坐在上首，接受晚辈的叩拜祝贺。然后全家围坐一桌吃长寿面。

有一年，我的外公过60岁大寿，那个时代能活到这个年龄就是高寿了。所以生日过得特别隆重，专门在饭店里庆寿，大厅里挂满了亲友们送的用绸缎被面做的'寿幛'。后来听大人说这些被面全家人用了许多年还用不完。庆典开始后主持人高声朗诵祝寿词称赞外公德高望重，治家有方。儿孙们排着队给老寿星叩头。礼毕，摆了几十桌酒席招待宾客和家人、还请了戏曲班子来唱堂会（一种到私家演的型式）。我们小孩子忙着看热闹。兴奋得当晚都睡不着觉。

那时，我们孩子过生日当然没有大人那么隆重，但也是不会被忽视的。记得妈妈从我记事起就教我，不但要记住自己的生日也要记住全家人的生日。小时候我们每年过生日，家里都做一套新衣服给我们穿。我七岁上小学那年，我过生日时，父母给我买了一套小西装，还有背带和领带，并带我到照相馆去拍了照片，我觉得神气极了。可惜这张照片没有保存下来。童年过生日那天早上起来，妈妈会给我们吃一个用冰糖煮的水波蛋，希望孩子生活的甜甜密密。吃寿面也是不可少的，是祝福孩子能长命百岁。这些美好的寓意充分表达了母亲对我们的爱。多年以后，一位长辈对我追述了我妈妈的一生说：'她短短的44年生命中，孕育了13个孩子，养护了9个儿女成人，她为你们献出了一切，不容易啊'！这番话对我震撼很大，我们的生日就是妈妈的受难日，每一个做儿女的都要记住妈妈养育我们所付出的辛苦，自己过生日别忘了妈妈的恩情！从此，我也永远记住了每年妈妈的生日-农历九月初八。

Excerpt from the e-mail sent by Léandre and Dominique's Chinese grandparents on 27 September 2010.

Summary of Key Points in Chapter 8

- Identity refers to our sense of who we are and our relationship to others. Our identity is not fixed; instead, it is constructed and reconstructed over time and in different contexts.
- Multilingualism provides a much more complicated reality for identity development. Thus, teens need to constantly negotiate their multiple identities.
- Identity negotiation happens on two levels: between the individual and others and within the individual regarding which of a number of possible identity positions they elect to take up.
- An examination of the period from the ages of 12 to 19 suggests that the following areas of Léandre and Dominique's identities were noticeable during adolescence: multilingualism (linguistic identity), multiculturalism (cultural identity), binationalism (national identity), biracialism (racial identity), local identity (St. Blaise), global identity (international travel) and name representation (effects of their names on their identity).
- Linguistic identity: The different languages used by Léandre and Dominique served different functions, for example:
  - English was treated as a neutral language.
  - French was treated as an emotional language.
  - Chinese was treated as a 'judgemental' language.
- Cultural identity: Language learning is a powerful device for activating and reinforcing associated cultural constructs and plays a critical role in the construction, maintenance and expression of a dynamic cultural self. There are some special characteristics in Léandre and Dominique's cultural development:
  - Special feelings towards Switzerland.
  - Firm association with the Chinese culture.
  - Multilingualism and multiculturalism deeply rooted in autobiographic memories.
  - Different representations of selves.
- National identity is complex. Generally, Léandre and Dominique tended to associate themselves with the nations for which they held passports.
- Both Léandre and Dominique had strong sentimental local connections with St. Blaise, Neuchâtel. They were also globally minded.
- People often judge a person's linguistic ability according to their racial categories.
- Léandre and Dominique's names often caused misunderstanding of their gender in the United States.
- Strategies for supporting multiple identity development during adolescence may include:
  - Multilingual and multicultural teens should be provided with opportunities to explore and with support.
  - Positive experiences encourage positive identity development.
  - Active engagement with heritage cultures is important.
  - Identity development is evolving.

Recommended Readings

Dewaele, J.-M. (2013) *Emotions in Multiple Languages*. New York, NY: Palgrave Macmillan.
González, N. (2005) *I Am My Language: Discourses of Women and Children in Borderlands*. Tucson: University of Arizona Press.
Pavlenko, A. and Blackledge, A. (eds) (2004) *Negotiation of identities in Multilingual Contexts*. Clevedon: Multilingual Matters.

Notes and References

[1] Excerpts from Dominique's class notebook.
[2] 炎黄子孙 (the descendants of emperors Yellow) is what Chinese call themselves.
[3] Reyes, A. (2007) *Language, Identity and Stereotype among Southeast Asian American Youth: The Other Asian*. Mahawah, NJ: Lawrence Erlbaum.
[4] Spernes, K. (2012) 'I use my Mother tongue at home and with friends-not in school!': Multilingualism and identity in rural Kenya. *Language, Culture and Curriculum* 25(2), 189–203.
[5] Kanno, Y. (2003) Imagine communities, school visions, and the education of bilingual students in Japan. *Journal of Language Identity and Education* 2 (4), 285–300.
Kanno, Y. and Stuart, C. (2011) Learning to become a second language teacher: Identities-in-practice. *The Modern Language Journal* 95 (2), 236–52.
[6] Lanza, E. and Svendsen, B.A. (2007) Tell me who your friends are and I might be able to tell what language(s) you speak: Social network analysis, multilingualism, and identity. *International Journal of Bilingualism* 11 (3), 275–300.
[7] Wang, Q. and Ross, M. (2007) Culture and memory. In H. Kitayama and D. Cohen (eds) *Handbook of Cultural Psychology* (pp. 645–667). New York, NY: Guilford Publications.
Wang, Q. (2008) Emotion knowledge and autobiographical memory across the preschool years: A cross-cultural longitudinal investigation. *Cognition* 108, 117–35.
[8] Giampapa, F. (2004) The politics of identity, representation, and the discourse of self-identification: Negotiating the periphery and the center (pp. 192–218). In A. Pavlenko and A. Blackledge (eds) (2004) *Negotiation of Identities in Multilingual Contexts*. Clevedon: Multilingual Matters.
[9] Harre, R. and van Lagenhove, L. (1999) *Positioning Theory: Moral Contexts of Intentional Action*. Oxford: Blackwell.
[10] Data analysis was based on 28-hour video recordings over a period of 7 years with 4 hours each year in addition to notes and conversations.
[11] The phrase 'manage identity' is borrowed from Rich, S. and Dais, L. (2007) Insights into the strategic ways in which two bilingual children in the early years seek to negotiate the competing demands in their identity in their home and school worlds. International *Journal of Early Years Education* 15 (1), 35–47.
[12] Norton, B. (2000) *Identity and Language Learning: Gender, Ethnicity, and Educational Change*. Harlow, UK: Longman/Pearson.
[13] Spernes, K. (2012) 'I use my Mother tongue at home and with friends-not in school!': Multilingualism and identity in rural Kenya. *Language, Culture and Curriculum* 25 (2), 189–203.
Lunga, V.B. (1994) Mapping African postcoloniality: Linguistic and cultural spaces of hybridity. *Perspectives on Global Development and Technology* 34, 291–326.
[14] Pavlenko, A. and Blackledge, A. (2004) New theoretical approaches to the study of negotiation of identities in multilingual contexts (pp. 1–33). In A. Pavlenko and A. Blackledge (eds) *Negotiation of Identities in Multilingual Contexts*. Clevedon: Multilingual Matters.
[15] Hoffman, E. (1989) *Lost in Translation*. New York, NY: Penguin Books.
[16] Wang, X.-L. (2008) *Growing Up With Three Languages: Birth to Eleven*. Bristol: Multilingual Matters.

17 Amato, P.R. (1994) Father-child relations, mother-child relations, and offspring psychological well-being in early adulthood. *Journal of Marriage and Family* 56 (4), 1031–42.
Bronte-Tinkew, J., Carrano, J., Horowitz, A. and Kinukawa, A. (2008) Involvement among resident fathers and links to infant cognitive outcomes. *Journal of Family Issues* 29 (9), 1211–44.
Dubowitz, H., Black, M.M., Cox, C.E., Kerr, M.A., Litrownik, A.J., Radhakrishna, A., English, D.J., Schneider, M.W. and Runyan, D.K. (2001) Father involvement and children's functioning at age 6 years: A multisite study. *Child Maltreatment: Journal of the American Professional Society on the Abuse of Children* 6 (4), 300–309.
Flouri, E. and Buchanan, A. (2002) The role of father involvement in children's later mental health. *Journal of Adolescence* 26 (1), 63–78.
Lamb, M.E. (2010) *The Role of the Father in Child Development* (5th edn). Hoboken, NJ: John Wiley & Sons.
Palkovitz, R. (2002) Involved fathering and child development: Advancing our understanding of good fathering. In C.S. Tamis LeMonda, and N. Cabrera (eds) *Handbook of Father Involvement: Multidisciplinary Perspectives*. Erlbaum, NJ: Routledge Academic.
Pancsofar, N. and Vernon-Feagans, L. (2006) Mother and father language input to young children: Contributions to later language development? *Journal of Applied Developmental Psychology* 27 (6), 571–87.
Parke, R.D. (1996) *Fatherhood*. Cambridge, MA: Harvard University Press.
18 Heath, S.B. (1983) *Ways with Words: Language, Life, and Work in Communities and Classrooms*. Cambridge: Cambridge University Press.
19 I used the word 'judgmental' in my book *Growing Up With Three Languages: Birth to Eleven*. In the current book, I have changed the word 'judgmental' to 'moral' because I think 'moral' more accurately describes the nature of Léandre and Dominique's language socialization process.
20 Chiu, C.-Y., Gelfand, M. Yamagishi, T., Shteynberg, G., and Wang, C. (2010) Intersubjective culture: The role of intersubjective perception in cross-cultural research. *Progress on Psychological Science* 1–12
21 Wang, Q. (2004) The emergence of cultural self-construct: Autobiographical memory and self-description in American and Chinese children. *Developmental Psychology* 40(1), 3–15.
Wang, Q. (2006) Relations of maternal style and child self-concept to autobiographical memories in Chinese, Chinese immigrant, and European American 3-year-olds. *Child Development* 77 (6), 1799–1814.
22 Data based on an analysis of 28-hour video recordings over a period of 7 years from ages 12 to 19 with 4 hours each year.
23 Spernes, K. (2012) 'I use my Mother tongue at home and with friends-not in school!': Multilingualism and identity in rural Kenya. *Language, Culture and Curriculum* 25 (2), 189–203.
24 Lunga, V.B. (1994) Mapping African postcoloniality: Linguistic and cultural spaces of hybridity. *Perspectives on Global Development and Technology* 34, 291–326.
25 Keysar, B. and Costa, A. (2012) Our moral tongue: Moral judgments depend on what language we are speaking. *New York Times Sunday Review*, 22 June 2014.
26 Dewaele, J.-M. (2013) *Emotions in Multiple Languages*. New York, NY: Palgrave Macmillan.
27 Kemmelmeier, M. and Cheng, B. (2004) Language and self-construal priming: A replication and extension in a Hong Kong sample. *Journal of Cross-Cultural Psychology* 35, 705–12.
Trafimow, D., Silverman, E.S., Fan, R.M.T. and Law, J.S.F. (1997) The effects of language and priming on the relative accessibility of the private self and the collective self. *Journal of Cross-Cultural Psychology* 28, 107–23.
28 Wang, Q. (2004) The emergence of cultural self-construct: Autobiographical memory and self-description in American and Chinese children. *Developmental Psychology* 40 (1), 3–15.
29 Conway, M.A. and Pleydell-Pearce, C.W. (2000) The construction of autobiographical memories in the self-memory system. *Psychological Review* 107 (2), 261–88.
30 Wang, Q. and Ross, M. (2007) Culture and memory. In H. Kitayama and D. Cohen (eds) *Handbook of Cultural Psychology* (pp. 645–67). New York, NY: Guilford Publications.

[31] Wang, Q. and Li, Y.J. (2010) 'My way or mom's way?' The bilingual and bicultural self in Hong Kong Chinese children and adolescents. *Child Development* 81 (2), 555–67.
[32] Ross, M., Xun, W.Q.E., Wilson, A.E. (2002) Language and the bicultural self. *Personality & Social Psychology Bulletin* 28, 1040–50.
[33] Wang, X.L. (2008) *Growing Up With Three Languages: Birth to Eleven*. Bristol: Multilingual Matters.
[34] Hong, Y.-Y., Wang, C., No, S, and Chiu, C.-Y. (2007) Multicultural identities. In S. Kitayama and D. Cohen (eds) *Handbook of Cultural Psychology* (pp. 323–45). New York: Guilford Press.
[35] E-mail on 3 May 2014.
[36] Wang, X.L. (2008) *Growing Up With Three Languages: Birth to Eleven*. Bristol: Multilingual Matters.
[37] Preece, S. (2009) Multilingual identities in higher education: Negotiating the 'mother tongue', 'posh' and 'slang'. *Language and Education* 24 (1), 21–39.
[38] Ideas derived from Malik, K. (2014) On brutishness and belonging. *New York Times*, 25 July 2014.
[39] Splitter, L.J. (2014) Myself in relation to others: Embracing our most intimate and our most globalized selves. In X.-L. Wang and R. Bernas, *People Without Borders: Becoming Members of Global Communities*. New York, NY: Untested Ideas Research Center.
[40] Mantero M. (2007) Toward ecological pedagogy in language education. In M. Mantero (ed.) *Identity and Second Language Learning: Culture, Inquiry, and Dialogic Activity in Educational Contexts*. Charlotte, NC: Information Age Publishing.
[41] Marcia, J.E. (1993) The relational roots of identity. In J. Kroger (ed) *Discussion on Ego Identity* (pp. 101–20). Hillsdale, NJ: Erlbaum.
Marcia, J.E. (1976) Identity six years after: A follow-up study. *Journal of Youth and Adolescence* 5, 145–50.
Marcia, J.E. (1967) Ego identity status: relationship to change in self-esteem, 'general maladjustment,' and authoritarianism. *Journal of Personality* 35, 118–33.
[42] Kroger, J. (2003) Identity development during adolescence. In G.R. Adams and M.D. Berzonsky (eds) *Blackwell Handbook of Adolescence* (pp. 205–26). Malden, MA: Blackwell Publishing.
[43] Norton, B. (2013) *Identity and Language Learning: Extending the Conversation*. Bristol: Multilingual Matters.

9 Multilingual Childrearing and Family Welfare

One day during breakfast, I asked Léandre (15; 4; 22) '你要几个儐子?' (How many oranges do you want?). Léandre inquired, '几只还是几个？'(What is the correct measurement word, 几只 or 几个?). I went on to have a lengthy conversation with him about Chinese measurement words (classifiers). Philippe, sitting next to Léandre, became increasingly annoyed and began to express his resentment, saying, 'Now, family breakfast time becomes the time for language lessons!' He left the breakfast table grouchily.

This episode points out an alarming issue about multilingual family communication, which often involves separate and exclusive conversations as a result of one-parent-one-language practice.[1] The purpose of this chapter is to discuss the importance of multilingual family welfare in the process of raising multilingual children and adolescents. It begins with a brief discussion about multilingual family-cohesion indicators: parental congruence on childrearing, quality of family communication, time allocated for heritage-language learning and leisure, and parental expectations for their children's heritage-language achievement. It then identifies some warning signs that commonly occur in multilingual families (such as the episode mentioned at the beginning of the chapter), which may jeopardise the welfare of multilingual families. The chapter concludes with practical strategies to help you continue your multilingual childrearing without sacrificing your family's wellbeing.

Heritage-Language Attainment and Family Wellbeing

Multilingual families typically reside in a place other than the parents' country/community of origin. Thus, they must construct their own unique identities and make their own unique family childrearing and language decisions in addition to coping with many other intricacies associated with raising children with more than one language and culture. These complex family characteristics will inevitably add more stress to everyday family life.

Factors that affect multilingual family wellbeing

Among family researchers, there have been different views on the exact dimensions of family wellbeing,[2] and there have also been ongoing debates as to how it should be measured.[3] Nevertheless, family cohesion, which is defined as the bonds that hold a family together,[4] has been consistently identified as a very important dimension of family wellbeing. Thus, the following four family-cohesion indicators that are pertinent to multilingual families will be addressed respectively: parental congruence on childrearing, quality of family communication, time allocation for heritage-language learning and leisure, and parental expectations for their children's heritage-language achievement.

Differences in parental childrearing beliefs and practices

Family research literature suggests that interparental congruence in childrearing is beneficial to children's development in general. Children from homes in which parents are more similar to one another in childrearing beliefs and practices tend to function well psychologically.[5] Higher quality parenting alliances are associated with parental involvement and engagements with their children.[6] Many studies have found that parental similarity leads to positive child development outcomes, such as social competence, whereas parental dissimilarity leads to negative child development outcomes.[7]

The common challenge facing multilingual families is that parents are likely to have different cultural and linguistic backgrounds, and thus they are more inclined to bring different **ethnotheories**[8] (values and practices of a culture) to their childrearing practices. These ethnotheories are often manifested in how parents interact with their children in the heritage-language socialisation process. Using reading and writing as an example, they can mean different things to different parents. If a parent was raised in a Western culture, such as that of North America or Europe, reading in the home environment may be regarded as an activity of enjoyment. In contrast, if a parent was raised according to the Confucian tradition, typically coming from East Asia, reading and writing may be treated as serious work.[9] Learning to read and write in some immigrant Chinese families is believed to follow a clear sequence: first, understand the meaning of the word, then learn how to pronounce it correctly, and finally repeat it, memorise it, carefully copy it and use it to make different sentences. Only when a child is able to prove competency in these aspects can they be given a book to read. According to such an ethnotheory, having immediate access to books devalues both the book and the principle of hard work. Children must work their way towards knowledge step by step, and the book is a reward for a child's conscientious achievements. A love of books comes after reading is learnt and not as a necessary prerequisite to it.[10]

When children in multilingual families are confronted with contrasting parental ethnotheories, some may eventually learn to negotiate between the different **cultural templates**[11] (cultural models) provided by their parents, while others may have difficulty in dealing with the incongruence of parenting practices and expectations and feel confused and trapped by the conflicting values and expectations between home and school/society.[12] Although there is little research at this time regarding how parental incongruence in childrearing can influence the development and wellbeing of a multilingual child, child research in general has shown that parental incongruence in childrearing values and practice is associated with children's behavioural and emotional problems[13] and issues with social competency.[14]

In my own family, my husband and I are from different cultural backgrounds. Philippe is from Switzerland and I am from China. Our beliefs about childrearing and heritage-language learning are quite different. Coming from the Confucian tradition, I believe in the *guanjiao* (管教) childrearing practice (guidance and education) and I consider parental guidance and children's efforts to be keys to success, including heritage-language learning success. Therefore, in my interactions with Léandre and Dominique, I tended to focus on supervising my children and urging them to spend time and work hard in learning Chinese. However, Philippe holds in a different childrearing view. He believes in self-exploration and child freedom. He tended to emphasise fun when teaching the boys French. Obviously, our children were exposed to incongruent beliefs and practices in learning their heritage languages. Thus, Philippe and I needed to constantly negotiate our differences and tried to reach common ground when helping our children develop their heritage languages.

Quality of family communication

Another area that may affect the multilingual family cohesion is the way that family members communicate with one another. For example, multilingual families often choose the **one-parent-one-language communication approach (OPOL)**; that is, each parent speaks his or her own heritage language to the children. Although this language practice has been shown to be effective in some children's multilingual development in cases where there is little or no community support[15] (my family is a case in point for the success of OPOL practice[16]), some argue that the OPOL approach may potentially create obstacles to family integration and cohesion.[17]

Communication involvement

In OPOL families, when one parent either does not understand the language of the other parent or has limited understanding of the spouse's language, the quality of family communication may be affected in the following aspects.

First, the parent who has little or no understanding of what is said among the other family members will miss much subtle yet valuable information carried in the conversation. Some families choose to relay or translate the conversation for the parent who does not understand the language being used.[18] Even though the translation and relaying process may be beneficial for children to learn how to express the same ideas in different languages and for parents from different linguistic and cultural backgrounds to use the opportunities to learn from each other,[19] such a communication process tends to break the natural, spontaneous conversation flow and can affect conversation topic maintenance and continuation. As a result, the topic under discussion will seldom evolve further. Moreover, such a communication pattern tends to encourage separate conversations among family members, and there is never a time when all the family members have a shared conversation together.

Second, when a parent who is constantly excluded from the conversation because of the inability to understand the 'other language' used in the family, the parent will either feel left out and 'marooned'[20] or simply feel indifferent about what has been said by the other family members.[21] For example, when Léandre and Dominique were younger, Philippe could guess the gist of our Chinese conversations using the contextual clues. However, when Léandre and Dominique reached adolescence, our Chinese conversation became more complex. As a result, Philippe could not understand our abstract conversations. I noticed when we had conversations in Chinese, he would read the newspaper or simply walk away. In the long run, such a negative emotional reaction or disengagement is likely to transfer to other areas of family life. This type of emotional transmission is referred to as **spillover**, which takes place when there is a direct transfer of mood, affect or behaviour from one setting to another.[22]

Finally, the OPOL family communication pattern may disengage the parent who does not understand the conversation. When one parent converses with the children, the other parent who has to wait for a turn to participate is likely to lose interest. Indeed, it is challenging for Philippe who does not have enough Chinese knowledge to participate in the conversation that I had with Léandre and Dominique. It is understandable that many times he felt left out in the conversation, and the vignette at the beginning of this chapter is a case in point. In a healthy family conversation, 'all family members participate in unrestrained interactions about a wide array of topics' and all 'family members are free to interact with one another as they share ideas, express concerns, and participate in decision making'.[23]

Direct communication

Children who are exposed to the OPOL communication style may fall into a habit of 'telling on the other parent' or 'gossiping about the other parent' in their presence, believing that the other parent will not know what is being said. Elsewhere,[24] I have reported that Léandre and Dominique, who were brought up with the OPOL method, had a tendency to complain about one parent to the other. If they were not happy with what their mother did to them (e.g. nagging), they would complain to their father that *'Maman m'agace'* (Mother is annoying me). Similarly, they would complain to their mother about their father: 'Father is bad to me' (爸爸不好). Such instances, if they occur frequently, are not healthy for the overall family relationship.

Challenges in OPOL communication

The family is a nexus of daily interchanges in which family members are affected and in turn, affect others.[25] The ability to communicate emotions and thoughts is crucial for this process. However, if a child's heritage-language acquisition environment is different from that of typical language acquisition (such as OPOL), there exist some challenges that may affect the parent-child relationship if not handled well.

The first challenge is the quality of parent-child communication. In a typical language-learning environment, children acquire a language by receiving multiple language inputs from various people such as parents, grandparents, other adults, teachers, peers and the media in different contexts. Together, these different people and communication settings provide a language-learning child with different communication models.[26] Children who are learning a language in such an environment tend to be more able to express complex thoughts, needs and emotions.

However, the children whose home-language input comes from limited sources (mainly from parents and sometimes from one parent) often have limited home-language communication ability. Even in a very carefully monitored linguistic environment, such as in our family, children have significantly less input than children whose input is from multiparty interlocutors.[27] As a result, some of these children may find it difficult to carry on extensive conversations with their parents in their heritage language. In families where the parents insist that their children use only the heritage language, conversations tend to be brief because of the children's low proficiency.

Most importantly, the children's lack of proficiency to use their heritage language to communicate with parents may affect the parent–child emotional availability, which has been termed 'the connective tissue' of children's healthy socioemotional development.[28] Research indicates that emotional availability highlights sensitivity and appropriate responsiveness to behaviour and emotions in everyday interactions, and it is related to attachment representations of parents[29] and attachment security in children.[30]

In addition, during adolescence, thorough and dynamic child–parent conversations are necessary for parents to understand the psychological and emotional needs of their children and provide adequate support. This parent-adolescent relationship is established through frequent communication, and such a relationship has long been deemed by researchers and clinicians as necessary for adolescent development and adaptation. Achieving a warm and close relationship, while still developing an individuated sense of self, is important in parent and adolescent exchanges.[31] Some parents and adolescents in multilingual homes may have difficulty in carrying out extensive exchanges due to their children's limited proficiency in their heritage language.

The second challenge of the OPOL practice is the lack of opportunities to fully participate in family conversation with both parents at the same time. Children who live in a family in which all family members are conversing in one common language tend to have more opportunities to participate in conversations with both parents and siblings, which allows children to learn the skills required to engage in conversations with others.[32] However, children from multilingual homes, particularly from OPOL families, have fewer opportunities to participate in conversations with both parents simultaneously. The lack of opportunities to fully participate in family conversation with both parents at the same time is another factor that may affect the quality of family communication dynamics.

The third challenge in the OPOL practice is the potential for a lack of communicative accountability on the part of the children. When multiple people are engaged in a conversation, there are different sources of challenges to the speakers.

In a multi-interlocutor conversation, different people are likely to question or contest a particular presentation of reality. A child or adolescent involved in such a conversation has to present arguments for his/her version of events or summon support for his/her interpretation and fill in many details.[33] In other words, the child is more accountable for clarifying his/her speech in such a conversational environment. However, if parents serve as the major conversational partners of children, as well as the major heritage-language providers in the home environment, they tend to become 'indulgent in ratifying their children's versions of events'[34] because they are familiar with the conversation context and are aware of their children's heritage-language limitations. As such, the children may not strive to make themselves understood, and deeper conversation may never happen among family members.

Allocation of time for leisure and heritage-language learning

It takes a great amount of time for a child to develop listening, speaking, reading and writing skills in one language. Needless to say, children who grow up with more than one language need even more time to develop these skills in multiple languages, especially in families where parents have to assume most of the responsibility for their children's heritage language development.

There is always a competition between the time needed for heritage-language learning activities and the time needed for leisure activities, such as sports and hobbies. As mentioned in Chapter 2, many heritage-language learning children and adolescents have to go to after-school programmes, attend weekend community heritage-language schools and carry out heritage-language learning activities (e.g. reading and writing) in addition to their regular school assignments. This extra work takes away from children and adolescents' time for leisure.

Leisure not only plays a recuperating role for children and adolescents' overall wellbeing,[35] but it also helps children function well academically and socially. Research has demonstrated that children who are more involved in leisure activities receive higher academic grades, are rated by their teachers as higher in academic competence and are more socially competent than peers who are less involved in such activities.[36]

Moreover, heritage-language learning also decreases parents' time for leisure, as multilingual childrearing involves a lot of invisible work and sacrifices.[37] If coping with the mundane routines of their everyday lives is already hard for parents, it will be even harder for them to find time to expose their children to their heritage language, particularly in regard to reading and writing, which involve an enormous amount of work.[38] It is indeed a struggle and even stressful for both parents and children in multilingual households to find time for heritage-language learning.

Thus, parents and children in these families have to pay a considerable price in order to keep up with their heritage language. Children have to trade leisure for heritage-language learning activities and parents have to sacrifice leisure time to teach the heritage language(s) to their children. When the stress of heritage-language learning mounts to a high level, both children and parents will feel overstretched, which might spill over into the other domains of family life and cause tension and conflicts between parents and children.

Parental expectations

Popular media, parenting advice books and parenting websites often portray multilingual childrearing as exalting. Many parents, without considering their own situation and circumstance, enthusiastically embrace the idea of raising multilingual children and put it into practice at all costs. To strive to make their children achieve a high proficiency in their heritage language, some parents even set unrealistic goals. For example, a mother's desire to make her 13-year-old son a balanced bilingual prompted her to teach 20 new heritage-language words daily, in addition to five pages of grammar exercises plus one heritage-language book per week.[39] This mother's plan was ambitious, to say the least, in her situation. Her son already had a full schedule for his schoolwork, sports and musical activities, and both parents had to work full time. This mother's ambition resulted in frustration for both her and her child.

Linguist Ingrid Piller has pointed out that the quest for 'perfectly balanced' multilingual children can result in both parental disappointment and children's sense of failure.[40] Forging ahead without adequate planning, proper assessment of family specific situations and support will certainly add stress to any family.

Strategies for promoting multilingual family welfare

Having identified the aforementioned challenges that can potentially threaten the multilingual family's welfare, and especially after having discussed the potential issues related to the OPOL practice, we should not feel discouraged from pursuing multilingual childrearing and abandon the OPOL practice. On the contrary, by recognising the potential issues, we can turn these challenges into opportunities to better promote our family's wellbeing. After all, many families who have taken the OPOL approach are successful in raising healthy and happy multilingual children.[41] Most importantly, being multilingual still has more advantages than disadvantages,[42] and 'knowing more has never been a disadvantage when compared to knowing less.'[43] Below are some strategies for you to consider.

Active planning

The key to promoting family wellbeing is communication. As Koerner and Fitzpatrick commented, 'Nowhere is the influence of family on individual behaviours more profound than in the area of communicative behaviours.'[44] Family communication is central in building positive relationships, resolving conflicts and strengthening family cohesion.

Multilingual family communication begins with childrearing planning.[45] As with any other important decisions parents make on behalf of their children, linguistic decisions will have consequences for their children's development, and the experiences provided by parents will make a profound mark on children's lives.[46] Serious and constant communications between parents should take place before any plans are implemented. I call this process **active planning**, which may include the following:

Clarify motives

It is important for you to communicate with your spouse or partner about the reasons why you want to pass down your heritage language to your children. You may want to ask yourselves such questions as whether it is for maintaining your heritage culture, for academic or general cognitive development, for future job opportunities, for well roundedness, for travelling or just for fad and fame? Frequent, extensive communication and reflection on these questions may help you clarify your motives, negotiate your differences and reach mutually agreeable childrearing decisions.

Evaluate parental ability and availability

After clarifying your motives for wanting to raise your children with your heritage language, it is very important for you to communicate with your partner about your own language competency and your ability and availability for helping your children's heritage-language learning. This is particularly necessary if you are the major source of your children's linguistic input. You must seriously assess your own language competence, as your language proficiency will directly influence your children's language proficiency. However, this does not mean that if you have a low level of proficiency in your heritage language (often as a result of not having had the opportunity to be educated), you cannot pass on the language to your children. Rather, it means that if you want your children to reach a certain level of heritage-language proficiency, additional support and input are essential.

Also, when there is little societal support in children's heritage-language development and when you are the major source for heritage-language input, you must prepare to invest considerable time and effort.[47] If you have various reasons that prevent you from spending time with your children, you will indeed face a serious challenge in raising your children with your heritage language. You must communicate with your partner and decide how you may be able to take on the challenge. If you are often absent, realistically estimating how much time you are able to devote to your children's heritage language and literacy learning on a daily or weekly basis can help you budget your time effectively. When you are conscious of your time constraints and communicate with each other, you tend to be more inclined to focus on the task and use every available minute.[48]

Alternatively, you may want to prioritise the important things that you must do in your lives. If you set your children's heritage-language literacy learning as one of your life's priorities, you will probably be able to find time creatively. For instance, often-absent and busy parents can make heritage literacy teaching and learning happen by using technology: talking and reading to your children through a webcam, Skype and FaceTime and using the internet, e-mails, and prerecorded video/audio.

If after seriously examining your availability, you conclude that you are unable to spend enough time teaching your children, you may want to find other options such as hiring a tutor, sending your children to a community heritage-language school, enrolling them in a school heritage-language after-school programme or an international school, asking extended family for help or seeking support from other parents who share the same linguistic background.

When you and your spouse or partner discuss these issues in your planning process, you are likely to think through your decisions, learn to budget your time and seek the necessary help to avoid frustration.

Decide a family communication system

It is also important for you to communicate with your spouse or partner and make a family language plan regarding what heritage language (if more than one) to use in the home environment, which parent will speak to the child in which language, and when the child will be introduced to the language(s).[49] Deciding on the family communication system at an early stage will be beneficial, preferably before the children are born.[50] There are at least three advantages in deciding on the family communication system before the children arrive. First, it gives parents time to think through the pros and cons of their choices and to modify them as many times as they want without having a direct impact on their children. Second, the communication system that parents use to talk to their children is likely to continue once it becomes a habit; therefore, having a communication system plan in place can help ensure its early attainment and avoid frustration later. Finally, the communication system parents decide to use is an important tool parents will rely on to carry out their plan.[51]

Even though the above strategies are recommended for deciding on a family communication system, it should not be set in stone. Circumstances do change and the family communication pattern can change as well, especially during adolescence. I met a French family in Beijing several years ago. The mother told me that they started off using the OPOL communication system with their children. When the children became teens, they all decided to converse in Chinese, which was the language they all felt comfortable speaking while they were living in China at that time.

Set achievable goals for heritage-language learning

It is also helpful for you to communicate with your spouse or partner about the goals and expectations of your children's heritage-language development. Parents have different purposes for raising children with more than one language: Some want their children to know their heritage language for religious reasons, some for academic reasons, others for economic reasons and still others for intergenerational communication reasons. These different purposes will require different levels of language proficiency.

Knowing what you and your children want to achieve in their heritage language will help you determine the efforts and resources you will invest. This will also help you be more focused in your efforts and become less frustrated and disappointed.

It is important to revisit and reevaluate the plans and goals you set for your children, and you should consider their developmental levels when setting these goals. Many plans and goals we set for Léandre and Dominique had to be changed because of circumstantial changes. For example, as I discussed in Chapter 7, I had to change my daily written communications (such as text messages and e-mails) with Léandre and Dominique to English rather than Chinese so that we could communicate with each other more effectively.

Negotiation between parents

Negotiating parental differences is also part of communication, and it can help us reach a consensus that is in the best interests of our children. Below are some useful tips regarding how negotiation can be carried out between parents.

Negotiating childrearing differences

As discussed earlier in the chapter, the heterogeneity in the makeup of multilingual families will result in a wide range of parenting beliefs and practices. These parenting differences (often shown, for example, in parental attitudes, behaviours and parenting styles when parents interact with their children in their heritage-language learning) will play a crucial role in children's overall development. Even though it is not easy to change one's beliefs, parents in multilingual families must consciously communicate their differences and negotiate them for their children's wellbeing. Research suggests that parents' ability to negotiate their differences and reach agreement in childrearing decisions leads to a positive family climate, which in turn positively influences children's social competence.[52]

Research also shows that parental differences are often adaptive.[53] Sometimes the seemingly conflicting parental beliefs about childrearing may actually share the same goals when examined carefully. For example, the authoritative parenting style (in which parents are nurturing, responsive and supportive yet set firm limits for their children) has been consistently reported to help children develop a sense of competence.[54] The authoritarian parenting style (in which parents are inflexible and harsh in controlling) is regarded in the literature as negative for children's development. At first glance, the authoritative and authoritarian parenting styles are different in orientation. Yet, cross-cultural research suggests that the authoritarian parenting style may sometimes be misunderstood. For example, psychologist Ruth Chao has argued that some Chinese American parenting behaviours may appear punitive but actually serve regulative and supportive functions.[55] Thus, if you and your spouse or partner are from different cultural and linguistic backgrounds, you may want to constantly communicate and negotiate your differences. Such negotiation may help you see your common goal. For instance, suppose you believe heritage-language reading and writing should be fun activities and your spouse believes they should be serious work, you may realise, through communication, that your goal is the same; that is, you both want to help your children learn well. With the common goal in sight, a middle ground in parenting practice can be negotiated between the two of you.

Sometimes when you and your spouse or partner cannot settle your differences or neither of you wants to compromise your beliefs, you may want to seek help from research information. With the availability of the internet, this is more possible than ever. For example, if you believe parental control in a child's heritage-language learning is important and your spouse or partner believes that a child-centred approach is more effective, you can negotiate your position through research information. In this case, literature suggests that child-centred language input provides greater opportunity for the child to become an active speaker of the heritage language.[56] Thus, research information may help facilitate the negotiation between parents about what approach to take when raising multilingual children.

Negotiating family communication

In families that practice the OPOL communication style, the frustration of not being proficient in the spouse's language or unable to participate in a family conversation with children and spouse presents difficulties for family communication. Nonetheless, you can overcome such communication difficulties if you are willing to explore different options.

First, the most effective way to deal with the communication barriers is for you to learn the language of the other parent.[57] Even if you develop only a passive knowledge of the spouse's language, this is better than nothing. This effort will help solve some of the problems discussed earlier in the chapter.

Second, we need to discuss our feelings openly and suggest what the other spouse can do to make him or her feel included if he or she does not understand our language. We can model this to our children as well, as frequent communication will help family relationships. Many studies have demonstrated that open family conversation enhances child wellbeing, even in the face of potentially difficult and stressful circumstances. If we encourage all family members to openly discuss a variety of issues, to weigh alternative perspectives and to respect each family member's freedom in doing so, we are likely to mitigate the stress[58] associated with multilingual childrearing.

Third, it may also be helpful to use a common language in family communication when all the members are present, such as during meal times. This communication pattern is called **one-context-one-language**. As long as this practice is done consistently, some families have been successful with it.

Finally, it is effective to use nonverbal clues to involve the other parent who does not understand your language in a conversation. For example, using frequent eye contact to maintain the attention of that parent.

Also, we can try to make our children's heritage-learning (such as reading and writing) an integral part of their family experience. For example, family members can share the events we read about in heritage-language newspapers or novels during dinner. The family members can also make heritage-language writing a family event. There are many occasions and opportunities when family members can work together to write in their heritage language(s): making family scrapbooks, family calendars, homemade books and multilingual family holiday greeting cards.[59] When all family members are involved in these activities, the family relationship will benefit.

Negotiating heritage-language socialisation strategies

Research has shown that when parents are warm and caring, share interests with their children, provide guidance and respect their children's needs for autonomy and privacy rather than being controlling, children tend to flourish in most of the aspects of child wellbeing: autonomy, environmental mastery, personal growth, positive relations with others, purpose in life and self-acceptance.[60] Therefore, it is important to communicate with our spouses or partners regarding our heritage-language socialisation strategies. Below are some ideas.

Children's wellbeing should always come first

Raising children with more than one language is not just a language issue; it is also a childrearing issue. Moreover, multilingual language acquisition is not only the learning of different linguistic systems but also of communicative competence as a child develops a social identity attached to the use of these languages.[61] How parents respond to their children's language use will have an impact on the children's development in the other areas. Therefore, the children's wellbeing should always come before anything else. Putting children's wellbeing first requires us to negotiate our different childrearing beliefs by doing the following:

First, we need to attend to children's emotional needs. Growing up with more than one language is challenging. Sometimes, conflicts between parents and children resulting from heritage-language learning can be emotional. Properly handling such conflicts may be crucial for children's emotional health. In order to ease tension and facilitate healthy emotional development in the heritage-language learning process, we can try to create a nurturing environment and make the process enjoyable. Being positive and supportive when interacting with children will make them feel encouraged in their heritage-language learning.

Second, we need to attend to children's developmental and individual needs. Children have different needs during different developmental stages. Some successful heritage-language teaching strategies used when a child was younger may not work when the child is older. Thus, using age-appropriate strategies to help children learn their heritage language is important. It might be helpful if we make an effort to understand the developmental characteristics and needs of our children through careful observations and conversations, and adequately change and adjust our strategies during our children's different developmental stages. The more we attend to the developmental needs of our children and the better we know our children, the more effective our heritage-language teaching strategies will be.

In addition, not all children are the same. Even siblings may show differences in their home-language learning styles and achievement. What an older sibling can do at a certain age in the home language should not be the yardstick for a younger sibling. Individual children have different developmental timetables and outcomes. Therefore, we need to attend to every child's needs and provide the best environment for each child to thrive at his or her own speed and potential.

Third, we need to balance heritage-language learning and other activities. Children will increasingly spend more time in school-related learning and extracurricular activities, such as sports and hobbies. The time spent on these activities will definitely compete with home-language literacy learning. Therefore, finding ways to balance the two is necessary.

We can consider a number of things to achieve the balance. We can ask ourselves whether we want to keep all the extracurricular activities in our children's lives or give up some activities to devote more time to heritage-language literacy learning. Giving up some extracurricular activities will leave space for heritage-language learning and reduce stress for both children and parents. Alternatively, we can reduce time spent on some extracurricular activities or rotate different activities. For example, Monday afternoon could be reserved for music lessons, Tuesday evening for heritage-language lessons and Wednesday afternoon for sports practice.

We can also try to incorporate our children's extracurricular activities into heritage-language learning. For example, if our children are interested in sports, we can use sports as a major attraction to help the children learn their heritage language. For example, we can download sports news in the heritage language for our children to read or encourage them to write about sports news with relatives in their heritage country. Additionally, we can talk about sports in the heritage language when we take their children to sports practice.[62]

Research has consistently shown that play and leisure can have an overall positive effect on children's physical, cognitive and social development.[63] Putting children's wellbeing first will help them develop a healthy personality and identity, while also developing multilingual abilities.

Communication should be the top priority in home-language learning

Learning a language is a process of learning how to communicate, and it is through communication that parents and children establish and strengthen their emotional bonds and that children learn the proper ways of using languages. However, because of the possible limitations of their linguistic abilities, heritage-language-speaking children will unavoidably make grammatical and vocabulary mistakes, and they will sometimes be unable to use the heritage language to express their thoughts and feelings (see Box 9.1 for an example). If we make a fuss about our children's errors or insist that our children use the heritage language instead of

> **Box 9.1 Example of Communication Break-Down**
>
> I told Léandre that he could pour the leftover tomato sauce in the garbage disposal. Léandre (15; 0; 24) hesitated and then said, '这是…' (this is…) and stopped talking because he did not know how to use the Chinese expression 浪费的行为 (behaviour of waste). The conversation broke down because of the limitation of his Chinese vocabulary.

helping them communicate, our children may simply 'shut themselves off.' In the long run, that kind of behaviour can be damaging to the parent-child relationship and consequently limit children's chances of learning their heritage language well. It is difficult for children to acquire active competence in their heritage language when there is little or no community support.[64] If we insist that our children speak the heritage language to us, this will lead to emotional strain or communication problems in the family.[65]

Thus, we may want to make communication between our children and ourselves a top priority in heritage-language teaching and learning. When children have difficulties expressing themselves in the heritage language or make mistakes, we can provide assistance and practice modelling (see Box 9.2). When children understand that parents are their conversation partners, they will feel encouraged to try to express their thoughts and feelings in the heritage language.

Moreover, we also need to attend to the issue of our children's affective filters. **Affective filters** (affects, feelings, emotions and moods) can affect a child and an adolescent's performance in the heritage language. Affective filters determine which language models to adopt, which part of the language will be attended to, when attempts at acquisition will stop and how fast a learner will learn the heritage language.[66]

> **Box 9.2 Example of Parental Heritage-Language Support**
>
> (Context see Box 9.1)
>
> **Mother**: Is this a <u>wasteful</u>? Yes, you are right. Yes, it is indeed not right to <u>waste</u>. Next time, I will cook less so that we will reduce <u>waste</u> (这是浪费的行为?你说的很对。是的,浪费的确是不好的行为。下次我少烧一点,这样我们就会减少浪费).
>
> **Léandre**: Yes, waste is a bad habit (是的。浪费是坏习惯).
>
> …
>
> [In this example, I helped Léandre learn the Chinese phrase 浪费的行为 (behaviour of waste) by having a natural conversation with him and at the same time, I helped him repair the conversation breakdown.]

If children or adolescents have anxiety about using their heritage language, that anxiety will block their ability to learn the language.

Heritage-language learning is a lifelong process

It is also important for parents to realise that language learning, whether it is one language or two or more, is a lifelong process. Understanding this, you will be able to regard your multilingual children's language learning as a process rather than as an end product. You will realise that the mistakes your children make while developing more than one language are an ordinary part of language learning and development. You will regard the mixing of languages as a common characteristic of children who grow up with more than one language. Consequently, you will be more motivated to work with your children rather than criticise them, and you will encourage you children to experiment and explore their heritage language(s). You will accept the different proficiencies that your children exhibit in their heritage-language achievement. You will also accept the different levels of proficiency that your children exhibit in their heritage language. Finally, and most happily, you will enjoy even the smallest achievement your children make in their heritage-language development.

Encourage autonomy in heritage-language learning

Research consistently shows that children, particularly adolescents, and their parents who exhibit autonomous behaviours within the context of parental guidance (moderate control) and warmth tend to demonstrate positive social and emotional development outcomes. [67]

Children and adolescents are not passive learners. They are dynamically contributing to their own development, including heritage-language development. If we observe our children carefully and listen to them attentively in order to understand their needs and wants, we can provide the best possible support for their heritage-language and multilingual development.[68]

Bolster children's self-confidence and support multilingual identity development

When children develop more than one language, they are also developing their identity. Children's multilingual experience will have a fundamental impact on how they feel about themselves. There is little research regarding how children's multilingual experience can affect their self-perception, however, according to Harter[69], children's sense of self has four important functions in their development. First, it helps them make sense of the things that happen to them (e.g. that kid next door always has play dates with me, and therefore, I must be likeable). Second, it motivates them to engage in behaviours to which others might respond favourably (e.g. if I can speak more than one language, other children will admire me). Third, it influences their reactions to events (e.g. I am really frustrated when I don't know how to express this idea in my home language). Finally, it allows them to envision the various future selves they might become (e.g. I want to be a successful writer). Once they begin to look seriously at a particular future self, it helps them make appropriate choices (e.g. I'd better write more if I want to become a successful writer). Children have a basic need to think of themselves as competent, likeable and worthy individuals, which is a means of achieving and maintaining a positive sense of self-worth. Research also suggests that a child who constantly experiences failure can develop a negative self-concept. Thus, one important way to help children develop a positive self-concept is to provide positive experiences in their language acquisition process. It is inevitable that children will make mistakes, and sometimes serious ones, when learning a language. However, you should not make them feel bad about the mistakes they make in learning their heritage language(s). Rather, you can help them realise that they are able to correct and avoid mistakes if they are willing to make an effort.

Moreover, as children enter school, their experience is further enriched by having to rise to the challenge of describing their school experience in their home languages. We may need to remember that our role is to facilitate the children's self-expression in the home languages but not to hinder them from talking about their school experience. Because children sometimes lack home-language vocabulary or make mistakes in the home languages, it is important that we make our children feel positive about the process. In other words, we should be supportive rather than critical about what our children say. Children's early experience in social interaction with parents and others can influence their self-development and that of their identity. If children experience success in what they do, then they will develop confidence about their abilities. On the other hand, if they constantly experience failure, they will develop doubts about themselves. The following are a few strategies for you to consider.

Attend to parents' own needs

Raising children with more than one language is challenging for children, but it is perhaps even more stressful (and frustrating at times) for parents. Thus, it is important that we take care of our own emotional needs so as to avoid letting negative reactions or stress affect the quality of our interactions with our children. It is expected that when we feel frustrated or stressed, our negative emotions will definitely spill over into our family life.

Find the source of the anxiety, frustration or anger

When we get angry with our children or become anxious or frustrated with them when helping them with their heritage-language learning, the first question we may want to ask ourselves is why we feel that way. Is it because we are trying to do too many things at the same time or are there other reasons? Finding the source of our own emotions can help us understand ourselves and then help us help our children. For example, early on in my children's home-language learning process (particularly in the reading and writing aspects), I found myself frequently angry and frustrated with them. When I reflected on the cause of such negative feelings, I found that I was trying to do too many things at the same time. For example, sometimes when I helped my children do their Chinese homework, I was also doing my own work. In such a situation, any slight 'resistance' from my children would trigger anger and frustration from me. Later, I learnt that I needed to prioritise my own work and my children's language activities. When I helped my children with their heritage-language learning, it should be my priority at that time. In doing so, I felt more relaxed and could devote my whole attention to my children. Naturally, my behaviour and mood were contagious to Léandre and Dominique. When they felt that I was there for them, they were in turn more cooperative with my requests.

Set small goals and take one step at a time
Another way to avoid parental stress is to set one goal at a time. In this way, we will feel less frustrated. If we expect too much and spread ourselves in too many directions, we are bound to be frustrated. If we have only one goal to achieve at one time, we tend to be more successful and less frustrated.

Keep parents' sanity
Keeping sane is very important for parents. One can't succeed without sanity. Engaging our children in many activities, such as heritage-language learning, we are often already overworked and stressed. Thus, giving ourselves a break once in a while can regenerate our energy and help us keep our sanity. It is all right to give oneself a break when feeling stressed. Missing a day or a week in home-language learning activities is not detrimental; in fact, it may actually help us recuperate. It is likely that happy parents will have happy children.

The bottom line

The bottom line is that if we are cognizant of the challenges associated with raising multilingual children and work on strategies to address them, our children can develop healthy personalities and identities while thriving as productive multilinguals.

Summary of Key Points in Chapter 9

- This chapter has highlighted four indicators that may threaten multilingual family well-being: parental differences in childrearing beliefs and practices, family communication quality, time allocation for heritage-language learning and leisure, and parental expectations concerning their children's heritage-language proficiency.
- There are some factors that will affect multilingual family wellbeing:
  - Differences in parental childrearing beliefs and practice.
  - Quality in family communication.

- Allocation of time for leisure and heritage-language learning activities.
- Parental expectations.
- To turn these issues into opportunities, parents can use the following strategies:
  - Active planning:
    - Clarify motives behind wanting children to learn a heritage language.
    - Evaluate parental heritage-language teaching ability and time availability in teaching the heritage language.
    - Decide on a family communication system and adjust it when necessary.
    - Set achievable goals for heritage-language learning.
  - Negotiation between parents:
    - Negotiate parental differences in childrearing beliefs and practice.
    - Negotiate family communication.
    - Negotiate heritage-language teaching strategies:
      - Children's wellbeing should always come first.
      - Communication should always be the priority of heritage-language learning.
      - Heritage-language development is a lifelong process.
      - Encourage autonomy in heritage-language learning.
      - Bolster children's confidence and support multilingual identity development.

Recommended Readings

Galvin, K.M., Braithwaite, D.O., Bylund, C.L. and Braithwaite, D. (2014) *Family Communication: Cohesion and Change*. Boston, MA : Pearson.

Notes and References

[1] One-parent-one-language (OPOL) practice is a family communication system in which one parent speaks to children exclusively in one language and the other parent speaks to children exclusively in a different language.

[2] Habermas, J. (1987) *The Theory of Communicative Action: Lifeworld and System*. Cambridge: Polity Press.

[3] Behnke, A. and MacDermid, S. (2004) Family well-being. http://wfnetwork.bc.edu/encyclopedia_template.php?id=235
Henry, M.I. (1996) Family well-being: Insights gained through the process of critical reflection. Paper presented at the American Association of Family and Consumer Sciences. Nashville, Tennessee, 29-30 June.

[4] Burt, R.S. (2000) The network structure of social capital: An annual series of analytical essays and critical reviews. In B.M. Staw and R.I. Sulton (eds) *Research in Organizational Behaviour* (pp. 345–23). Amsterdam, NL: Elsevier.
Huijnk, W., Verkuyten, M. and Coenders, M. (2010) Intermarriage attitude among ethnic minority and majority groups in the Netherlands: The role of family relations and immigrant characteristics. *Journal of Comparative Family Studies* 41 (3), 389–414.
Verkuyten, M. and Zaremba, K. (2005) Inter-ethnic relations in a changing political context. *Social Psychology Quarterly* 68, 375–86.

Jetten, J., Spears, R. and Manstead, A.S.R. (1997) Strength of identification and intergroup differentiation: The influence of group norms. *European Journal of Psychology* 27, 603–09.

[5] Deal, J.E., Halverson, C.F. and Wampler, K.S. (1989) Parental agreement on child-rearing orientations: Relations to parental, marital, family, and child characteristics. *Child Development* 60, 1025–1034.

Lanz, M., Scabini, E., Vermulst, A. and Gerris, J.R.M. (2001) Congruence on child rearing in families with early adolescent and middle adolescent children. *International Journal of Behavioral Development* 25 (2), 133–9.

[6] Fagan, J. (2014) Adolescent parents' partner conflict and parenting alliance, fathers' prenatal involvement, and fathers' engagement with infants. *Journal of Family Issues* 35 (11), 1415–39.

[7] Lindsey, E.W. and Mize, J. (2001) Interparental agreement, parent-child responsiveness, and children's peer competence. *Family Relations* 50, 348–54.

[8] Harkness, S. and Super, C.M. (2006) Themes and variations: Parental ethnotheories in western cultures. In K.H. Rubin and O. Boon Chung (eds) *Parental Beliefs, Parenting, and Child Development in Cross-Cultural Perspective*. 61–80. New York: Psychology Press.

[9] Wang, X.-L. (2011) *Learning to Read and Write in the Multilingual Family*. Bristol: Multilingual Matters.

[10] Gregory, E. (2008) *Learning to Read in a New Language*. Los Angeles: Sage.

[11] Rosaldo, R. (1989) *Culture and Truth: The Remaking of Social Analysis*. 140. Boston: Beacon Press.

[12] Ying, Y.-W., Coombs, M. and Lee, P.A. (1999) Family intergenerational relationship of Asian American adolescents. *Cultural Diversity and Ethnic Minority Psychology* 5, 350–67.

[13] Vaugh, B.E., Block, J.H. and Block, J. (1988) Parental agreement on child rearing during early childhood and the psychological characteristics of adolescents. *Child Development* 59, 1020–33.

[14] Lindsey, E.W. and Mize, J. (2001) Interparental agreement, parent-child responsiveness, and children's peer competence. *Family Relations* 50, 348–54.

[15] De Houwer, A. (1990) *The Acquisition of Two Languages: A Case Study*. Cambridge: Cambridge University Press.

Hoffmann, C. (1985) Language acquisition in two trilingual children. *Journal of Multilingual and Multicultural Development* 6 (6), 479–95.

Hoffmann, C. (2001) Toward the description of trilingual competence. *International Journal of Bilingualism* 5 (1), 1–17.

Leopold, W.F. (1939) *Speech Development of a Bilingual Child: A Linguist Record*. Evanston, IL: The Northwestern University Press.

Ronjat, J. (1913) *Le dévelopement du language observé chez un enfant bilingue*. Paris: Champion.

Saunders, G. (1988) *Bilingual Children: From Birth to Teens*. Clevedon: Multilingual Matters.

Taeschner, T. (1983) *The Sun is Feminine: A Study of Language Acquisition in Bilingual Children*. Berlin: Springer-Verlag.

Wang, X.-L. (2008) *Growing Up With Three Languages: Birth to Eleven*. Bristol: Multilingual Matters.

[16] Wang, X.-L. (2008) *Growing Up With Three Languages: Birth to Eleven*. Bristol: Multilingual Matters.

[17] Zierer, E. (1977) Experiences in the bilingual education of a child of pre-school age. *IRAL* 15, 143–8.

[18] Wang, X.-L. (2008) *Growing Up With Three Languages: Birth to Eleven*. Bristol: Multilingual Matters.

[19] Wang, X.-L. (2008) *Growing Up With Three Languages: Birth to Eleven*. Bristol: Multilingual Matters.

[20] Barron-Hauwaret, S. (2004) *Language Strategies for Bilingual Families: The One-Parent-One-Language Approach*. Clevedon: Multilingual Matters.

[21] Wang, X.-L. (2008) *Growing Up With Three Languages: Birth to Eleven*. Bristol: Multilingual Matters.

[22] Almeida, D.M., Wethington, E. and Chandler, A.L. (1999) Daily transmission of tensions between marital dyads and parent-child dyads. *Journal of Marriage and Family* 61 (1), 49–61.

[23] Koerner, A.F. and Fitzpatrick, M.A. (2002) Toward a theory of family communication. *Communication Theory* 12, 70–91.
[24] Wang, X.-L. (2008) *Growing Up With Three Languages: Birth to Eleven*. Bristol: Multilingual Matters.
[25] Larson, R.W. and Almeida, D.M. (1999) Emotional transmission in the daily lives of families: A new paradigm for studying family process. *Journal of Marriage and Family* 61 (1), 5–20.
[26] Dickinson, D.K. and Tabors, P.O. (2001) *Beginning Literacy With Language: Young Children Learning at Home and School*. Baltimore, MD: Paul H. Brookes.
Snow, C.E. (1991) The theoretical basis for relationships between language and literacy in development. *Journal of Research in Childhood Education* 6, 5–10.
[27] Wang, X.-L. (2008) *Growing Up With Three Languages: Birth to Eleven*. Bristol: Multilingual Matters.
[28] Easterbrooks, A.M., Biesecker, G. and Lyons-Ruth, K.A. (2000) Infancy predictors of emotional availability in middle childhood: The role of attachment and maternal depression. *Attachment and Human Development* 2, 170–87.
Chaudhuri, J.H., Easterbrooks, A.M. and Davis, C.R. (2009) The relation between emotional availability and parenting style: Cultural and economic factors in a diverse sample of young mothers. *Parenting: Science and Practice* 9, 277–99.
[29] Biringen, Z., Matheny, A., Bretherton, I., Renouf, A. and Sherman, M. (2000) Maternal representation of the self as parent. *Attachment and Human Development* 2, 218–32.
Ziv, Y., Aviezer, O., Gini, M., Sagi, A. and Koren-Karie, N. (2000) Emotional availability in mother-infant dyad as related to the quality of infant-mother attachment relationship. *Attachment and Human Development* 2, 149–69.
[30] Biringen, Z., Matheny, A., Bretherton, I., Renouf, A. and Sherman, M. (2000) Maternal representation of the self as parent. *Attachment and Human Development* 2, 218–32.
Oyen, A.-S., Landy, S. and Hilburn-Cobb, C. (2000) Maternal attachment and sensitivity in an at-risk sample. *Attachment and Human Development* 2, 203–17.
[31] Beveridge, R.M. and Berg, C.A. (2007) Parent–adolescent collaboration: An interpersonal model for understanding optimal interactions. *Clinical Child and Family Psychology Review* 10 (1), 25–52.
[32] Blum-Kulka, S. and Snow, C.E. (2002) Editors' introduction. In S. Blum-Kulka and C.E. Snow (eds) *Talking to Adults: The Contribution of Multiparty Discourse to Language Acquisition* (pp. 1–12). Mahwah, NJ: Lawrence Erlbaum Associates, Publishers.
Heath, S.B. (1983) *Ways With Words: Language, Life, and Work in Communities and Classrooms*. Cambridge: Cambridge University Press.
[33] Blum-Kulka, S. and Snow, C.E. (2002) Editors' introduction. In S. Blum-Kulka and C.E. Snow (eds) *Talking to Adults: The Contribution of Multiparty Discourse to Language Acquisition* (pp. 1–12). Mahwah, NJ: Lawrence Erlbaum Associates, Publishers.
[34] Blum-Kulka, S. and Snow, C.E. (2002) Editors' introduction. In S. Blum-Kulka and C.E. Snow (eds) *Talking to Adults: The Contribution of Multiparty Discourse to Language Acquisition* (pp. 1–12). Mahwah, NJ: Lawrence Erlbaum Associates, Publishers.
[35] Holder, M.D., Coleman, B. and Sehn, Z.L. (2009) The contribution of active and passive leisure to children's well-being. *Journal of Health Psychology* 14 (3), 378–86.
[36] Fletcher, A.C., Nickerson, P. and Wright, K.L. (2003) Structured leisure activities in middle childhood: Links to well-being. *Journal of Community Psychology* 31 (6), 641–59.
[37] Okita, T. (2002) *Invisible Work: Bilingualism, Language Choice and Childrearing in Intermarried Families*. Amsterdam: Benjamins.
Wang, X.-L. (2008) *Growing Up With Three Languages: Birth to Eleven*. Bristol: Multilingual Matters.
[38] Wang, X.-L.(2011) *Learning to Read and Write in the Multilingual Family*. Bristol: Multilingual Matters.

[39] Wang, X.-L. (2011) *Learning to Read and Write in the Multilingual Family*. Bristol: Multilingual Matters.
[40] Piller, I. (2002) *Bilingual Couples Talk: The Discursive Construction of Hybridity*. Amsterdam: John Benjamins.
[41] Wang, X.-L. (2008) *Growing Up With Three Languages: Birth to Eleven*. Bristol: Multilingual Matters.
Barron-Hauwaret, S. (2004) *Language Strategies for Bilingual Families: The One-Parent-One-Language Approach*. Clevedon: Multilingual Matters.
[42] Baker, C. (2007) *A Parents' and Teachers' Guide to Bilingualism* (3rd ed). Clevedon, UK: Multilingual Matters.
[43] Bialystok, E. (2002) Acquisition of literacy in bilingual children: A framework for research. *Language Learning* 52 (1), 159–99.
[44] Koerner, A.F. and Fitzpatrick, M.A. (2002) Toward a theory of family communication. *Communication Theory* 12, 70–91.
[45] Cuero, K. and Romo, H.D. (2007) Raising a multicultural multilingual child. Paper presented at the Annual Meeting of the American Sociological Association, New York, 10 August.
[46] Baker, C. (2007) *A Parents' and Teachers' Guide to Bilingualism* (3rd ed). Clevedon, UK: Multilingual Matters.
[47] Okita, T. (2002) *Invisible Work: Bilingualism, Language Choice and Childrearing in Intermarried Families*. Amsterdam: Benjamins.
[48] Wang, X.-L. (2011) *Learning to Read and Write in the Multilingual Family*. Bristol, UK: Multilingual Matters.
[49] Baker, C. (2007) *A Parents' and Teachers' Guide to Bilingualism* (3rd edn). Clevedon: Multilingual Matters.
Cunningham-Andersson, U. and Andersson, S. (1999) *Growing Up With Two Languages*. New York: Routledge.
Takeuchi, M. (2006) *Raising Children Bilingually Through The 'One Parent-One Language' Approach: A Case Study Of Japanese Mothers In The Australian Context*. New York: Peter Lang.
Wang, X.-L. (2008) *Growing Up With Three Languages: Birth to Eleven*. Bristol: Multilingual Matters.
[50] Janssen, C. and Pauwels, A. (1993) *Raising Children Bilingually in Australia*. Melbourne: Language and Society Center, Monash University.
Wang, X.-L. (2008) *Growing Up With Three Languages: Birth to Eleven*. Bristol: Multilingual Matters.
[51] Wang, X.-L. (2008) *Growing Up With Three Languages: Birth to Eleven*. Bristol: Multilingual Matters.
[52] Sotomayor-Peterson, M. (2009) Parental cultural values, co-parental, and familial functioning in Mexican immigrant families: Its impact on children's social competence. *Dissertation Abstracts International Section A: Humanities and Social Sciences* 69 (8-A), 3342.
[53] Chao R. (2001) Extending research on the consequences of parenting style for Chinese Americans and European Americans. *Child Development* 72, 1832–43.
Ispa, J.M., Fine, M.A., Halgunseth, L.C., Harper, S., Robinson, J., Boyce, L., Brooks-Gunn, J. and Brady-Smith, C. (2004) Maternal intrusiveness, maternal warmth, and mother-toddler relationship outcomes: Variations across low-income ethnic and acculturation groups. *Child Development* 75 (6), 1613–31.
Spera, C. (2005) A review of the relationship among parenting practices, parenting styles, and adolescent school achievement. *Educational Psychology Review* 17 (2), 125–46.
Varela, E.R., Vernberg, E.M., Sanchez-Sosa, J.J., Riveros, A., Mitchell, M. and Mashunkashey, J. (2004) Parenting style of Mexican, Mexican American, and Caucasian-non-Hispanic families: Social context and cultural influences. *Journal of Family Psychology* 18 (4), 651–57.
[54] McPherson, G.E. (2009) The role of parents in children's musical development. *Psychology of Music* 37 (1), 91–110.

Pomerantz, E.M. and Dong, W. (2006) Effects of mothers' perceptions on children's competence: The moderating role of mothers' theories of competence. *Developmental Psychology* 42 (5), 950–61.

Pomerantz, E.M. and Eaton, M.M. (2001) Maternal intrusive support in the academic context: Transactional socialization processes. *Developmental Psychology* 37, 174–86.

Pomerantz, E.M., Grolnick, W.S. and Price, C.E. (2005) The role of parents in how children approach achievement: A dynamic process perspective. In A.J. Elliot and C.S. Dweck (eds) *Handbook of Competence And Motivation* (pp. 259–78). New York: Guilford.

Steinberg, L., Lamborn, S.D., Darling, N., Mounts, N.S. and Dornbusch, S.M. (1994) Over-time changes in adjustment and competence among adolescents from authoritative, authoritarian, indulgent, and neglectful homes. *Child Development* 63, 754–70.

[55] Chao, R.K. (1994) Beyond parental control and authoritarian parenting style: Understanding Chinese parenting through the cultural notion of training. *Child Development* 65 (4), 1111–19.

Chao, R.K. (2000) Cultural explanations for the role of parenting in the school success of Asian-American children. In R.D. Taylor and M.C. Wang (eds) *Resilience Across Contexts: Family, Work, Culture, And Community* (pp. 333–63). Mahwah, NJ: Lawrence Erlbaum Associates.

Chao, R.K. (2001) Extending research on the consequences of parenting style for Chinese and European Americans. *Child Development* 72 (6), 1832–43.

[56] Dopke, S. (1992) *One Parent One Language: An Interactional Approach*. Amsterdam: John Benjamins.

[57] Barron-Hauwaret, S. (2004) *Language Strategies For Bilingual Families: The One-Parent-One-Language Approach*. Clevedon: Multilingual Matters.

[58] Schrodt, P. and Ledbetter, A.M. (2007) Communication processes that mediate family communication patterns and mental well-being: A mean and covariance structures analysis of young adults from divorced and nondivorced families. *Human Communication Research* 33, 330–56.

[59] Wang, X.-L.(2011) *Learning to Read and Write in the Multilingual Family*. Bristol: Multilingual Matters.

[60] Huppert, F.A., Abbott, R.A., Ploubidis, G.B., Richards, M. and Kuh, D. (2010) Parental practices predict psychological well-being in midlife: Life-course associations among women in the 1946 British birth cohort. *Psychological Medicine* 40, 1507–18.

Ryff, C.D. (1989) Happiness is everything, or is it? Explorations on the meaning of psychological well-being. *Journal of Personality and Social Psychology* 57, 1069–81.

Ryff, C.D. and Keyes, C.L.M. (1995) The structure of psychological well-being revisited. *Journal of Personality and Social Psychology* 69, 719–27.

[61] Lanza, E. and Svendsen, B.A. (2007) Tell me who your friends are and I might be able to tell you what language(s) you speak: Social network analysis, multilingualism, and identity. *International Journal of Bilingualism* 11 (3), 275–300.

[62] Wang, X.-L.(2011) *Learning to Read and Write in the Multilingual Family*. Bristol: Multilingual Matters.

[63] Fletcher, A.C., Nickerson, P. and Wright, K.L. (2003) Structured leisure activities in middle childhood: Links to well-being. *Journal of Community Psychology* 31 (6), 641–59.

[64] Romaine, S. (1989) *Bilingualism*. Oxford: Blackwell Publisher Ltd.

Romaine, S. (1995) *Bilingualism*. Oxford: Blackwell Publisher Ltd.

[65] Noguchi, M.G. (1996) The bilingual parent as model for the bilingual child. *Seisaku Kagaku* 245–61. Kyoto: Ritsumeikan University.

[66] Brown, S. and Attardo, S. (2008) *Understanding Language Structure, Interaction, and Variation: An Introduction to Applied Linguistics and Sociolinguistics for Nonspecialists*. Michigan: University of Michigan Press.

[67] Allen, J.P., Hauser, S.T., Bell, K.L. and O'Connor, T.G. (1994) Longitudinal assessment of autonomy and relatedness in adolescent-family interactions as predictors of adolescent ego development and self-esteem. *Child Development* 65, 179–94.

Barber, B.K. (1996) Parental psychological control: Revisiting a neglected construct. *Child Development* 67, 3296–319.

Conger, R.D., Neppi, T., Kim, K.-J. and Scaramella, L.V. (2003) Angry and aggressive behavior across three generations: A prospective, longitudinal study of parents and children. *Journal of Abnormal Child Psychology* 31 (2), 143–60.

[68] Wang, X.-L. (2009) Ensuring sustained trilingual development through motivation. *The Bilingual Family Newsletter* 26 (1), 1–7.

[69] Harter, S. (1996) Teacher and classmate influence on scholastic motivation, self-esteem, and level of voice in adolescence. In J. Juvonen and K. Wentzel (eds) *Social Motivation: Understating Children's School Adjustment* (pp. 11–42). New York: Cambridge University Press.

10 Pulling It Together: Concluding Thoughts

During one of Léandre's weekly FaceTime[1] conversations with me four weeks after he entered college, he told me that he was considering taking a Chinese-language class. He reasoned at length to elucidate why it was important for him to read and write Chinese well. Also, in the second semester of his freshman year of college, Léandre told his father that he had registered for a French film class, which was taught entirely in French. Upon hearing Léandre's desire to continue with his heritage-language learning, both Philippe and I were beside ourselves with joy and triumph. We were relieved that our years of relentless efforts had finally borne fruit. Our experience with Léandre made us realise that as long as parents instil the right attitude in their children and use the right strategies to support them in their heritage-language development, children are likely to be self-motivated to follow the path to multilingualism, even though the road may be bumpy along the way.

This concluding chapter will pull together the important information conveyed throughout the book and present a panoramic view of multilingual childrearing. Essential take-away messages are provided to help you reflect on your own multilingual childrearing experience. To broaden the discussion on multilingual parenting, this chapter also briefly touches upon multilingual childrearing in special circumstances which have not been addressed previously in this book and which may be of interest for some parents. These special topics include how single parents and monolingual parents raise multilingual children; how parents help children with special needs develop multilingual abilities; and how parents continue to support their children's heritage-language development when their children leave home for college or other independent living situations. The chapter ends on an upbeat note: Although it is challenging to raise multilingual children and teenagers, it is definitely a worthwhile endeavour.

Essential Take-Away Messages

Throughout the book, you have the opportunity to read about my account of raising multilingual adolescents, which include achievements as well as challenges. It is clear that appropriate parental strategies are essential to help teens maintain their heritage language(s) and develop multilingual identities. Here, I reiterate several important messages for you to use as a reminder in your future multilingual childrearing practice.

Supporting your teens' development should be the priority

Although the focus of this book is on raising multilingual teens, it is, in fact, also a book about raising children. It is clear whatever we do as parents will have a profound impact on our children. Therefore, it is important to make the support of your teens' overall development a priority while interacting with them in their heritage-language attainment. As shown throughout the book, supporting teens' identity, social and cognitive development can be incorporated in the heritage-language learning activities. If we constantly remind ourselves that raising a multilingual child is only part of raising a whole person, we will interact with our teens in a holistic way.

Setting goals and planning focused efforts

Setting achievable goals for your children's heritage-language and multilingual development is critical to help them succeed and reduce their frustration. This is especially important during adolescence when teens are engaged in many other activities. To begin, you may want to ask yourself the following questions:

- What proficiency level do I want my teens to achieve in the areas of heritage-language speaking, reading and writing?
- Do I have the ability, support and resources to help my children achieve these goals? If not, how can I get help?

With these questions in mind, you are likely to set more realistic goals and make feasible plans.

Setting short-term and long-term heritage-language learning goals

When setting goals for your children's heritage-language learning, you may want to consider two kinds of goals: short term and long term. Your short-term goals can be weekly or monthly, and your long-term goals can be yearly or based on developmental stages (e.g. early childhood, elementary school, middle school and high school). Also, in setting short-term and long-term goals, it may be effective to write down concrete heritage-language learning goals that you can work on with your children. Most importantly, you should remind yourself and your children of the heritage-language learning goals and plans by posting them in a place that you frequent, such as on the refrigerator door. This kind of visual reminder can help you follow through with your plans. Some parents who attended my parenting workshops shared that writing down plans and frequently

> **Box 10.1 Quote From A Parent About Planning**
>
> Before this workshop, I wasn't serious about planning my kid's Polish language learning. I did one thing one day and tried another on other days. I didn't really know what I was doing, how much progress she made, and didn't know where we were going… Since I began to write down my child's Polish learning goals and to plan the action steps, I have become more organised and more clear about what we need to do…and my child also understands better what she needs to learn…I definitely see the importance of planning in helping children learn their home language…
>
> Armelia

visiting them was a very helpful strategy that helped them to keep their plans in check. Box 10.1 is a quote from Armelia,[2] mother of a 13-year-old girl from New Jersey, USA.

Setting up achievable heritage-language learning goals

Although setting heritage-language learning goals is important, setting achievable goals is even more essential. If your goals for your children's heritage-language learning are too ambitious, you and your children are likely to be frustrated and disappointed. Box 10.2 is a reminder.

This mother's aspiration for her children's heritage-language learning is certainly admirable; however, her demands are not realistic for at least two reasons. First, expecting children who live in a non-Chinese-speaking environment to reach the same language and literacy proficiency as children who live in a Chinese-speaking environment is unrealistic. Language development, especially literacy development such as reading and writing, requires sufficient exposure and constant

> **Box 10.2 Example of Unreasonable Expectations on Heritage-Language Learning**
>
> Being an Asian, I believe in making an effort in learning and I hold the same belief for my three children's Chinese-language learning. Because my kids live in the US, they don't have opportunities to use Chinese. I send them all to a Chinese language school and I expect them to be fluent in reading and writing Chinese and to keep the same Chinese level like the kids at the same age in China…I give my kids lots of Chinese exercises daily and they spend most of their Saturdays and Sundays going through Chinese drills in addition to spending 3 hours in the Chinese language school…[3]

> **Box 10.3 Example of Parental Self-Reflection**
>
> …I not only failed in making my children learn Chinese. I scared them away from it…Knowing what I know now, I would have started modestly and focused on setting up goals that they could achieve…[4]

practice. Despite the type of Chinese-language learning opportunities from the children's weekly Chinese school and daily exercises provided by the mother, her children live in an English-speaking environment and their exposure to Chinese is insufficient. Second, there is a time-constraint issue. Obviously, her children go to school and have other school-related assignments and social activities. The mother reflected on her practice at the end of my parent workshop and had a revelation (see Box 10.3).

This mother's experience serves as a reminder of the importance of setting achievable heritage-language learning goals.

Setting heritage-language learning goals together with your children

It is also important that children participate in setting heritage-language learning goals and making plans. Communicating the goals and plans to your children or teens can help you realise your goals and plans more effectively. It is also vital to get your children's input when you set goals and make plans. Sometimes, you will be surprised by how understanding and thoughtful your children can be in the process. For instance, Léandre (15; 2; 3) told me that instead of asking him to write Chinese idioms during snack time, I should focus on helping him understand Chinese idiom usage. He commented that if I explained the idioms to him with related stories, he would concentrate and enjoy them because he liked learning the stories related to each idiom while enjoying his snack. Indeed, he made a very useful suggestion for me to help him learn. With his busy school schedule, it was more realistic for me to talk about Chinese idiom usage with him than it was for me to ask him to write about idioms.

Differentiating heritage-language learning goals

When setting heritage-language learning goals and making plans, you might want to be mindful of differentiating the plans and goals for your children's social language and literacy development. **Social language** is the language used in everyday communication, and **literacy** means reading, writing and other critical literacy and digital literacy abilities. These two kinds of development need different supporting strategies. The ideal goal for heritage-language development is, of course, to help our children develop competence in all areas; however, because the heritage-language learning environment is different from the typical language-learning environment, it is likely that heritage-language literacy development will be more challenging. Based on my experience, focusing on building the foundation of heritage-language literacy may be a more realistic goal for many families. In other words, even though it is often challenging for heritage-language learners to develop competency in their heritage-language literacy, such as reading and writing, it is important to develop essential heritage-language literacy skills that will help them further develop competency when future opportunities arise. For instance, Mrs Chen's son acquired basic writing skills in Chinese (such as the stroke order of Chinese characters, punctuation-mark usage and sentence structure) in his childhood and adolescence. Even though he could not really read and write Chinese well at high-school graduation, he had built basic Chinese literacy skills that he was able to develop further when his company assigned him to work in China. Thus, it is likely that for many heritage-language learning teens, developing basic literacy skills in heritage-language literacy is a more realistic goal than achieving actual competency in heritage-language reading and writing.

Modifying your plans based on circumstances

It is crucial that you adjust your plans and change your strategies based on circumstances when things do not work out. In some cases, abandoning your plan in the best interests of your children and yourself is necessary. For example, in my two children's Chinese writing development, my original goal was to help them develop age-appropriate writing ability in Chinese. However, during their teenage years, I realised that to force my original plan on them was not realistic. Chinese writing requires lots of practice and time. With the boys' busy schedules, which I outlined in Chapter 2, a choice had to be made between Chinese writing development and other activities in the teens' lives. Thus, in their mid-adolescent years (when they were around 15 years old), I decided that I would focus more on oral Chinese language development and use talking as the main medium for Chinese literacy teaching. I used this strategy during meal times and travel time in the car to enhance Chinese language and literacy abilities that would be useful for the boys' later Chinese literacy development.

Because I adjusted my plans, the kids felt more relaxed and more eager to engage in conversations that led to their Chinese-language and literacy development. Frankly speaking, I also felt less stressed; that is, I did not feel the need to always 'spoil' the fun during snack or meal time by pulling out Chinese language exercise sheets and asking the children to work on them. Instead, I could use situational contexts to provide relevant Chinese language-related information verbally. If you want to know more about how to plan heritage-language and heritage-language literacy development, please refer to Chapter 3 in my book *Learning to Read and Write in the Multilingual Family*.[5]

Focusing on your family's situation

Finally, when setting up goals and making plans for your children, it is important to consider your own family situation. Different families have different situations.

Because multilingual families are complex, it is not an exaggeration to say that no multilingual families look exactly alike. For some families, multilingual development is a necessity, and for other families, it is a choice. No matter which route your family takes, considering your own circumstance will help you attend to your children's needs. There is so much information, and sometimes misinformation, out there that one can easily get confused with different advice from lay people and experts. One thing is crucial: It is always wise to critically filter what we see and hear. Listen to others' advice, including expert advice, critically and cautiously. This does not mean, however, that you need to run afoul of those who have good intentions to help you. Some tips may work for one family but may not work for another. Using others' experiences to help you reflect on your own may be a better approach.

Communicating parenting differences with children

In Chapters 2 and 9, I mentioned that parents from multilingual families are often from different linguistic and cultural backgrounds. Parental childrearing beliefs and practices in teaching and learning may conflict with each other. In addition, parental beliefs may be different from those of the mainstream culture. These inconsistencies in belief systems and childrearing practices may cause parental conflicts in how heritage language should be taught and learnt in the family environment. In Chapter 9, I provide some concrete strategies for how to handle parental conflicts in multilingual childrearing. In this section, I would like to revisit this issue by focusing on communicating parenting differences with your children.

Using my own family as an example, I believe in praising children's efforts and playing down their abilities. Therefore, in my interactions with them, I often stress how much effort they have put into doing something (including their Chinese-language learning) instead of focusing on whether or not they do it well. My husband Philippe, however, believes otherwise. He thinks that if children are already doing well, it does not matter whether they make an effort or not; rather, he values the end result over the process. The truth is that neither of us is really wrong in our beliefs, and belief systems are often hard to change. The key is how we discuss our beliefs with our children, help them understand our perspectives, take into consideration their responses to our beliefs and parenting styles and negotiate and adjust our parenting practices accordingly when necessary.

Perhaps we can focus on balancing parental desires and aspirations for our children with our children's reaction to our strategies. In practice, what this means is that we need to discuss our beliefs with our children frequently and give them room to respond to what we believe and what we do. If they resist what we do, we should communicate again. Adolescence is a good time to carry out conversations like this because of adolescents' cognitive advancement and perspective-taking ability. In the process of interacting and negotiating with each other, parents and children both need to give and take. Such a family dynamic is healthy as nobody dominates the decision-making process.

Ultimately, children are resilient in general. In a typical family environment, they will not get confused by their parents' different beliefs and parenting styles as long as parents communicate with their children about their beliefs consistently, just as children do not get confused when learning different languages. The success in parenting is to communicate with our children about our beliefs openly and explain why we interact with them the way we do. In fact, I think my two children only became increasingly more flexible in responding to my husband's and my parenting differences, and as a result, they also carry such flexibility outside our home environment into their school environment. Thus, the bottom line is that exposing children to different parenting beliefs and styles can be positive, given that constant communication is involved.

Increasing conversation length by providing situationally appropriate heritage-language input

Because heritage-language learning and developing conditions are different from the typical language-learning environment, it is essential for children and adolescents to receive good-quality heritage-language input to optimise their chances of becoming multilingual.

Good-quality input is particularly vital for heritage-language-learning children and adolescents because their heritage-language environment is limited to a few people and often only to one parent. Thus, well-thought-out and purposeful language usage and modelling needs to be carried out in the situationally appropriate conversation context. Box 10.4 presents an example of what good-quality situationally appropriate heritage-language input looks like.

In this example, the conversation topic is like that of any daily conversation. I took advantage of this situational-prompted conversation to teach Léandre and Dominique the authentic Chinese expressions 集中注意力 (focused or concentration), 分散注意力 or 注意力分散 (distraction), and 质量 (quality). At that point, neither Léandre nor Dominique used these expressions in an authentic Chinese way.

Some may question whether parents should turn everyday conversation into language teaching. Here is my take (subject to debate) on this issue. Because of the challenges of heritage-language teaching and learning, as shown in this book, I actually see several advantages of this kind of parent-child interactive dynamic in situationally appropriate contexts. First, the conversation length is increased. I have calculated the typical conversational turns between non-language-related and typical conversation between my two teens and heritage-language-related conversation. Language-related conversations definitely have more turns, as there are six turns in this conversation instead of three turns in normal conversation during adolescence.[7] More turns means more interactions, and more interactions mean more opportunities to use heritage language. During the adolescent period,

> **Box 10.4 Example of Situationally Appropriate Heritage-Language Input**
>
> Léandre (16; 2; 2) was doing his PSAT[6] practice exercises in the kitchen. The rest of the family was chatting. Léandre complained that he was distracted from what he was doing.
>
> **Léandre:** Can you lower your voice? I cannot concentrate. (能不能小声点？)
>
> **Mother:** We are sorry. Can you do it upstairs? (对不起。 你可不可以上楼去做？)
>
> **Léandre:** Ok. (好) [Reluctantly collecting his practice sheet.]
>
> **Mother:** You will be distracted if you do it here. (你在这里做注意力会分散。)
>
> If you go upstairs, you will be focused and you will not be distracted. (你上楼去做你的练习，你会集中注意力，你不会分散注意力。)
>
> Dominique, did you hear that? (昵可，你听道了吗？)
>
> **Dominique:** What? (什么？)
>
> **Mother:** Did you hear what I just said to Léandre? He will be more focused and not be distracted if he does his PSAT exercises upstairs. (你听到我对理昂说什么了吗？ 他如果上楼做他的 PSAT，他会集中注意力，他不会分散注意力).
>
> **Dominique:** Focused and not distracted. (集中注意力，不会分散注意力。)
>
> **Mother:** Yes, concentrated and not distracted. (对，集中注意力，你不会分散注意力。)
>
> By the way, the quality of his work will also be good. (对了，他做的质量也会好).
>
> **Mother:** Léandre, do you agree that the quality of your work will be good if you are concentrated and less distracted? (理昂，你同不同意，如果你集中注意力，不分散注意力，你做的质量会好？)
>
> **Léandre:** Maybe. (可能。)

lengthening the conversation between parents and teens is positive in parent-child relationships and heritage-language learning.

Second, language-related conversation can lead to conversations about other aspects of life. For example, this conversation topic led to a conversation about Léandre's stress about having to do his regular class assignments and prepare for PSAT later that afternoon. This gave me a good understanding of how to help him cope with stress.

Third, this is also an occasion for parents to assess teens' heritage-language development. Through interactions with Léandre in this context, I knew that he needed to learn more Chinese expressions to express his thoughts. In other words, because parents rarely (almost never) test their children's heritage-language development in the home environment, activities such as this will help us get a sense of our children's heritage-language developmental levels by carrying on purposeful yet also enjoyable conversations in the context.

Finally, conversations like this not only give parents an opportunity to model heritage-language use but also allow siblings to get heritage-language input, as can be seen in how I involved Dominique in the conversation.

Using heritage language consistently in communication

The language or languages used to communicate with your children need to be consistent. Indeed, both research and observation show that to achieve heritage-language proficiency, consistent input tends to yield better results. Some researchers even go further by suggesting that heritage-language-speaking parents should perhaps resist any temptation to communicate in mainstream language with their children just because they are able to do so.[8]

Maximising heritage-language exposure through a variety of resources

In a typical language-learning environment, parents are not the only people who provide language input for their children. The variety of input from different resources helps a language learner learn. However, heritage-language-learning children often lack this kind of variety in input sources. Thus, you may want to make an effort to expand the input for your children.

Input from grandparents, relatives and heritage-language community

Research has consistently shown that intergenerational transmission of heritage languages is the most effective way to preserve and even revive languages. Thus, grandparents and relatives are potentially great resources for children to acquire, maintain and develop their heritage-language proficiency and knowledge of heritage culture.[9] Even if grandparents and close relatives may live apart from your family, they can provide valuable heritage-language input for your children. Thanks to the advancement of communication technology, it is possible that grandparents and relatives can influence your children's heritage-language development via e-mails, Skype, FaceTime and webchat. As shared in previous chapters, the virtual interactions between Léandre and Dominique and their Chinese grandparents have helped both children's Chinese-language development and cultural knowledge. I especially find it useful for our children to hear the family stories and anecdotes recounted in these web conversations. Moreover, Léandre and Dominique learnt many idioms and colloquialisms from their Chinese grandparents, which they would not have learnt from me, their major Chinese-language input.

Input from media and technology

Multimedia technology is prevalent in our lives. Nowadays, there are many ways that children can receive heritage-language input through multimedia technology, such as YouTube videos, television shows, news reports, music and video games. Although there is conflicting information about whether young children can learn language from media such as television,[10] older children can certainly benefit from multimedia input. Dominique, for example, has learnt many French colloquial expressions by listening to French popular music. Thus, encouraging children to explore heritage-language multimedia during adolescence is a positive way to combine heritage-language learning and adolescent natural inclination.

Input from travelling to heritage-language-speaking countries

Our experience with our children suggests that spending time in the heritage-language-speaking countries and other environments in which the heritage language is spoken has been very effective for Léandre and Dominique. Each time Léandre and Dominique spend a summer in their heritage-language-speaking countries or environment, we observe a visible progress in their heritage languages. Elsewhere, I mentioned that Léandre and Dominique used to comment that they needed a vacation when they found that they had made mistakes in their heritage languages.[11]

Of course, international travelling requires money and time. As a result, many families may find travel difficult. I suppose that every family can make their own decision regarding what they want to prioritise and where to spend their financial resources. International travel not only helps children's language exposure but also promotes their overall development of a global mindset. I have shared my thoughts on international travel in an edited book I put together with Dr Ronan Bernas, *People without Boarders: Becoming Members of Global Communities*. I share an excerpt with you in Box 10.5.

Making one of the languages solid while developing other languages

Throughout this book, I have indicated that knowing more than one language is an advantage for children and adolescents. However, the reality about multilingualism is there are also various degrees of competence in children's different languages. Based on our experiences and observations, I believe that having a solid knowledge of at least one language, meaning to be competent in speaking, reading and writing, is beneficial to children's overall communicative confidence.

In our own childrearing practice and life circumstance, English is the language that Léandre and Dominique have had the most chances in which to develop their overall competence in speaking, reading and writing. As a family, we decided that they would receive continuous education after high school and develop a fuller degree of competence in English. With a solid foundation in one language, they will feel confident as language users.

> **Box 10.5 Broadening One's Horizon Through International Travel**[12]
>
> Although international travel is not the only thing for children to develop a global mindset, it does help broaden children's horizons. As Mark Twain so famously put it, 'Nothing so liberalizes a man and expands the kindly instincts that nature put in him as travel and contact with many kinds of people' (1867). Some people may not have financial resources for international travels; budget travel can be an alternative to get in touch with real people in the real world. Often for those who do travel internationally, it may mean sacrifices at the expense of other aspects in life. I know a Finnish couple who live in a very small apartment and are very frugal in their daily expenses. But every year, they manage to bring their daughter to one or two different countries through budget travel. They said the choice for them was clear whether to have a big house or to travel. They chose the latter.
>
> International travel has also been the priority of our family. My husband and I have made sure that our two children grew up travelling by tightening our belts on other things. Over the years, we have seen how our two children have benefitted from their international travels, especially in their views and approaches to issues. For example, I have recently read a college course paper written by our older son Léandre on the future of the European Union. I was impressed with his take in looking at the economic austerity issue. He reinterpreted Nietzsche's two morals in the modern context and expressed his views on the responsibility of rich nations in relation to less wealthy nations. His arguments were fair and balanced, and he could explore the issue from different perspectives. The examples that he used were from his observations through travelling.

Our decision was influenced by the stories we heard from some multilingual people about their feeling of their 'inadequate proficiencies' in their different languages. Box 10.6 is Anna's lament.

To avoid the sentiment felt by multilinguals like Anna, our family had a discussion about where Léandre and Dominique would go for their post-high-school education, because for a while Léandre and Dominique were contemplating applying to non-English-speaking colleges in continental Europe. In our discussions, I conveyed my thinking about making one language (in their case, English) solid. Léandre and Dominique argued that their English was already good. I said that even though their English was excellent, they needed more opportunities to develop into more mature English language communicators, especially in reading and writing. I convinced them that college was a good place for them to further develop their English literacy and academic literacy abilities. In the end, they both agreed.

Overall, making one of your children's languages solid is something I would like you to think about seriously. Whatever you decide to do, please make sure that your children will not share Anna's sentiment. When I communicated with Anna, I found her English was excellent. I also found that the issue is not really whether

> **Box 10.6 Anna's Comments on Her Own Multilingual Competence[13]**
>
> ...I was brought up speaking four different languages: Russian, Polish, English and Czech. During my school years, I travelled all over the world and learnt many more languages. Honestly, I don't feel confident with any of my languages, especially in reading and writing. I make mistakes in almost all my languages...I wish I had one language that I can function confidently...

her English (or other languages) is good or not. Instead, the real issue is how she feels about her own language ability, and it seems that her low self-confidence in her own language abilities is really the problem. As parents, we may want to pay attention to this issue.

Focusing on communication

Heritage-language learning is important, but communication with our children and teens is even more important. During the adolescent period, communication between parents and teens is essential. I mentioned in Chapter 7 that it is important to be flexible and allow teens to write in the language in which they are most competent and comfortable for the purposes of communication. If we insist that our teens communicate with us in their heritage language(s), especially in writing, they might stop communicating with us. As I discussed in Chapter 7, I have let Léandre text me in English since he went to college. I found it is a lot easier for him (and for me also) to communicate more frequently if we communicate in English, as it usually takes me a lot longer to write in Chinese.

Moreover, because heritage-language-learning teens do not live in the heritage-language-dominant environment, their heritage-language proficiency may be limited and they may make mistakes. Thus, we must learn the art of correcting mistakes; that is, we need to learn how to correct our children's mistakes without interfering with our communication with them, and we need to learn how to correct their mistakes without discourage their heritage-language learning.

Incorporating paralanguage learning into heritage-language learning

When helping your children develop their heritage language(s), it is crucial to consider paralanguage in the heritage culture as an integral part of heritage-language learning process. **Paralanguage** refers to communication that is other than spoken, such as gestures, kinesics (body language), facial expressions, tone/voice use, proxemics (e.g. the physical distance between people), time concept and space arrangement. Paralanguage has been referred to as the 'hidden aspects' of communication. I have commented elsewhere[14] that it would be unimaginable for someone to speak Italian without making some Italian gestures and facial expressions. Learning the paralanguage in the heritage culture while learning heritage language will help your children communicate effectively with heritage-language speakers.

Children learn their paralanguage in their ambient culture through observations and practices. However, heritage-language-learning children and adolescents typically do not have the opportunity to acquire heritage-culture paralanguage. To get an idea on how to help children develop paralanguage simultaneously with their heritage language, please refer to my book *Growing Up With Three languages: Birth to Eleven*.[15]

Understanding individual differences in heritage-language development

Although there is a general language development (heritage-language development included) trend for children with typical development, individual differences are ubiquitous. Different children have different talents, personalities and aptitudes. Therefore, avoiding comparing your child with another, including siblings, will help you see your child's strengths and areas for improvement. During the adolescent period, teens are very sensitive to others' judgemental comments; sometimes even implicit comments can make them feel bad. Box 10.7 is an example from Joseph, a parent who has two English-Hebrew bilingual teenagers.

If you observe differences among your children or other peers in terms of their heritage-language development gap, the best thing to do is perhaps to focus on the child's strengths and figure out his or her particular circumstances. While it is natural for parents to compare their children to one another or to others, it is perhaps better to focus on your child's individuality and help your child to develop his or her potential to the fullest degree. Recognising your child's individuality means that you will find effective ways to help your child grow. For example, Dominique has a very good memory (he said that he had 'photographic memory'); he could remember complicated Chinese characters faster than Léandre, whereas Léandre had a better Chinese-language instinct than Dominique. Thus, I pointed out their individual strengths and focused on the areas in which they needed help. As a result, Léandre and Dominique never felt that they needed to compete with each other and they had a quite good self-assessment about their own strengths and areas that needed improvement.

Assessing heritage-language and multilingual achievements in your children's contexts

Language competency is usually assessed through standardised tests. I have shown some in Appendix A. Although the standardised tests can provide a useful norm for

---

Box 10.7 Inappropriate Comparison between Children[16]

My older son was fluent in Hebrew. By age 13, he could read religious texts in Hebrew. But my younger son could not even read the basic Hebrew text at the same age. So, one day, I said to him, 'Your brother could read a lot better than you at your age. You should be ashamed of yourself.' My comment hurt my younger son deeply. He was actually never motivated to improve his Hebrew. In a recent conversation with him (he is now 22), he told me that he remembered my comment and had always felt inferior to his older brother...

us, they may not capture the real heritage-language proficiency of heritage-language-learning children and teens who are learning their heritage language(s) in a variety of home contexts. Therefore, I would like to argue that standardised tests may not completely measure children's heritage-language competency because of their unique heritage-language learning environment. I believe that using situational contexts, such as children's narratives and real-life language use, is perhaps a more accurate way to assess your children's heritage-language competence and progress than using standardised tests. Hence, the measures I described at the end of Chapters, 3, 4, 5, 6 and 7 may be helpful for you to understand your children's heritage-language abilities in different areas.

Reflecting on parental practices

To ensure our children's heritage-language learning success, frequently reflecting on our own practice is vital. Over the years, I have taken notes about my interactions with my two children. These notes have helped me reflect on my parenting practice. When I recently reviewed my notes over the last 19 years, I realised that there were many things I would have forgotten if I had not written them down. Most importantly, these notes helped me think about my successes and failures and find more suitable ways to support my children in their heritage-language attainment and multilingual identity development. Through constant self-reflection, I have observed my growth as a parent over the years. Box 10.8 is an example of a reflection template that I found useful.

You can come up with your own template and entry style. The point is to record what you do and your children's reaction and use that to guide your subsequent interactions with them. If you keep up the habit of reflecting on your daily interactions with your children, you will see the benefit.

Box 10.8 Example of A Reflection Template

Date: 12/3/2010
Context: During lunch, Dominique complained that I always wanted to talk about Chinese measurement word use.
Interactions: Discussed why it was important to talk about measurement words.
Thoughts and reflection: Next time I need to find a different way of involving Dominique and try to increase his motivation. Maybe I can incorporate 'teaching' in the actual use of these measurement words.
Follow-Up: (12/15/10) I used the measurement words 罐 (can), 袋 (bag), and 锅 (pot) when Dominique asked me to cook pasta for him. I asked him to give me one <u>can</u> of tomato sauce (一罐番茄酱) and one <u>bag</u> of pasta (一袋意大利面). I told him that I will then heat a <u>pot</u> of water (烧一锅水). I think it worked well by incorporating teaching these measurement words in natural interactions.

Thinking medially

Heritage-language and multilingual development is often portrayed as a one-way endeavour; that is, many people believe it only involves the efforts of parents. In fact, up until this point, I may have given you the unintended impression that I am writing a book to help parents make their children multilingual. To recant this impression, I would like to introduce medial thinking in parenting (including language teaching), which will encourage us to rethink the role both parents and children (adolescents included) play in the process of multilingual development.

Medial thinking is also called middle-voiced thinking.[17] The middle voice was originally a grammatical notion. It is interesting to use this notion as a way to think about the dynamics between parents and children in terms of heritage-language learning and multilingual development. Most modern languages have lost the middle voice and have kept only the active and the passive voice, as in 'Tom learns Spanish' (active voice) and 'Tom is asked by his parents to learn Spanish' (passive voice). In ancient Greek, there is a third voice called the 'middle voice,' which indicates that the action is performed with special reference to the subject (the doer, or the agent). The closest English equivalent of middle voice is something like, 'Tom *got blamed* by his parents for not learning Spanish.' According to the French linguist Émile Benveniste,[18] in the common active/passive distinction, the stress is on the subject (the doer or the agent) as opposed to the object or the patient (the receiver); that is, 'Who does what, what is being done by whom?' By contrast, in the middle voice, the focus is on the location of the subject (doer) with respect to the action of the verb. Whereas in the active voice the subject is outside the verb, as if dominating the action, in the middle voice the subject (the doer) is encompassed within the action. A doer is still engaged in the action, but the important question is no longer what the doer does or who the doer is, but rather where the doer is located. The key here is location. In the middle voice, the subject of a verb is within the action of the verb. To put it plainly, although Tom was blamed by his parents, he was also responsible for the blame for what he did not do. The event involved both (parents and Tom), not just one party.

This medial thinking can help us visualise the process of heritage-language maintenance and multilingual development; that is, *both* parents and adolescents play a role in the process. It forces us to focus on the whole process rather on either parents or adolescents alone. Medial thinking also encourages us to treat multilingual development as a dynamic process of *both* and *more* (i.e. both parents and adolescents contribute to the multilingual development process, and adolescents elaborate, construct, reconstruct and re-create their heritage language[19] in their language-learning environment) rather than a process of *either/or* (i.e. either parents alone or adolescents alone determine the multilingual development). Below is an example to illustrate what it means to think and act medially.

When Léandre was in middle school, he never did his Chinese homework immediately after he came home from his Chinese-language school on Saturdays.

He would always want to play instead. As a believer in 'work first, then play,' I, of course, tried to encourage him to finish his Chinese homework first and then play. I cannot remember how many times both his father and I told him that playing is much more fun without having work hanging over one's head. But he still procrastinated in doing his Chinese homework (and other homework as well). He came to his father and me one day and explained why he wanted to play first and then do his homework: 'When I do my homework first, it takes me two hours to do what I can do in 20 minutes in the evening.' It took us a while to make sense of what he meant, but we finally understood what he was saying. If he played first, it would leave him little time to do his homework and force him to do it when he was completely focused, whereas if he started early, he would idle and waste time; consequently, he would end up having no time to play at all. His reasoned procrastination baffled us. We were sceptical at first, but it turned out that his explanation was not an excuse; he got his homework done and done well. Seeing his results, we stopped insisting that he do his homework immediately after school.

The moral of this story is that, although Léandre's approach did not convince us, as we continue to avoid procrastinating our own tasks, we learnt from this thinking that being involved in the learning of a heritage language is a medial process. We wanted Léandre to do his homework the same way we would do it ourselves; however, we realised that it was not just our will against his will. It was not us alone wanting him to comply. In fact, Léandre himself did not object to completing the Chinese homework. He was willing to do it, only later. We came to realise that he and we (his parents) were involved in a medial process. We were agents, among many others, on opposing sides of the question of when Léandre should do his Chinese homework. The mediality of the conflict between us lay in the fact it was a process of multiple agents encompassing and changing both him and us.

As a medial process, heritage-language learning is beyond the opposition between active and passive, subject and object, or agent and patient. It does not involve either/or undertakings but both-and-more events. Rather than something one does to someone, they become something one is involved in together. That is, although parents tend to be on the giving side and children (adolescents included) on the receiving end, mediality amounts to more than swapping the roles between adolescents and parents. If we think 'in the middle voice,' we can see that by helping our children learn the heritage language, we, as parents, become not only more knowledgeable but also different persons and that by raising multilingual children, we grow ourselves.

Thus, raising multilingual children and adolescents is, in fact, also parent development. Raising multilingual children and adolescents is a process not only *in* which but also *of* which parents participate. The nuance between the two constructions 'in' and 'of' is compelling. It is a process that affects and changes everybody involved, both parents and adolescents. I would like us to use medial thinking in our interactions with our children.

Being an advocate for multilingualism and heritage-language maintenance

In this book and other places,[20] I have shared with readers my family stories of raising multilingual children by emphasising how parents can provide support for their children in their heritage-language and multilingual development at the family level. However, raising multilingual children is not just a private matter.[21] Depending on parents alone to shoulder the tasks of helping their children maintain their heritage language(s) without societal support is not enough to create an environment in which multilingual children can achieve their highest potential. It takes a village to raise a child,[22] and it also takes a community and society to raise a multilingual child. Many factors in a child's environment, such as the immediate and extended family, neighbourhoods, schools, parents' work places, mass media, community services, political systems and cultural beliefs work together to contribute to a child's development,[23] multilingual development included.

Therefore, it is important for parents to join the efforts for heritage-language preservation in public education and promote democratic access to multilingualism.[24] Moreover, to truly encourage multilingualism and heritage-language maintenance, parents must help to create a society that adopts a collaborative and inclusive approach to multilingual education. Unless heritage language is given a society prestige, such as making its learning financially and socially rewarding,[25] and until heritage language is given the same power and prestige as the mainstream or dominant language, its maintenance is rarely sustained beyond two generations.[26]

There are many ways that you can get involved and become active. Based on your different abilities and talents, you can choose a particular level to start your efforts: from classroom and school to community and government. Even the smallest step can make an important difference for promoting the cause. Together with others, you can help create a more supportive social and academic environment for bilingual and multilingual children, and such action can be particularly helpful to economically underprivileged children who might not otherwise have access to multilingual education.[27] In fact, in some regions and countries, heritage languages have now been revitalised and are taught in state-funded schools as a result of the efforts of concerned citizens.[28]

Challenging Issues of Raising Multilingual Children in Special Circumstances

Before I end the book, I would like to share some thoughts about raising multilingual children in special circumstances.

Single parents

Raising multilingual children is difficult, and raising multilingual children as a single parent is even more challenging. However, as tough as it can be, it is possible as long as parents use the right strategies. Research has shown that single parents are able to promote both languages in the home when they are actively involved with their children's language development.[29] However, what is most challenging if you are a single parent is that your former or deceased spouse spoke to your children in a different language before, and you do not speak that language or have any knowledge about that language. If this is the case, you may want to try the following:

- Send your children to heritage-language school.
- Hire language tutors if you have the financial means.
- Keep in touch with the ex-spouse or his/her family and relatives and use their linguistic resources via communication technology such as Skype, FaceTime and webchat.

The key is to make sure that your children have enough heritage-language input. Box 10.9 illustrates Mina's accounting of her successful story, which may serve as an inspiration for you if you are a single parent who aspires to raise multilingual children.

Monolingual parents

Can monolingual parents raise multilingual children? Yes, it is possible. Although it is tough, it can be achieved if parents provide adequate targeted language (the specific language being learnt) input. Many monolingual expatriates and sojourners have multilingual children because of the linguistic environment in which their children live. Nevertheless, it is extremely challenging for monolingual parents who want to raise monolingual children when multilingual input is available neither at home nor outside. In this case, the first and most important thing you need to ask

Box 10.9 Example of Single-Parent Raising Multilingual Children

My husband left my 10-year-old son and me six years ago. Before he left, he spoke Turkish to my son. I had no knowledge about it. At that point, my son could already converse in Turkish fluently with my ex-husband and his relatives. But he did not know how to read Turkish. With my ex leaving us, my son's Turkish was in jeopardy. I did not do anything first and later I decided that it would be a pity to let my son lose his Turkish. Through a friend, I found a Turkish lady who was willing to meet my son once a week and tutored him for reading and writing. She also had weekly phone chats with my son as well. This was very helpful. I got in touch with my son's aunt who was also happy to take my son for summer vacation for about 3 years consecutively...Now my son is approaching 16, he is well-versed in Turkish, and he can communicate quite well in Turkish both in speaking and writing...I think it is possible for single parents to raise bilingual and multilingual children. But, one needs to work on it...

yourself is why you want to your children to be multilingual and whether or not you have the resources and support your children need to be multilingual. After you make sure that you are clear about your motives, you need to actively plan how to make it possible by using purposeful measures, such as sending your children to language schools, hiring private language tutors, learning the target language together, using media resources and encouraging online exchanges with other native speakers of the target language(s).

No matter what monolingual parents try to do, they must make sure that their children receive sufficient target-language input from proper sources to ensure acquisition. Without adequate target-language input, your children are unlikely to acquire a target language. Even though, as a monolingual parent, you are not able to provide target-language input for your children, your major role in the process of your children's multilingual development is to provide them with support and secure resources. One encouraging thing is that there are many people in the world who became bilingual and multilingual without bilingual or multilingual parents. More importantly, even if your children know a little about other languages, they are better off than if they know nothing.

Children with special needs

Parents of children and teens with cognitive and language disabilities such as Down syndrome, **specific language impairment** (SLI)[30] and autism are often counselled away from multilingualism. The common advice is that multilingualism will hinder these children's language development further and the language input should be restricted to a single language. The common myths are:

- Exposing children and teens with cognitive and language disabilities to more than one language will make their language delay even worse.
- A new language should not be introduced to children or teens with cognitive and language disabilities because they already experience a delay in their first language.
- Parents should stop speaking heritage language(s) to their children with cognitive and language disabilities and should concentrate on one language (often mainstream or school language) development.
- It is too difficult for children and teens with cognitive and language disabilities to handle more than one language.

As a result, when some parents find out that their children have disabilities, they feel they should stop speaking their home language to their children and begin to switch to the mainstream language, even if they are not proficient or comfortable in the mainstream language themselves.

There are several potential problems when parents decide to stop speaking their home language with their children with cognitive and language disabilities:

- If parents try to speak a language with which they are not comfortable, it can jeopardise parent-child connection and interaction. This can lead to great emotional and psychological difficulties for parents and children, as language is strongly linked to emotion, affect and identity.[31]
- Children who speak a home language are at risk for incomplete learning or loss of their home language.[32] This can affect how well children learn a new language, as a strong foundation in the home language benefits new-language learning.
- Children's links to their home culture can be compromised.[33]
- Relationships with these extended family members who do not speak the mainstream language can suffer.[34]

The misconceptions about the multilingual development of children with cognitive and language disabilities are not supported by research. Although these children face language-learning challenges, they are not greater than monolingual children with the same language impairment.[35] It is possible that they can become multilingual. Research suggests that negative effects of multilingualism are not found in children with cognitive and language disabilities. These children generally do not have any extra delay or difficulties when compared to monolingual children with similar language difficulties. Moreover, young children with SLI who are learning more than one language at the same time do not demonstrate any greater difficulties in their two languages as compared to monolingual children with the same disability.[36] Furthermore, those children with SLI who simultaneously develop more than one language demonstrate the same challenges as monolingual children with SLI but do not show any extra burden or difficulties.[37] For example, a study comparing children with Down syndrome being raised in bilingual homes with monolingual children with Down syndrome found that the bilingual children performed at least as well as the monolingual children with Down syndrome.[38] In addition, a study indicates that when the vocabularies of English-Chinese bilingual children with autism and monolingual children with autism were compared, bilingualism did not have a negative effect on the children's language development, as both groups had similar vocabulary scores.[39]

Thus, it is clear that children with cognitive and language impairments can learn more than one language within the limit of their impairment,[40] as long as there is support in their home, school and community. Multilingual experts have made the following suggestions:

Children with cognitive and language impairment and their parents should share a common language so that they can communicate a wide variety of family values, experiences, care and concern.[41]

- Children with specific language impairment living in families where knowing two, or more, languages is useful and important should be given every opportunity to acquire two languages.[42]
- Bilingual children need continuous and regular exposure to both languages to ensure their complete acquisition.[43]

- Special consideration should be given to home languages. It is advisable to provide more exposure to home languages than majority languages in the home to offset the lack of exposure to these languages in the community.[44]
- The major goal of therapy for young bilingual children with cognitive and language impairment should be helping to hone their skills in their home language.[45]

Thus, there are many benefits for parents in communicating with their children with cognitive and language disabilities in their home language.[46]

Multilingual development after children leave home

There is almost no literature currently available regarding the role of parents in their children's multilingual development after their children leave home for college and the workforce. Traditionally, parenting advice books stop after the teen years. However, as any parent knows, parents are always parents; parenting does not stop when our children leave our homes. Although we may lose 'control' of what we can do with our children, we are always there to help them. Since the adolescent years in modern societies have extended beyond the traditional teenager years, parents continue to assume the responsibilities of supporting their children after they leave home. Thus, parents can take advantage of their children's further heritage-language development.

In our experiences with Léandre, we found that conversations via communicative technologies, such as texting, FaceTime and e-mails, have helped him continue with his heritage-language development. Although the interaction does not happen on daily basis, the weekly interactions are still quite effective. If the first 18 years he spent with us were spent building the foundation for his heritage-language development, his weekly interactions with us while in college will allow him to maintain and continue with his heritage-language development.

Thus, parents can make plans as to how to help their children further develop their heritage language(s) by doing the following:

- Plan what you want to teach or expose your children to when they no longer live with you on a regular basis. I found that planning is still helpful. For example, Léandre still makes mistakes in using Chinese measurement words (classifiers) when I have virtual conversations with him. Therefore, in my FaceTime conversations with him, I purposefully repeated those measurement words. For him, it was just a conversation. For me, a language lesson was in session according to my plan to enrich his Chinese measurement word vocabulary and usage.
- Encourage heritage-language literacy development via e-mails and texting. Living apart from children can be an opportunity for them to develop their reading and writing skills in their heritage languages. Philippe has been doing that with our children. The written exchanges between the boys and Philippe have greatly enhanced the children's French literacy competence.

Taken together, it is indeed possible for parents to continue to help their children with their heritage-language development. As one would say, a parent's job never ends.

Concluding Remarks

In this book, I have shared my family's experience in raising multilingual children and teens in particular. It is important to stress that our way is not the only way, but it is one way that has worked for us. Heritage-language development, including multilingual development, is a complex process. There are different ways to achieve multilingualism.[47] As shown in this book, multilingual development and heritage-language learning are not easy endeavours; there are many challenges, frustrations and even problems, such as those outlined in Chapter 9. However, there is also much excitement and joy involved in raising multilingual children. Through reflecting on my children's multilingual development journey, I have realised that our efforts and frustration, and our children's struggles, have all been worthwhile considering the advantages that they have gained in the process. I hope that this book has helped you understand the reality of multilingual childrearing and encouraged you to move forward with confidence. I look forward to sharing Léandre and Dominique's continued multilingual development when they leave home for college and the workplace in my next book, tentatively titled *Continuing with Three Languages: Young Adulthood*. I will now leave you with an encouraging note: try your best and enjoy your children and the multilingual childrearing process.

I wish you all the best in your endeavours to bring up multilingual children!

Summary of Key Points in Chapter 10

This chapter presents several take-away messages for parents.

- Support your children's development and make it a priority in your interactions with them.
- Set goals for your teens' heritage-language development:
    - Set short-term and long-term goals.
    - Set achievable goals.
    - Set goals together with your teens.
    - Differentiate between heritage-language development goals: social vs. literacy.
    - Modify goals based on circumstances.
    - Focus on your own family situation .
- Communicate parental differences with your teens.
- Increase conversation length by providing situational appropriate heritage-language input.
- Use heritage language consistently in communication.
- Maximise heritage-language exposure via a variety of resources, for example:

- - Input from grandparents and relatives.
  - Input from media and technology.
  - Input from travelling to heritage-language-speaking countries and regions.
- Make one language solid while developing all other languages.
- Focus on communication when developing heritage language(s).
- Incorporate paralanguage learning in heritage-language learning.
- Be mindful of individual learning differences.
- Access heritage-language achievements in your children's particular context rather than using standardised tests.
- Reflect on parental practices.
- Think medially and treat multilingual development as a dynamic process of *both* and *more* (i.e. both parents and adolescents contribute to the multilingual development process, and adolescents elaborate, construct, reconstruct and re-create their heritage language in their language-learning environment) rather than a process of *either/or* (i.e. either parents alone or adolescents alone determine multilingual development).
- Be an advocate for multilingualism.
- It is also possible for single parents, monolingual parents and parents with children with cognitive and language disabilities to raise multilingual children, as long as adequate strategies and support are provided.
- Furthermore, it is also possible for parents to continue to help their children's heritage-language and multilingual development after their children leave home.
- Although the path to multilingualism may be challenging, it is a worthwhile effort when the advantages are weighed.

Recommended Readings

Baker, C. (2014) *A Parents' and Teachers' Guide to Bilingualism* (4th edn). Bristol: Multilingual Matters.
Grosjean, F. (2012) *Bilingual Life and Reality*. Cambridge, MA: Harvard University Press.
Scott, C. and Windsor, J. (2000) General language performance measures in spoken and written narrative and expository discourse of school-age children with language learning disabilities. *Journal of Speech, Language, and Hearing Research* 43, 324–39.

Notes and References

[1] FaceTime is a video call on an Apple cell phone.
[2] Workshop discussion excerpts (2 November 2012).
[3] Workshop discussion excerpts (2 November 2012).
[4] E-mail communication (12 May 2014).
[5] Wang, X.-L. (2011) *Learning to Read and Write in the Multilingual Family*. Bristol: Multilingual Matters.
[6] PSAT is the test that helps students to practice for the SAT exam.
[7] Data were calculated based on randomly sampled 24-hour videos between the ages of 15 and 16.
[8] Brown, C.L. (2011) Maintaining Heritage Language Perspectives of Korean Parents. *Multicultural Education* 19 (1), 31–37.

[9] Park, E. (2006) Grandparents, grandchildren, and heritage language use in Korean. In K. Kondo-Brown (ed.) *Heritage Language Development: Focus on East Asian Immigrants* (pp. 57–85). Amsterdam: John Benjamins Publishing Company.

[10] Close, R. (2004) Television and language development in the early years: A review of the literature. National Literacy Trust, retrieved from http://www.literacytrust.org.uk/assets/0000/0429/TV_early_years_2004.pdf

[11] Wang, X.-L. (2008) *Growing Up With Three Languages: Birth to Eleven*. Bristol: Multilingual Matters.

[12] Wang, X.-L. and Bernas, R. (2014) *People Without Borders: Becoming Members of Global Communities*. New York, NY: Untested Ideas Research Center.

[13] Workshop discussion excerpts (22 February 2013).

[14] Wang, X.-L. and Bernas, R. (2014) *People Without Borders: Becoming Members of Global Communities*. New York, NY: Untested Ideas Research Center.

[15] Wang, X.-L. (2008) *Growing Up With Three Languages: Birth to Eleven*. Bristol: Multilingual Matters.

[16] Wang, X.-L. (2008) Growing Up With Three Languages: Bir*th to Eleven*. Bristol: Multilingual Matters.

[17] Eberhard, P. (2004) *The Middle Voice in Gadamer's Hermeneutics: A Basic Interpretation With Some Theological Implications*. Tübingen, Germany: Mohr Siebeck.

Eberhard, P. and Wang, X.-L. (2010). A middle-voiced understanding of diversity. *The International Journal of Diversity* 10 (4), 295–305.

[18] Benveniste, E. (1971) *Problems in General Linguistics* (pp. 148–149). University of Miami Press.

[19] Romanine, S. (1989) The role of children in linguistic change. In I.E. Breivik and E.H. Jahr (eds) *Language Change. Contributions to the Study of Its Causes*. Berlin: Mouton de Gruyter.

[20] Wang, X.-L. (2008) *Growing Up With Three Languages*: Birth to Eleven. Bristol: Multilingual Matters.

Wang, X.-L. (2011) *Learning to Read and Write in the Multilingual Family*. Bristol: Multilingual Matters.

Wang, X.-L. (2014–2015) Multilingual family welfare. In T.K. Bhatia and W.C. Ritchie (eds) *The Handbook of Bilingualism and Multilingualism*. Malden, MA: Wiley-Blackwell Publishing.

Wang, X.-L. (2011) Teaching children to read and write in more than one orthography: Tips for parents. *Multilingual Living*, September 26, 2011 Issue.

Wang, X.-L. (2010) Acquiring Chinese simultaneously with other languages: Effective home strategies. In J. Cai, J. Cen, and C. Wang (eds) *Teaching and Learning Chinese: Issues and Perspectives* (pp. 175–96). Charlotte, NC: Information Age Publishing.

Wang, X.-L. (2009) Ensuring sustained trilingual development through motivation. *The Bilingual Family Newsletter* 26 (1), 1–7.

Wang, X.-L. (2009). Making communication the priority of multilingual learning. *Multilingual Living Magazine*.

[21] Piller, I. (2005) Book review of *Language Strategies for Bilingual Families: The One-Parent-One-Language Approach* by Suzanne Barron-Hauwaret. Clevedon: Multilingual Matters (2004). *The International Journal of Bilingual Education and Bilingualism* 8 (6), 614–17.

[22] An African proverb.

[23] Bronfenbrenner, U. (1979) *The Ecology of Human Development: Experiments by Nature and Design*. Cambridge, MA: Harvard University Press.

Bronfenbrenner, U. (2005) *Making Human Beings Human: Bioecological Perspectives on Human Development*. Thousand Oaks, CA: Sage.

[24] Piller, I. (2005) Book review of *Language Strategies For Bilingual Families: The One-Parent-One-Language Approach* by Suzanne Barron-Hauwaret. Clevedon: Multilingual Matters (2004). *The International Journal of Bilingual Education and Bilingualism* 8 (6), 614–17.

25 Sakamoto, M. (2006) Balancing L1 maintenance and L2 Learning: Experiential narrative of Japanese immigrant families in Canada (pp. 34–56). In K. Kondo-Brown (ed.) *Heritage Language Development: Focus on East Asian Immigrants*. Amsterdam: John Benjamins Publishing Company

26 Sakamoto, M. (2006) Balancing L1 maintenance and L2 Learning: Experiential narrative of Japanese immigrant families in Canada (pp. 34–56). In K. Kondo-Brown (ed.) *Heritage Language Development: Focus on East Asian Immigrants*. Amsterdam: John Benjamins Publishing Company

27 Wang, X.-L. (2008) *Growing Up With Three Languages: Birth to Eleven*. Bristol: Multilingual Matters.

28 Harrison, B. (1998) The development of an indigenous language immersion school. *Bilingual Research Journal* 22, 297–316.

29 Obied, V.M. (2010) Can one-parent families or divorced families produce two-language children? An investigation into how Portuguese-English bilingual children acquire biliteracy within diverse family structures. *Pedagogy, Culture and Society* 18 (2), 227–43.

30 Children and teens with specific language impairments often have no other developmental difficulties (for example, motor skills, cognitive/thinking skills and social skills are all developing normally) except language-related difficulties.

31 De Houwer, A. (1999) Two or more languages in early childhood: Some general points and practical recommendations. Centre for Applied Linguistics. Available online at: http://www.cal.org/resources/digest/earlychild.html

32 Paradis, J. (2010) The interface between bilingual development and specific language impairment. *Applied Psycholinguistics* 31, 227–52.

33 Wong-Fillmore, L. (1991) When learning a second language means losing the first. *Early Childhood Research Quarterly* 6, 232–346.

34 Wong-Fillmore, L. (1991) When learning a second language means losing the first. *Early Childhood Research Quarterly* 6, 232–346.

35 Paradis, J., Genesee, F. and Crago, M. (2011) *Dual Language Development and Disorders: A Handbook on Bilingualism and Second Language Learning*. Baltimore, MD: Paul H. Brookes Publishing Co.
Hambly, C. and Fombonne, E. (2011, September 22) The impact of bilingual environments on language development in children with autism spectrum disorders. *Journal of Autism and Developmental Disorders*. [E-publication ahead of print].

36 Paradis, J. (2010) The interface between bilingual development and specific language impairment. *Applied Psycholinguistics* 31, 227–52.

37 Paradis, J., Crago, M., Genesee, F. and Rice, M. (2003) Bilingual children with specific language impairment: How do they compare with their monolingual peers? *Journal of Speech, Language, and Hearing Research* 46, 1–15.
Gutierrez-Clellen, V., Simon-Cereijido, G. and Wagner, C. (2008) Bilingual children with language impairment: A comparison with monolinguals and second language learners. *Applied Linguistics* 29, 3–20.

38 Kay-Raining Bird, E., Cleave, P., Trudeau, N., Thordardottir, E., Sutton, A. and Thorpe, A. (2005) The language abilities of bilingual children with Down Syndrome. *American Journal of Speech-Language Pathology* 14, 187–99.

39 Petersen, J., Marinova-Todd, S.H. and Mirenda, P. (2011) An exploratory study of lexical skills in bilingual children with Autism Spectrum Disorder. *Journal of Autism and Developmental Disorders* DOI: 10.1007/s10803-011-1366-y.

40 Genesee, F. (2009) Early childhood bilingualism: Perils and possibilities. *Journal of Applied Research in Learning 2 (Special Issue)* 2, 1–21.

41 Kohnert, K., Yim, D., Nett, K., Kan, P.F. and Duran, L. (2005) Intervention with linguistically diverse preschool children: A focus on developing home languages(s). *Language, Speech and Hearing Services in Schools* 36, 251–63.

42 Genesee, F. (2009) Early childhood bilingualism: Perils and possibilities. *Journal of Applied Research in Learning 2 (Special Issue)* 2, 1–21.

43 Genesee, F. (2009) Early childhood bilingualism: Perils and possibilities. *Journal of Applied Research in Learning 2 (Special Issue)* 2, 1–21.
44 Genesee, F. (2009) Early childhood bilingualism: Perils and possibilities. *Journal of Applied Research in Learning 2 (Special Issue)* 2, 1–21.
45 Kohnert, K., Yim, D., Nett, K., Kan, P.F. and Duran, L. (2005) Intervention with linguistically diverse preschool children: A focus on developing home languages(s). *Language, Speech and Hearing Services in Schools* 36, 251–63.
46 De Houwer, A. (1999) Two or more languages in early childhood: Some general points and practical recommendations. Centre for Applied Linguistics. Available online at:http://www.cal.org/resources/digest/earlychild.html
Wong-Fillmore, L. (1991) When learning a second language means losing the first. *Early Childhood Research Quarterly* 6, 232–346.
Kohnert, K., Yim, D., Nett, K., Kan, P.F. and Duran, L. (2005) Intervention with linguistically diverse preschool children: A focus on developing home languages(s). *Language, Speech and Hearing Services in Schools* 36, 251–63.
47 Thomas, C. (2012) *Growing Up With Languages: Reflection on Multilingual Children*. Bristol: Multilingual Matters.

Appendix: Examples of Standardised Language Assessments

- **CDIs**
  - (MacArthur-Bates Communicative Developmental Inventories) asks parents to check off words their child says or signs, including vocabulary relating to things in the home, people, action words, description words, pronouns, prepositions, question words, sentences and grammar.
- **CELF-3**
  - (Clinical Evaluation of Language Fundamentals – Third Edition) measures abilities in word meanings, word and sentence structure, recall and retrieval of spoken language.
- **FLIT**
  - (Figurative Language Interpretation Test) is a multiple-choice, standardised test consisting of two equivalent 50-item forms that can be used to pre- and post-test students' figurative language progress. It can be administered in groups or individually during a regular 50-minute class period.
- **GMRT**
  - (Gates-MacGinitie Reading Test) assesses reading achievement.
- **LAB-R**
  - (Language Assessment Battery – Revised) assesses reading, writing, listening, comprehension and speaking in English and Spanish.
- **LAC-R**
  - (Lindamood Auditory Conceptualisation Test – Revised) assesses the ability to perceive and conceptualise sound units and the changes in their number and relationship in spoken syllables and words.
- **MLAT**
  - Measures metalinguistic awareness.

- **NAP**
  - (Narrative Assessment Protocol) measures and monitors preschool children's use of semantic and syntactic forms by using a wordless picture book, *Frog, Where Are You?* by Mercer Mayer. It is a cost-effective way to measure young children's narrative microstructure.
- **OWLS**
  - (Oral and Written Language Scales) measures listening, comprehension, oral expression and written expression.
- **PPVT-III**
  - (Peabody Picture Vocabulary Test – Third Edition) measures receptive vocabulary achievement and verbal ability.
- **SALT**
  - (Systematic Analysis of Language Transcripts) is a language-sampling tool that measures expressive language production such as utterance formulation, word finding, semantics and pragmatics.
- **TOPA**
  - (Test of Phonological Awareness) measures the ability to isolate individual phonemes in spoken words.
- **TWS**
  - (Test of Written Spelling) measures spelling ability.
- **WMLS-R**
  - (Woodcock-Muñoz Language Survey – Revised) measures cognitive-academic language proficiencies.
- **WLPB-R**
  - (The Woodcock Language Proficiency Battery – Revised) measures bilingual language proficiency.
- **WRAML**
  - (Wide Range Assessment of Memory and Learning) assesses verbal and visual memory skills in situations involving both immediate recall and acquisition of new information.

For more information about standardised language assessment, go to http://www.asha.org/assessments.aspx, which was put together by the American Speech-Language-Hearing Association.

Glossary

Abstract words: words that do not have concrete meanings (e.g. *myth* and *emancipation*).

Active planning: the process of planning for children's heritage-language learning through serious and constant communications between parents.

Adolescence: a transitional period from middle childhood to adulthood.

Adolescent egocentrism: an adolescent belief that they are the centre of attention and that others are highly attentive to their behaviour and appearance.

Adverbial conjuncts: a type of adverbial adjunct that is used to join two independent clauses to make a compound sentence (e.g. *moreover, however, accordingly, hence, similarly, consequently, therefore* and *furthermore*).

Adverbial disjuncts: a type of adverbial adjunct that is used to comment on a speaker's or writer's attitude towards, or descriptive statement of, the propositional content of the sentence (e.g. *in my opinion, to be honest, frankly* and *perhaps*).

Affective: emotion relating to moods, feelings, and attitudes

Affective filters: a complex of negative emotional and motivational factors (such as anxiety, self-consciousness, boredom, annoyance and alienation) that may interfere with language learning.

Agency: the capacity of individuals to act independently and to make their own free choices.

Alphasyllabary: a segmental writing system in which consonant–vowel sequences are written as a unit: Each unit is based on a consonant letter and vowel notation is secondary, such as such as the Korean *hangul*.

Amalgamation: a combination of forward and backward transfer.

Appositive: a noun, a noun phrase or a noun clause that is placed next to another noun to remake it or to describe it in another way.

Aptitude: mental ability

Articles: words that are used with nouns to indicate the types of references being made by the nouns, such as *a* or *the* in English.

Autobiographical memory: the ability to recall episodes, experiences and events in an individual's life.

Backward transfer: use of heritage-language narrative strategy to process mainstream language.

Clausal density: the average number of clauses (main and subordinate clauses) per T-unit.

Cognates: words in different languages that share the same etymology; they tend to have similar form and meaning but not always pronunciation (e.g. *activate* in English and *activer* in French).

Cognition: intellectual ability.

Common underlying proficiencies: proficiency in one language can be transferred to another one.

Communication block: to stop communicating because of lack of vocabulary or other skills needed for communication.

Compounding morphemes: combinations of two or more root words that generate new meanings (e.g. *classroom*).

Compound words: words that are formed by adding two or more words together (e.g. *grapefruit* and *schoolteacher*).

Contextual abstraction: using context clues to determine the meaning of unfamiliar words.

Contrasting phoneme: words that have one different phonological element, such as *bad-bed*; *let-lit*; *pan-pen*; *pat-bat*; *pin-bin*; and *rot-lot*.

Conversational cooperative strategies: people cooperate to achieve mutual conversation.

Creole: originating from a mixture of two or more languages, creole is developed from a pidgin (a simplified version of a language that develops as a means of communication between two or more groups that do not have a language in common). Creoles differ from pidgins because creoles have been nativised by children as their primary language, with the result that they have features of natural languages that are normally missing from pidgins, which are not anyone's first language.

Critical literacy: the ability to read beyond lines by critiquing texts in different formats, challenging the status quo and questioning authorities.

The CQSP strategy (clarification, questioning, summarisation and prediction): a strategy used for processing both narrative and expository texts.

Crosslinguistic synonyms: the same thing referred to in more than one way in different languages, such as *cup*, *tasse* and 杯子 in English, French and Chinese.

Cultural templates: cultural models for behaving in a certain way.

Deductive teaching: explaining rules first and following this with exercises.

Dental sibilants: sounds made with a hissing effect.

Dependent clause: subordinate clauses or nonclausal structures that are attached to it or embedded within it.

Derivational morphology or derivational words: a single root word or root form can generate a large number of derived forms by having a prefix or a suffix added to it (e.g. adding *–ness* to *slow* becomes *slowness*).

Direct teaching: directly teaching the meaning of words.

Direction of transfer: the transfer from a stronger language to a less strong language versus from the less strong language to a stronger language.

Discourse with a big D: highlights different cultural, social and linguistic groups' practices in using language based on their beliefs and values.

Discussion-based instruction (DBI): a reading comprehension strategy that focuses on using dialogues to explore ideas and develop understanding of different types of texts.

Distributed characteristic of multilingual word learning: Multilingual children may have vocabulary discrepancies in different languages (i.e. they may have more words in one language and less words in another language)

Emblems: conventional gestures.

Emotion-laden words: words that do not refer to emotions directly but instead express emotion (such as *loser*) or elicit emotions from the interlocutors (such as *malignancy*); these are represented, processed and recalled differently from concrete words (e.g. *cup* and *chair*).

Emotion words: words that directly refer to particular affective states (such as *scared* and *anxious*) or processes (such as *worry*).

Emotional intelligence: the ability to identify and manage one's own emotions and the emotions of others.

EmPOWER method: a method that encourage learners to proceed by first reading the instructions carefully (E), then making a plan that is based on a communicative purpose that will help them get started (MP), organising their ideas graphically using templates specific to the intended genre (O), working from the plan to represent the idea with written language (W) and evaluating and reworking the draft with the purpose and audience in mind (ER).

Ethnotheories: values and practices of a culture.

Explanation reading training (ERT): using explicit and direct instruction to show the purpose and function of different strategies.

Expository text: text to explain and inform.

Expressive lexicon: vocabulary that one can use in communication.

Extensive reading: an approach that requires that a reader read quickly and in large quantities.

Factive verbs: verbs that presuppose the truth (e.g. *notice* and *see*).

False cognates: words in different languages that have overlapping orthographic (spelling) or phonological (sound) properties but have little or no semantic (meaning) overlap.

False friends (see **false cognates**)

Fan fiction: a text written by fans of an original work in which they add their own version of creativity and twist to the original piece.

Fast-mapping cognitive ability: the mental process whereby a new concept is learnt based only on a single or limited exposure to given information.

Figurative language: language is used in nonliteral and abstract ways.

First language: language that is acquired from birth.

Fixed mindset: regarding success or failure based on innate ability.

Formal operational thought: taking logical inferences merely through verbal representations.

Forward transfer: using mainstream-language narrative strategies to process the heritage-language narrative.

Fossilisation: a language phenomenon in which a language learner enters into a plateau and does not make any progress. Because it is difficult to determine when the language-learning process has ceased, this phenomenon is now often referred to as **stabilisation.**

Frontal lobe: responsible for judgement and decision making.

Genderlect: a particular speech or conversation style used by a particular gender.

Growth mindset: regarding one's success and failure based on one's effort.

Growth spurts: a rapid increase in height and sometimes also in weight.

Heteroglossia: the presence of two or more voices within a text.

Heterophones: words that are spelt the same but have different pronunciations and meanings, such as *row* (propel with oars) and *row* (argument).

Heteronyms (see **heterophones**)

High point analysis (HPA): measurement of the narrative macrostructure or the story grammar.

Higher functional load: the importance of a phoneme in the phonemic inventory of a language.

Homographs: words that are spelt the same and may sound alike (e.g. *row a boat* vs. *row of homes*) or they may sound different from each other (e.g. *record player* vs. *record a speech*).

Homophones: words that sound alike and may be spelt alike or differently but have different meanings, such as *bear* (animal) and *bear* (tolerate) and *mean* (unkind) and *mean* (average).

Honorifics: linguistic features that mark relative social status and index social difference.

Hypertext: also referred to as digital text, multimedia text, electronic text, web text, the internet-based system of communication or new literacies. These texts are characterised by multisequential text patterns, which present readers with an array of information options online. They are also highly interactive, allowing readers to make choices based on personal interest or purpose. In hypertext reading, the reader's purpose and choices, rather than the author's, determine the reading sequence, whereas in conventional text reading, the author determines the reading sequence.

Imperfect subjunctive: the French imperfect subjunctive is a literary verb form used in formal writing.

Incidental exposure: learning the new meaning of words in context by looking for cues and drawing from background knowledge.

Independent clause: main clause.

Indirect feedback: a process that results from error/contrastive analysis on the part of the parent, who hints at the type of error the child may have made but does not provide explicit instruction.

Inductive teaching: rules are inferred in the examples.

Inference or inferencing: the ability to draw conclusions by connecting related information that may be implicit.

Inflectional morphemes: word endings that indicate case, verb tense, gender or syntax in an alphabetic language.

Intensive reading: slow and careful reading.

Intentional conversation: conversation planned by the parent to teach a heritage language.

Interlanguage: new language learners' own version of a target language.

Intersentential: between-sentence connective words (e.g. *furthermore, consequently, however, moreover* and *rather*).

Intrasentential: within-sentence words (e.g. *although, but, since, unless, whenever*).

K-W-L chart: a chart that is used to help children build background knowledge. K stands for what they already know before the reading, W stands for what they want to know about the reading, and L stands for what they have learnt after the reading.

Lexias: specific blocks of text.

Lexical complexity: use of multisyllabic words.

Lexical density: use of a variety of lexical items, such as nouns, verbs, adjectives and adverbs.

Lexical diversity: use of different types of words.

Lexical inferencing: a strategy that teaches children how to search for key words that allow them to understand the text better and the kinds of inferences that can be made from these words.

Lexicon: words.

Limbic system: responsible for emotions, reward-seeking, novelty, risk-taking and sensation-seeking behaviours.

Literate lexicon: words used in more advanced reading materials, such as abstract nouns (*freedom, challenge*), mental state verbs (*assume, explain*) and derivatives (*relationship, respectful*).

Loan blending: borrowing words from another language for communication.

Marked: difficult features in a language.

Marked sounds: difficult sounds in a language.

Masking phenomenon: language learners either do not know or only have partial knowledge about the vocabulary, but they do not reveal their lack of knowledge.

Maze: false start, hesitation, repetition or a reformulation of a sentence.

Measurement words (or classifiers): words used along with numerals to define the quantity of a given object (such as one 篇 essay) in Chinese.

Mental lexicon: mental storage of words that can be activated by a language user.

Metacognitive conversations: in-depth, reflective conversations in which both parents and teens become aware of their own thinking.

Metalinguistic ability: awareness of the rules and features of a language.

Metalinguistic feedback (see **indirect feedback**)

Metalinguistic reflection: reflecting and commenting on language-related issues.

Minimal pair (see **contrasting phoneme**)

MLU (mean length of utterance): the average number of words used in utterances.

Morphemes: the smallest meaningful unit, such as *s* in *works*.

Morphological: word structure.

Morphological analysis: analysis of the components of words and use that information to infer meaning of the entire word; e.g. to learn the word *talkativeness* by analysing the parts *talkative-* and *–ness*.

Morphological awareness: the ability to reflect upon and manipulate morphemes (the smallest phonological unit that carries meaning) and to use word formation rules to construct and understand morphologically complex words.

Multilingual bootstrapping hypothesis: a theory according to which the more advanced language system will boost the development of the less advanced one.

Multimodality: the modes of representation beyond print, including such things as the visual, auditory, gestural and kinesthetic.

Multipass approach: a method that is useful to support expository-text comprehension. This approach consists of three passes: survey, size-up and sort-out. In the survey pass, children look for information about the main ideas and organisation by reading the text title and introduction, reviewing the relationship to adjunct paragraphs, reading subtitles, looking at illustrations and captions, reading summary paragraphs and paraphrasing the information. In the size-up pass, children skim the text to seek specific information for answering questions at the end of chapter or questions they have formulated in their minds. In the sort-out pass, children test themselves by reading each question at the chapter's end and checking off those they can answer immediately. If they cannot answer the questions easily, they return to the text section where the answers might be found and read until they can answer the questions.

Multisensory structured learning (MSL) approach: a method that utilises several sensory channels simultaneously and synthesises stimuli coming from these channels.

Narrative assessment protocol (NAP): measurement of the narrative microstructure.

Narrative scoring scheme (NSS): measurements of narrative macrostructure and evaluation of more advanced elements of the narrative quality beyond story grammar such as literal language and lexical, conjunctive and referential cohesive devices, as well as metacognitive and metalinguistic verbs.

Narrative texts: texts that describe things.

Nonfactive verbs: verbs that express uncertainty about the truth (e.g. *guess* and *believe*).

Nonword repetition (NWR): NWR task that requires repeating novel phonological forms such as *woogalamic* or *noitauf*. It mimics one of the most basic and important language-learning mechanisms: immediate repetition of unfamiliar words.

Nonwords: in language studies, researchers often use nonwords (or nonsense words) to test children and adolescents' understanding of the morphological rules.

Novel conceptual combination: individuals who are exposed to more than one language and culture tend to have more than one set of cultural tools to interpret the world. These tools can foster competent behaviours in multiple cultures. For instance, an individual who has extensive knowledge and experiences in cultures A and B may be able to retrieve ideas from cultures A and B spontaneously and place them in juxtaposition and, through creative insights, integrate the two into a novel idea.

One-parent-one-language (OPOL): each parent speaks his or her own heritage language to the children.

Online affinity spaces: virtual space where informal learning takes place.

Online production: immediate and on-the-spot communication.

Opaque compounds: when the meaning of the compound is not closely related to one or both constituent morphemes, such as *jailbird*.

Orthographic structure knowledge: knowledge that semantic and phonetic radicals are located in specific places in Chinese characters.

Orthographic systems: writing systems.

Overextension: extending the meaning of a word.

Paralanguage: communication that is other than spoken, such as gestures, kinesics (body language), facial expressions, tone/voice use, proxemics (e.g. the physical distance between people), time concept and space arrangement.

Persuasive writing: writing used to convince others.

Phonemes: the smallest meaningful sound unit of a language.

Phonetic inventory: all the sounds in a language.

Phonological: sound system.

Phonological translation: the ability to hear a word in one language and to render that word – not its meaning but its phonological form – in the other language.

Phonotactic constraints: rules governing possible sound sequence.

Phonotactic knowledge: knowledge of the constraints in the sequencing of sounds and the phonological rules.

Pinyin: the phonetic system for transcribing the pronunciations of Chinese characters into the Latin alphabet.

Polysemous words: words that have multiple meanings.

Possessive pronouns: nouns that demonstrate ownership, such as *mine* and *ours* in English.

Poststructuralist view: identity may include notions of the self as imposed, assumed or negotiated.

Pragmalinguistic failure: when the pragmatics used by a speaker are systematically different from those of native speakers of the heritage language or when speech-act strategies are inappropriately transferred from the mainstream language to the heritage language.

Pragmatics: how language is used in a proper social context.

Predictive inferences: the strategy that helps language learners to focus on sentence meaning by searching for key words surrounding covered sentences.

Prosody: stress, intonation, pitch, rate and rhythm.

Puberty: biological changes such as sexual maturity.

Reading apprenticeship model: a teaching method for adolescent literacy development, which is based on an understanding of literacy as a social, cultural and cognitive activity, mediated by settings, tasks, purposes and other social and linguistic factors.

Receptive lexicon: vocabulary that one can understand but not necessarily use in communication.

Reflective positioning: our own attempts at self-representation.

Registers: communication style in a particular context.

Relative clauses: clauses that start with relative pronouns such as *that*, *which* and *who*.

Retroflex sounds: sounds that are articulated with the tip of the tongue curled upwards and back against or near the juncture of the hard and soft palates.

Schemata: a mental framework or concept that helps organise and interpret information.

Script inferencing: inferencing from written texts.

Selective attention: when more than one language coexists, one of the languages must be constantly inhibited to prevent ongoing intrusion.

Self-efficacy: the belief about one's ability to do things.

Self-regulation: a form of self-control or self-monitoring in the learning process, which consists of strategies such as setting standards and goals for oneself and engaging in self- motivated learning.

Shared book reading: reading together with children and talking about the reading.

Social language: the language used in everyday communication.

Sociopragmatic failure: communicative failure in appropriate social and cultural contexts.

Specific language impairment (SLI): language impairment that delays the mastery of language skills in children who have no hearing loss or other developmental delays.

Speech act: a type of communication function in which speakers apologise, greet, request, promise, congratulate, complain, invite, compliment or refuse.

Spillover: direct transfer of mood, affect or behaviour from one setting to another.

Stabilisation (see **fossilisation**)

Story grammar: the elements of a story, such as an introduction, events, a resolution and a coda.

Story recounting: a scaffolding process in which parents and adolescents coconstruct stories/narratives.

Strategy-based instruction (SBI): a method that teaches reading comprehension by focusing explicitly on teaching strategies to aid comprehension.

Structure strategy training (SST): a method that teaches language learners how to use paragraphing and signalling cues to figure out the overall organisation of the information they are reading.

Subordination index (see **clausal density**)

Syncretic language use or communication: language learners draw multiple resources from their respective languages and cultures and form their nuanced and creative way of communication.

Syncretic literacy: multilinguals use creative forms of literacy practices and transform their literacy experiences by blending their existing pool of languages and cultures.

Syntax or syntactic: word order or sentence.

Terminable unit (T-unit): consists of one main clause plus any subordinate clause that is attached to or embedded in it.

Theme comprehension strategy: the ability to derive a more general message from a passage of text to help reading comprehension.

Theory of mind: the ability to read others' minds.

Thinking aloud: verbalising one's thinking.

Tier-one words: the basic and frequent words that rarely require purposeful instruction because they are embedded in the everyday environment (e.g. *clock* and *walk*).

Tier-three words: words that are not frequently used or are limited to a specific domain and are quite technical and sophisticated (e.g. *isotope* and *lathe*).

Tier-two words: words that appear frequently (e.g. *coincidence, absurd, industrious* and *fortunate*).

Translanguaging: multilingual speakers' shuttling between their different languages for communication purposes.

Transparent compounds: Compounds in which the meaning of the compound is predictable from the meaning of the constituent morphemes, such as *birthday*.

Unified competition theory: according to which multilinguals are sensitive to phonological properties that are common across languages.

Utterances: units of thoughts and ideas.

Vowel-shifting rules: the rules that account for vowel alternation, such as *divine-divinity, sane-sanity* and *extreme-extremity*.

Weakeners: discourse markers that are also called 'intensifier' or 'hedge' words, such as *sort of* and *I think*.

Wh-question generation: a strategy that encourages language learners to generate their own queries about the text by asking questions (*who, where, when* and *why*).

Wordle (www.wordle.net): a website for generating **word clouds** (a cluster of words) from text that you provide; the clouds show words that appear more frequently in that text.

Author Index

Abbott, R., A., 131
Adams, G.R., 52
Aldrich, N.J., 210
Alegria, J., 131
Alejandra, C.A., 22
Alfieri, L., 210
Almeida, D.M., 260
Altarriba, J., 104
Amato, P.R., 239
Anderson, R.C., 129, 131, 209
Andersson, S., 129, 131, 209
Arafeh, S., 212
Archibald, L.M.D., 73
Ashburner, J., 22
Attardo, S., 54
August, D., 71
Aviezer, O., 260

Baba, J., 166
Bailey, A.L., 213
Baker, C., 4, 11, 23, 166, 261, 286
Baker, W.J., 103, 129
Bamberg, M., 165
Barber, B.K., 262
Barr, R., 104
Barron-Hauwert, S., 259
Basboll, H., 54
Basnight-Brown, D.M., 104
Bavin, E.L., 210
Bayley, R., 165
Beck, I.L., 103
Bedore, L.M., 73
Behnke, A., 258
Bell, K.L., 262
Bellugi, U., 165
Benko, S., 61, 212
Bereiter, C., 211
Berg, C.A., 260
Berk, L.E., 53
Berman, R.A., 130
Bernas, R., 240, 273, 287
Berninger, V., W., 131

Berwing, B., 103
Berzonsky, M.D., 52
Beveridge, R.M., 260
Bhatia, T.K., 23
Bialystok, E., 3, 22, 23, 24, 54, 211, 261
Biemiller, A., 103
Biesecker, G., 260
Bingham, G.E., 167
Biringen, Z., 260
Black, M.M., 239
Blackledge, A., 158, 166, 210, 238
Blaye, A., 23
Bleses, D., 54
Block, J.H., 259
Blum-Kulka, S., 260
Bohman, T.M., 73
Boon Chung, O., 259
Boyce, L., 261
Boyd, F.B., 210
Brady-Smith, C., 261
Breivik, I.E., 287
Bretherton, I., 260
Bromley, K., 104
Bronfenbrenner, U., 287
Bronte-Tinkew, J., 239
Brooks-Gunn, J., 261
Brooks, P.J., 210
Brown, C.L., 286
Brown, H.D., 151, 165, 166, 167, 213
Brown, S., 54, 114, 262
Bruck, M., 131
Buchanan, A., 239
Burt, R.S., 258
Byers-Heinlein, K., 71

Cabrera, N., 239
Cai, J., 287
Caldas, S.J., 22
Cambournes, B., 213
Caravolas, M., 54
Caraway, T.H., 167
Carlisle, J., 129

Carlo, M.S., 211
Carrano, J., 239
Casanave, C.P., 211
Castano, E., 213
Cazden, C.B., 105
Cenoz, J., 23, 166
Chandler, A.L., 260
Chao, R.K., 261
Chaudhuri, J.H., 260
Chen, X., 131, 209
Cheng, B., 239
Cheng, C., 130
Chiu, C.-Y., 23, 239, 240
Chung, O.B., 259
Chung, W.-L., 131
Cleave, P., 288
Close, R., 287
Cobo-Lewis, A.B., 72
Coenders, M., 258
Cohen, A.D., 23, 54
Cohen, D., 23, 239, 240
Cohen, E., 72
Cohen, J., 103, 211
Cohen, K. 211
Coiro, J., 209
Cole, P., 166
Coleman, B., 260
Conger, R.D., 263
Connor, U., 211
Content, A., 131
Conway, M.A., 239
Coombs, M., 259
Cortes, R.S., 23
Costa, A., 239
Coutya, J., 23
Cox, C.E., 239
Crago, M., 288
Craik, F.I.M., 22, 23
Crease, A., 166
Crinion, J.T., 22
Crowther, R., 104
Cuero, K., 261
Cummins, J., 22, 104, 209, 211
Cunningham-Andersson, U., 261
Curdt-Christiansen, X.-L., 32, 53, 209
Curtis, M.E., 104
Curtis, S., 54
Curwood, J.S., 212

Dais, L., 238
Damrad-Frye, R., 165

Danzak, R.L., 209
Darling, N., 262
Davis, C.R., 260
De Groot, A.M.B., 72
De Houwer, A., 103, 166, 259, 288, 289
De Vries Guth, N., 53
Deal, J.E., 259
Demeulenaere, H., 73
Derwing, B., 126, 129, 131
Dewaele, J.-M., 238, 239
Di Cristo, A., 72
Diaz, C.J., 212
Dibaj, F., 23
Dibuz, P., 209
Dickinson, D.K., 103, 165, 167, 260
Dodd, B., 72
Dong, W., 262
Dopke, S., 262
Dornbusch, S.M., 262
Doughty, C.J., 103
Dressler, C., 130
Dubowitz, H., 239
Duran, L., 288, 289
Durgunoglu, A.Y., 130, 209, 211
Durkin, K., 104
Duthie, J.K., 129, 131
Dweck, C.S., 44, 54, 262

Easterbrooks, A.M., 260
Eaton, M.M., 262
Eliers, R.E., 72
Elliot, A.J., 262
English, D.J., 239
Erway, C.C., 71
Eslami, Z., 104
Evaod, A., 129

Fagan, J., 259
Fine, M.A., 261
Fitzgerald, J., 208, 209, 211
Fitzpatrick, M.A., 247, 260, 261
Fletcher, A.C., 260, 262
Fletcher, P., 103, 129
Flouri, E., 239
Fombonne, E., 288
Foorman, B., 131
Forster, K.I., 24
Frackowiak, R., 22
Francis, D., 131
Francis, N., 130, 211
Friesen, D.C., 22

Frost, R., 24
Fuligni, A.J., 23

Gaffney, J.S., 131, 209
García, E., 23
García, H., 23
García, O., 158, 167
Garman, M., 103, 129
Garrett, P., 72
Gass, M., 103
Gee, J.P., 14, 23, 212
Gelfand, M., 239
Geluck, P., 22, 225
Genesee, F., 130, 166, 288, 289
Gerris, J.R.M., 259
Geva, E., 130
Ghosn, I.K., 213
Giampapa, F., 238
Gildea, P.M., 103
Gillam, R.B., 73
Gini, M., 260
Gleason, J.B., 61, 72
Goffman, L., 71
Goldstein, B., 165
Goldstein, H., 104
Goldman, S.R., 170, 185, 210
Gollan, T.H., 24
González, N., 165, 238
Gorter, D., 166
Graham, S., 208
Grech, H., 72
Green, L., 129
Greenberg, Z.I., 23
Greenleaf, C., 210
Greenspan, S.I., 212
Gregory, E., 209
Grice, P., 166
Grolnick, W.S., 262
Grosjean, F., 130, 286
Guion, S., 72
Guo, J., 209, 212
Gutierrez-Clellen, V., 288

Habermas, J., 258
Hakuta, K., 22
Halberda, J., 104
Halgunseth, L.C., 261
Hall, S.G., 25, 53
Halverson, C.F., 259
Hambly, C., 288
Hammer, C.S., 165

Hancin-Bhatt, B.J., 130
Hanley, R., 54
Harkness, S., 259
Harper, S., 261
Harre, R., 238
Harrison, B., 288
Harter, S., 255, 263
Haun, D., 72
Hauser, S.T., 262
Heath, S.B., 239
Henry, M.I., 258
Herman, P.A., 104
Hesketh, L.J., 129, 131
Hewitt, R., 71
Hilburn-Cobb, C., 260
Hinchman, K.A., 104
Hinds, J., 211
Hirsch, E., 211
Hirst, D., 72
Hoefnagel-Höhle, M., 72
Hoff, E., 71, 72, 73, 165, 209
Hoffman, E., 238
Hoffmann, C., 22, 259
Holder, M.D., 260
Hong, Y.-Y., 23
Hornberger, N.H., 211, 212
Horowitz, A., 239
Horowitz, R., 23, 54
Hu, C.-F., 131
Huang, H., 54
Huang, S., 104
Huijnk, W., 258
Hulstijn., W., 71
Hunt, K.W., 132
Huppert, F.A., 262
Huttenlocher, J., 131

Ingram, D., 73
Ispa, J.M., 261

Jackson, W.C., 104
Jahr, E.H., 287
James, C., 72, 201
Janik, V., 103
Janssen, C., 261
Jetten, J., 259
Johansson, V., 105
Johns, A.M., 22, 53
Johnson, H., 188, 210
Jones, B., 166
Jones, K., 22, 53

Jones, L., 53
Jørgensen, J.N., 103
Juelis, J., 129
Justice, L.M., 71, 103, 129, 165
Juvonen, J., 263

Kamil, M.L., 104, 130
Kan, P.F., 288, 289
Kanno, Y., 238
Kaplan, R.B., 211
Kay-Raining Bird, E., 288
Kell, T., 212
Kelley, A., 104
Kemmelmeier, M., 239
Kent, R., 71
Kerr, M.A., 239
Keyes, C.L.M., 262
Keysar, B., 72, 239
Kidd, D.C., 213
Kieffer, M.J., 131
Kim, K.-J., 263
Kinukawa, A., 239
Kitayama, H., 238, 239
Kitayama, S., 23, 240
Klecan-Aker, J.S., 167
Koda, K., 130
Koerner, A.F., 247, 260, 261
Kohnert, K., 104, 288, 289
Kolokonte, M., 103
Komaroff, E., 165
Kondo-Brown, K., 52
Kontra, E.H., 73
Koren-Karie, N., 260
Kornos, J., 73
Krashen, S.D., 11, 210
Kress, G., 209
Kroger, J., 240
Krohn, R., 71
Kroll, J., 72
Ku, Y., 129
Kubota, R., 211
Kucan, L., 103
Kuh, D., 262
Kuo, L., 128, 129
Kupersmitt, J., 165
Kwan, E., 54

Lam, K., 129
Lamb, M.E., 239
Lamborn, S.D., 262
Lammers, J.C., 212

Landy, S., 260
Lanz, M., 259
Lanza, E., 165, 238, 262
Larson, R.W., 260
Latman, V., 22
Law, J.S.F., 239
Ledbetter, A.M., 262
Lee, C.A., 209
Leichtman, M.D., 165
LeMonda, C.S.T., 239
Lenhart, A., 212
Lenski, S., 211
Leopold, W.F., 259
Lesaux, N., 131
Lester, M., 132
Lev-Ari, S., 72
Levin, I., 129
Levin, J.R., 104
Lewin, T. 208
Lewis, G., 166
Lewis, M., 53,
Leybaert, J., 131
Li, G.-F., 54
Li, H., 131
Li, P., 130
Li, Y.J., 240
Li, W.-L., 131
Liberman, D., 131
Lindsey, E.W., 259
Liontas, J.I., 164
Litman, C., 210
Litrownik, A.J., 239
Long, M.H., 103
Long, S., 209
Lopez, L.M., 165
Losh, M., 165
Lugo-Neris, M.J., 104
Luk, G., 22, 23, 54
Lunga, V.B., 238, 239
Luo, Y.C., 129, 131
Lyons-Ruth, K.A., 260

Maasen, B., 71
MacArthur, C.A., 208, 209, 211
MacDermid, S., 258
Macgill, A., 212
MacSwan, J., 103, 211
MacWhinney, B., 60, 72
Magnified, A.M., 212
Mahony, D.L., 129
Makin, L., 212

Malgady, R.G., 22
Malik, K., 240
Malus-Abramowitz, M., 131
Mansfield, T.C., 129, 131
Mansour, S., 167
Manstead, A.S.R., 259
Mantero, M., 240
Marchand-Martella, N.E., 208
Marcia, J.E., 231, 240
Marencin, N., 167
Marinova-Todd, S.H., 288
Marquardt, T.P., 130
Marslen-Wilson, W., 131
Martínez-Flor, A., 54
Martella, R.C., 208
Martello, J., 212
Martin, F.N., 130, 131
Martin-Jones, M., 22, 53
Martin, M.M., 24
Mashunkashey, J., 261
Matheny, A., 260
McAlister, K.T., 103, 211
McCabe, A., 165, 167
McCutchen, D., 129
McDaniel, M.A., 104
McDermott, P.A., 209
McGee, A., 188, 210
McKay, S.L., 211
McKeown, M.G., 103, 104
McLaughlin, B., 211
McNabb, M.L., 173, 208, 209
Mcpherson, G.E., 261
McQuillan, J., 210
Mechelli, A., 22
Meisel, J.M., 130
Miller, G.A., 103
Miller, J.F., 129
Mills, M.T., 167
Mirenda, P., 288
Mitchell, M., 261
Mize, J., 259
Moats, L., 129
Modderman, S.L., 208
Morgan, J., 166
Mosenthal, P.B., 104
Mounts, N.S., 262
Mourssi, A., 212

Nagy, W.E., 104, 130, 131
Nelson, N.W., 210, 212
Neppi, T., 263

Nett, K., 288, 289
Neuman, S.B., 103, 104
Nickerson, P., 260, 262
Nijakowska, J., 73
Nippold, M.A., 53, 92, 103, 104, 105, 108, 111, 112, 128, 129, 130, 131, 134, 165, 167, 208, 212
Nir-Sagiv, B., 209, 212
Noguchi, M.G., 262
Noppeney, U., 22
Norton, B., 232, 238, 240
Novy, D., 131
Nuske, N.J., 210
Nuttall, C., 210

O'Connor, T.G., 262
O'Doherty, J., 22
Obied, V.M., 288
Oh, J.S., 23
Okita, T., 260, 261
Oller, D.K., 72, 103
Ordóñez, C.L., 211
Owens, K.B., 53
Owens, R.E., 71, 130, 165, 208
Oyen, A.-S., 260

Paap, K.R., 23
Packard, J.L., 131, 209
Padilla, R., 23
Palkovitz, R., 239
Pan, S., 208
Pancsofar, N., 239
Paradis, J., 288
Park, E., 166, 287
Parke, R.D., 239
Pasquarella, A., 129, 131
Pauwels, A., 261
Pavlenko, A., 94, 95, 104, 238
Pedrazgo, S., 53
Pence, K.L., 71, 103, 130, 165, 208
Perkins, K., 213
Perry, N.E., 53
Peters, H., 71
Petersen, H.M., 208
Petersen, J., 288
Piller, I., 247, 261, 287
Pleydell-Pearce, C.W., 239
Ploubidis, G.B., 262
Polat, N., 73
Pomerantz, E.M., 262
Portes, A., 23, 53

Poulin-Dubois, D., 23
Power, M.A., 211
Pratt-Fartro, T., 25, 53
Preece, S., 240
Pressley, M., 104
Price, C.E., 262
Price, C.J., 22

Quinlan, T., 129

Radhakrishna, A., 239
Ran, A., 53
Rapaport, S., 129
Ravid, D., 129
Reilly, J., 165
Remi, G., 211
Renouf, A., 260
Reyes, A., 238
Rice, M., 288
Richards, M., 262
Riera, M., 50, 51, 52, 54, 234
Rindal, U., 72
Ritchie, W.C., 23
Riveros, A., 261
Robinson, J., 261
Rodriguez, B.L., 165
Rogler, L.H., 23
Rolstad, K., 103
Romaine, S., 262
Romo, H.D., 261
Ronjat, J., 259
Rosaldo, R., 259
Rosenblum, G.D., 53
Rosenfield, S., 210
Rubin, K.H., 259
Rumbaut, R.G., 23, 53
Runyan, D.K., 239
Ryff, C.D., 262

Sagi, A., 260
Saiegh-Haddad, E., 130
Sakamoto, M., 21, 24, 33, 53, 288
Sanchez-Sosa, J.J., 261
Santrock, J.W., 53
Saunders, G., 259
Scabini, E., 259
Scaramella, L.V., 263
Scardamalia, M., 211
Scarpino, S.E., 165
Schatz, M., 213
Schauffler, R., 53

Schecter, S., 165
Schneider, M.W., 239
Scholfield, P., 72
Schrodt, P., 262
Schwartz, M., 165, 166
Schwiebert, C., 129
Scott, C.M., 130, 132, 210, 286
Scott, J.A., 104
Seeff-Gabriel, B., 73
Sehn, Z.L., 260
Selinker, L., 103
Senechal, M., 131
Shanahan, T., 130
Shaul, Y., 165, 166
Sheridan-Thomas, H.K., 104, 209, 210, 212
Sherman, M., 8, 260
Shire, B., 104
Shteynberg, G., 239
Shu, H., 131
Silliman, E.R., 210
Silverman, E.S., 239
Simon-Cereijido, G, 288
Simpson, J., 23
Slobin, D.I., 53, 209, 212
Smith, A., 71, 212
Smith, C., 129
Snow, C.E., 72, 211, 260
Soler, E.A., 54
Sotomayor-Peterson, M., 261
Souza, A.L., 71, 72
Spears, R., 259
Spera, C., 261
Spernes, K., 238, 239
Spiegel, C., 104
Splitter, L.J., 240
Stackhouse, J., 73
Staw, B.M., 258
Steinberg, L., 262
Stokes, S.L., 130, 132
Strömqvist, S., 164, 165, 166
Stuart, C., 238
Sullivan, J.H., 23, 164, 166, 210
Sulton, R.I., 258
Summers, C., 73
Super, C.M., 259
Sutherland-Smith, W., 209
Sutton, A., 288
Svendsen, B.A., 238, 262

Tabors, P.O., 23, 260
Taeschner, T., 259

Taft, M., 131
Takeuchi, M., 261
Tatum, A.W., 209
Taturn, A.W., 210
Taylor, R.D., 262
Telley, S.A., 53
Tenenbaum, H.R., 210
Terry, N.P., 162, 167
Thomas, C., 289
Thordardottir, E., 288
Thorpe, A., 288
Thurber, B.B., 209
Tierney, J., 104
Tochelli, A.L., 210, 212
Trafimow, D., 239
Trudeau, N., 288

Vach, W., 54
Van Borsel, J., 73
Van Lagenhove, L., 238
Van Lieshout, P., 71
Varela, E.R., 261
Vasilyeva, M., 131
Vaugh, B.E., 259
Vaughan, K., 131
Verbruggen, F., 211
Verhoeven, L., 130, 164, 165, 166
Verkuyten, M., 259
Vermeulen, K., 131
Vermulst, A., 259
Vernberg, E.M., 261
Vernon-Feagans, L., 239
Volk, D., 209

Wagner, C., 288
Wampler, K.S., 259
Wang, C., 23
Wang, M.C., 130, 239, 262

Wang, Q., 165, 238, 239, 240
Wang, X.-L., 24, 54, 72, 103, 129, 166, 208, 210, 212, 225, 238, 240, 259, 260, 261, 262, 263, 286, 287, 288
Waterfall, H., 131
Waters, G., 131
Wei, L., 167
Wells, B., 73
Wentzel, K., 263
Wethington, E., 260
White, S., 131
White, T.G., 131
Wiesel, E., 104
Wilkinson, L.C., 213
Williams, C., 166
Williams, F., 105
Willson, V., 104
Wilson, A.E., 240
Windsor, J., 130, 286
Wong-Fillmore, L., 289
Woolfolk, A., 53
Wright, K.L., 262
Wu, X.-C., 209
Wulfeck, B., 165

Xun, W.Q.E., 240

Yamagishi, T., 239
Yang, C., 130
Yim, D., 289
Ying, Y.-W., 259

Zaremba, K. 258
Zehr, M., 72
Zhang, H., 131
Zhou, X.-L, 131
Zierer, E., 259
Ziv, Y., 260

Subject Index

Abstract words, 94, 293
Active planning, 247, 248, 258, 293
Adolescence, 25, 293
Adolescent egocentrism, 28, 301
Adverbial conjuncts, 113, 293
Adverbial disjuncts, 113, 293
Affective, 43, 293
Affective filters, 254, 293
Agency, 42, 43, 293
Alphasyllabary, 36, 293
Amalgamation, 140, 293
Appositive, 130, 293
Aptitude, 11, 21, 294
Articles, 115, 294
Autobiographical memory, 223, 224, 294

Backward transfer, 141, 294

Clausal density, 126, 294
Cognates, 79, 294
Cognition, 45, 294
Common Underlying Proficiencies, 193, 294
Communication Block, 180, 294
Compound words, 75, 109, 294
Compounding morphemes, 107, 294
Contextual abstraction, 86, 87, 91, 294
Contrasting phoneme, 68, 294
Conversational Cooperative Strategies, 151, 294
Creole, 21, 294
Critical literacy, 20, 169, 172, 203, 204, 295
CQSP strategy (Clarification, Questioning, Summarization, and Prediction), 185, 295
Cross-linguistic synonyms, 78, 295
Cultural templates, 242, 295

Deductive teaching, 48, 295
Dental sibilants, 56, 295
Dependent clause, 110, 126, 295
Derivational morphology or derivational words, 107, 295
Direct teaching, 47, 48, 86, 87, 192, 295
Direction of transfer, 119, 295

Discourse with A Big D, 14, 295
Discussion-Based Instruction (DBI), 184, 186, 295
Distributed characteristic of multilingual word learning, 295

Emblems, 159, 160, 295
Emotion-laden words, 94, 96, 295
Emotion words, 94, 295
Emotional intelligence, 205, 295
EmPOWER method, 200, 296
Ethnotheories, 242, 296
Explanation Reading Training (ERT), 185, 296
Expository text, 99, 110, 169, 170, 188, 206, 296
Expressive lexicon, 78, 296
Extensive reading, 189, 190, 296

Factive verbs, 92, 296
False cognates, 79, 97, 296
False friends, 79, 97, 296
Fan fiction, 195, 196, 296
Fast-mapping cognitive ability, 87, 296
Figurative language, 135, 136, 152, 154, 156, 198, 296
First languages, 57, 296
Fixed mindset, 44, 296
Formal operational thought, 27, 296
Forward transfer, 140, 296
Fossilization, 84, 296
Frontal lobe, 27, 297

Genderlect, 134, 136, 152, 297
Growth mindset, 44, 297
Growth spurts, 27, 297

Heteroglossia, 158, 186, 297
Heteronyms, 64, 297
Heterophones, 64, 297
High Point Analysis (HPA), 160, 161, 297
Higher functional load, 69, 297
Homographs, 76, 297
Homophones, 6, 65, 76, 297

Honorifics, 154, 297
Hypertext, 169, 171, 172, 173, 203, 297

Imperfect subjunctive, 116, 297
Incidental exposure, 75, 298
Independent clause, 124, 126, 298
Indirect feedback, 197, 298, 299
Inductive teaching, 48, 298
Inflectional morphemes, 101, 107, 298
Intensive reading, 189, 190, 298
Intentional conversation, 46, 47, 48, 68, 81, 97, 156, 174, 298
Interlanguage, 84, 139, 298
Intersentential, 124, 298
Intrasentential, 75, 124, 298

K-W-L chart, 189, 298

Lexias, 172, 298
Lexical complexity, 75, 102, 298
Lexical density, 75, 102, 298
Lexical diversity, 75, 101, 102, 298
Lexical inferencing, 187, 188, 298
Lexicon, 16, 74, 79, 77, 78, 82, 85, 86, 91, 94, 95, 97, 101, 123, 136, 137, 298
Limbic system, 27, 298
Literate lexicon, 92, 299
Loan blending, 80, 81, 85, 299

Marked, 48, 299
Marked sounds, 69, 299
Masking phenomenon, 101, 299
Maze, 120, 299
Measurement words (or classifiers), 14, 47, 115, 116, 141, 155, 277, 284, 299
Mental lexicon, 86, 89, 124, 137, 299
Metacognitive conversations, 45, 299
Metalinguistic ability, 6, 19, 92, 135, 141, 198, 299
Metalinguistic feedback, 197, 299
Metalinguistic reflection, 141, 157, 299
Minimal pair, 68, 299
MLU (Mean Length of Utterance), 109, 110, 299
Morphemes, 69, 101, 107, 109, 120, 121, 299
Morphological, 108, 120, 122, 124, 299
Morphological analysis, 100, 299
Morphological awareness, 118, 119, 121, 122, 123, 299
Multilingual bootstrapping hypothesis, 117, 299
Multimodality, 96, 203, 299
Multipass approach, 188, 300

Multisensory Structured Learning (MSL) approach, 67, 300

Narrative Assessment Protocol (NAP), 160, 161, 292, 300
Narrative Scoring Scheme (NSS), 160, 162, 300
Narrative texts, 169, 300
Nonfactive verbs, 92, 124, 300
Nonword repetition (NWR), 69, 300
Nonwords, 69, 70, 125, 126, 300
Novel conceptual combination, 6, 300

One-parent-one-language (OPOL), 243, 300
Online affinity spaces, 196, 301
Online production, 77, 301
Opaque compounds, 109, 301
Orthographic structure knowledge, 123, 301
Orthographic systems, 36, 37, 176, 122, 301
Overextension, 82, 85, 301

Paralanguage, 275, 276, 301
Persuasive writing, 85, 109, 113, 171, 198, 206, 301
Phonemes, 55, 56, 301
Phonetic inventory, 56, 69, 301
Phonological, 55, 57, 58, 61, 64, 66, 67, 68, 69, 70, 301
Phonological translation, 59, 60, 301
Phonotactic constraints, 61, 70, 301
Phonotactic knowledge, 61, 70, 301
Pinyin, 65, 301
Polysemous words, 91, 92, 124, 301
Possessive pronouns, 115, 301
Pragmalinguistic failure, 149, 150, 151, 301
Pragmatics, 140, 155, 302
Predictive inferences, 187, 188, 302
Prosody, 56, 57, 302
Puberty, 27, 302

Reading apprenticeship model, 189, 302
Receptive lexicon, 78, 302
Reflective positioning, 215, 302
Registers, 28, 198, 302
Relative clauses, 110, 171, 302
Retroflex, 59, 302

Schemata, 47, 48, 302
Script inferencing, 188, 302
Selective attention, 3, 302
Self-efficacy, 233, 302

Self-regulation, 200, 302
Shared book reading, 187, 302
Subordination index, 110, 303
Sociopragmatic failure, 149, 150, 152, 302
Specific Language Impairment (SLI), 282, 283, 302
Speech act(s), 150, 303
Spillover, 244, 303
Stabilization, 84, 303
Story grammar, 134, 141, 161, 162, 170, 303
Story recounting, 159, 303
Strategy-Based Instruction (SBI), 184, 185, 303
Structure Strategy Training (SST), 185, 303
Syncretic language use or communication or syncretic writing, 138, 139, 202, 176, 303
Syncretic literacy, 177, 303
Syntax or Syntactic, 70, 110, 113, 193, 303

Terminable unit (T-unit), 109, 303
Theme comprehension strategy, 170, 303
Theory of mind, 205, 303
Thinking aloud, 188, 189, 303
Tier one words, 80, 93, 303
Tier three words, 80, 93, 304
Tier two words, 80, 93, 304
Translanguaging, 157, 158, 186, 187, 304
Transparent compounds, 109, 304

Unified Competition Theory, 60, 304
Utterances, 109, 161, 304

Vowel-shifting rules, 56, 304

Weakeners, 150, 304
Why-question generation, 188, 304
Wordle, 96, 304